D1292784

Refugee and Immigrant Health

A Handbook for Health Professionals

We live in an age of constantly shifting populations, as immigrants and refugees seek a safe haven from war, famine, and poverty. The healthcare of these dispossessed people is now a stark challenge not only in zones of conflict but in those wealthier countries that have offered sanctuary. The book is based on the authors' combined 40-plus years of work as clinicians and teachers in refugee and immigrant health. It is written with clinicians and students in mind and is thus practical, yet theory based, so it can be used in the field and as a teaching text. The book bridges physical health (highlighting infectious disease risks), mental health, and spiritual issues, while encompassing population-specific information on history of immigration, culture and social relations, communications, religions, pregnancy and childbirth, end-of-life issues, and health screening. It also details health beliefs and practices of over 30 ethnic groups commonly found as refugees or immigrants from more than 40 countries.

Charles Kemp has worked in refugee health for more than 20 years. He teaches courses in community health and hospice/palliative care at Baylor University and works as a family nurse practitioner in the Agape Clinic, serving immigrants and refugees in inner-city Dallas, Texas. He is author of two books, more than 50 articles for professional journals, and 30 papers for professional meetings. He also maintains websites on cross-cultural health, infectious diseases, and hospice care.

Lance Rasbridge, a medical anthropologist, coordinates the Refugee Outreach Program of Parkland Hospital, Dallas, Texas, which he cofounded in 1991. Previously he was a lecturer in Southeast Asian Studies, at the University of Texas at Dallas. He served on the initial Metroplex Refugee Network board, was past president of Refugee Services of Texas, and currently presides over the Center for Survivors of Torture.

Refugee and Immigrant Health

A Handbook for Health Professionals

Charles Kemp, F.N.P., F.A.A.N. and
Lance A. Rasbridge, Ph.D.

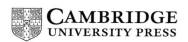

CAMBRIDGE
UNIVERSITY PRESS

PUBLISHED BY THE PRESS SYNDICATE OF THE UNIVERSITY OF CAMBRIDGE
The Pitt Building, Trumpington Street, Cambridge, United Kingdom

CAMBRIDGE UNIVERSITY PRESS
The Edinburgh Building, Cambridge CB2 2RU, UK
40 West 20th Street, New York, NY 10011–4211, USA
477 Williamstown Road, Port Melbourne, VIC 3207, Australia
Ruiz de Alarcón 13, 28014 Madrid, Spain
Dock House, The Waterfront, Cape Town 8001, South Africa

http://www.cambridge.org

First published 2004

Printed in the United Kingdom at the University Press, Cambridge

Typefaces Minion 10.5/14 pt. and Formata   *System* LATEX 2$_\varepsilon$ [TB]

A catalogue record for this book is available from the British Library

Library of Congress Cataloguing in Publication data
Kemp, Charles, 1944–
Refugee and immigrant health: a handbook for health professionals / Charles Kemp and Lance A. Rasbridge.
   p.   cm.
Includes bibliographical references and index.
ISBN 0 521 82859 7 (hardback) – ISBN 0 521 53560 3 (paperback)
1. Transcultural medical care – Handbooks, manuals, etc.   2. Immigrants – Health and hygiene – Handbooks,
manuals, etc.   3. Refugees – Health and hygiene – Handbooks, manuals etc.   4. Minorities – Medical
care – Handbooks, manuals, etc.   I. Rasbridge, Lance A. (Lance Andrew)   II. Title.
RA418.5.T73K45   2004   362.1 – dc22   2003069744

ISBN 0 521 82859 7 hardback
ISBN 0 521 53560 3 paperback

To those seeking refuge and to those giving refuge

In Memoriam
Sergio Vieira de Mello, 1949–2003
United Nations diplomat whose light brought hope to the countless
displaced and oppressed from Bangladesh, Cyprus, Mozambique, Peru,
Lebanon, Cambodia, the Balkans, East Timor, and finally Iraq. Let it shine.

Contents

Part III　Appendices

Contributors

If no author is listed for a chapter, the authors are Charles Kemp and Lance A. Rasbridge

Rachel H. Adler, Ph.D.
The College of New Jersey

Timothy Benner, Ph.D.
Southern Methodist University

Sonal Bhungalia, R.N.
Columbia University

Jennifer Foster Broekema, R.N.
Baylor University

Bi-Jue Chang, R.N., M.S., C.C.R.C.
Baylor University Medical Center

Mindy Early, R.N.
Baylor University

Zbys Fedorowicz, B.D.S., L.D.S., R.C.S. (Eng)
Bahrain Quality Society

Wael Wagih Hamed, F.R.C.S., M.Sc., M.D.
Cairo University

M. Douglas Henry, Ph.D.
University of North Texas

Charles Kemp, F.N.P., F.A.A.N.
Baylor University Louise Herrington School of Nursing

Manja Lee, R.N.
Parkland Health and Hospital System

Tracey Mackling, R.N.
Baylor University

Jennifer Murray, R.N.
Baylor University

Brenda Newell, R.N.
Baylor University

Lance A. Rasbridge, Ph.D.
Parkland Health and Hospital System

Nitaya Thammasithiboon, R.N., A.P.R.N., F.N.P., B.C.
Baylor University

Kathryn Ryczak, R.N.
Baylor University

Stephanie Van De Kieft, R.N.
Baylor University

Margaret Young, R.N.
Baylor University

Preface

Beginning with the first waves of bewildered Southeast Asian rice farmers arriving to the inner city in the early 1980s, up through the recent group of Somali Bantus, many never having seen a toilet or even a staircase, we are entering our third decade of witnessing, and indeed participating in the resettlement of refugees and immigrants. And what a long, strange trip it has been! We offer this book in a spirit of respect for the people who have passed through, for their strength, their dignity, their struggles, their failures, their triumphs.

An early caution: In the second section of the book we present a large amount of culture-specific information in which complex beliefs and practices are reduced to generalities. Not everything presented on a specific culture or group applies to every member of that culture or group. Expecting individuals or even populations to conform to information presented on a culture leads directly to stereotyping and misperception. The culture-specific information is given as a means of *beginning* to understand people from a particular culture. From this beginning, we build understanding of individuals, families, and cultures.

The book is part of our ongoing efforts to increase understanding of refugee and immigrant health specifically, and cross-cultural health generally. The book is organized philosophically and conceptually on building cultural competence (see Chapter 1) and is divided into two Parts corresponding to the two components or sets of skills necessary to achieving full cultural competence.

- Generic cultural competence is knowledge and skills applicable to any patient or community cross-cultural encounter. To this end the first Part of the book looks at broad issues related to refugee and immigrant health in particular and cross-cultural health in general.
- Specific cultural competence is knowledge and skills applicable to patients and communities from specific cultural backgrounds. The second Part of the book examines specific populations in terms of background, history of immigration,

culture and social relations, communications, religion, health beliefs and practices, pregnancy and childbirth, end of life, and health problems and screening. The populations discussed were selected on the basis of recent history of significant immigration to the West. Information came both from the literature and from participant observation and was reviewed by community experts when possible.

All the chapters are authored by Charles Kemp and Lance Rasbridge except where noted.

A brief word about us, the authors: Charles Kemp, a family nurse practitioner, teaches courses in community health and end-of-life care at Baylor University Louise Herrington School of Nursing, works at the Agape Clinic serving refugees and immigrants, and gardens in his spare time. Lance Rasbridge, a medical anthropologist, is the co-ordinator for the Refugee Outreach Program for the Dallas County Hospital District, is involved in community development in Cambodia, and finds peace in building furniture.

Acknowledgements

Special thanks to Parkland Health and Hospital System and the dedicated Refugee Outreach Program team, from whom I learn every day; to my parents, who provided not only role models but opportunities; and to my wife, Diane and son, Dylan for unwavering love and support.   – L. A. R.

Deepest appreciation to the volunteers and staff at Agape Clinic, especially Bobbie Baxter, Lupe Springer, and Leslie Kemp; to the Agape patients and the Old East Dallas community; to my colleagues at Baylor, especially Judy Lott, Phyllis Karns, Kathryn Leonard, Patti Cade, and Becky Robbins; to my students; to the men in my Bible study, Open Ring Class, and our teacher, Dan Foster; to the congregations of First Presbyterian Church; Grace United Methodist Church, and GraceLife Fellowship; to the men and women of East Dallas Police Storefront (you too, Gilbert); to the United States Marine Corps; to faculty and staff at St. Marks School of Texas, especially Arnold Holtberg; and to Jeff Wiseman. And above all, my love, respect, and gratitude to my wife, Leslie and my son, David.   – C. K.

Neither this book nor the website on which it is based would be possible without support from the Texas Department of Health and Sam Householder. We are grateful for the support.   – L. A. R. and C. K.
                http://www3.baylor.edu/~Charles_Kemp/refugee_health.htm

Note on the photographs

Most of the photographs in this book were taken by our friend and colleague, Judy Walgren. Judy, Victoria Loe, and Gayle Reaves shared the 1994 Pulitzer Prize for international reporting for a series of 14 stories that examined the epidemic of violence against women across the world. Judy also wrote and took the photographs for *The Lost Boys of Natinga: A School for Southern Sudan's Young Refugees*. She is involved with a project addressing the problem of child labor (Child Labor and the Global Village: Photography for Social Change at www.childlaborphotoproject.org/index.html) and she continues in other ways to bring light into the darkness. Judy can be contacted at www.jujuphoto.com/.

Part I

Issues and background

1

Toward a cultural understanding of refugee and immigrant health

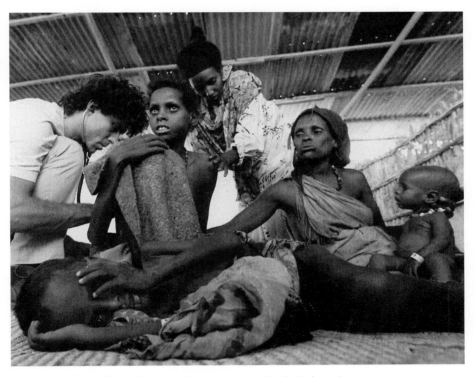

Camp outpatient clinic. (Photograph by courtesy of Judy Walgren.)

Refugee and Immigrant Health: A Handbook for Health Professionals, Charles Kemp and Lance A. Rasbridge. Published by Cambridge University Press. © C. Kemp and L. A. Rasbridge 2004.

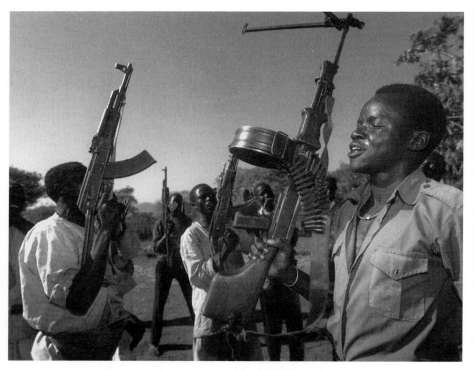

Violence is always close to refugees. (Photograph by courtesy of Judy Walgren)

Introduction

The movement of peoples and populations has been a constant in the course of human evolution, and humans as a species demonstrate remarkable plasticity and resiliency in adapting to new environments. In modern times, the circumstances of why people relocate are as varied as the cultures from which they come, but one aspect of migration is universal – immigrants carry with them more than just suitcases.

From the health perspective, immigrants and refugees of all kinds bring with them diverse epidemiological profiles based on different environments and endemicities of disease in their areas of origin. Sometimes their illness picture is a direct result of the experience of emigration, especially for refugees. They also arrive with widely divergent past experiences with Western medicine. But most of all, refugees and immigrants bring with them their cultural beliefs and practices, including those involving health and illness, which frequently contrast greatly with host country norms. Apart from the epidemiology, the study of health among refugees and immigrants is really a study in culture, the domain of anthropology, because while illness and disease may be universal, the definition of health, the interpretation of symptoms, and remedies and treatments to promote and restore health are very much culturally defined. Sensitizing healthcare professionals to these cultural differences is the main goal of this book.

Cultural competence

Cultural competence is the ability to "perform and obtain positive clinical outcomes in cross-cultural encounters" (Lo & Fung, 2003, p. 162). Within this broad definition, there are two related sets of competencies (Dunn, 2002; Lo & Fung, 2003):

(a) Generic cultural competence is knowledge and skills applicable to any patient or community cross-cultural encounter. This competency is gained through being involved in cross-cultural encounters on a regular basis; observing and evaluating patient, community, and provider (one's own) responses to cross-cultural encounters; seeking and learning general knowledge and skills related to cross-cultural health care; and maintaining a basic attitude of respect for and openness to other cultures.

(b) Specific cultural competence is knowledge and skills applicable to patients and communities from specific cultural backgrounds. This competency is gained through learning about other cultures *and* one's own culture from "participant–observer" patient and community encounters, from other sources such as the literature, and from personal or other professional endeavors to expand the knowledge base regarding specific cultures. The capacity to communicate on a deep level with persons who speak languages other than the native language of the host country is part, but far from all of this competence. The use of interpreters is necessary, but their interactions must also be observed and understood to insure that relationships are truly therapeutic.

Although most healthcare providers think in terms of individual competency, it is important that institutions also work toward cultural competence (Shaw-Taylor, 2002).

Cultural competency in health care is of profound importance on several levels. Perhaps the most obvious, sensitivity to the customs of others to even a minor degree conveys respect, and with respect, compliance on medicines and regimens is more likely to follow. When dealing with refugees and immigrants, the communicable disease risks alone speak volumes toward the critical needs of detection, prophylaxis, and treatment. Increased rapport with patients contributes positively to this endeavor, and not taking this additional step of accommodation risks driving this vulnerable population underground, resulting in serious public health consequences. Moreover, cultural misunderstandings can lead to misdiagnoses (see Galanti, 1997).

With cultural competence comes learning and the acceptance that different beliefs and practices are neither inferior nor more correct than one's own values: the anthropological concept of cultural relativism. Western providers have much to learn from the vast world of healing as practiced around the globe. Even the Western notion of health itself can be reevaluated in this expanded focus, notably, the idea only recently valued in the West that health encompasses spiritual, familial, and community wellness in addition to the mere absence of disease. Finally, cultural sensitivity invokes compassion and empathy, an attempt to treat the whole patient by putting his or her present health state in the context of the broader historical events, which for an immigrant or refugee runs the spectrum from cultural uprootedness to severe psychological and physical trauma.

One important caveat: the intent of this book is not to stereotype all persons from a given culture as prescribing to each and every characteristic outlined; indeed, there frequently can be more intracultural variation within an ethnic group than exists intercultural variability. The ethnic chapters are solely generalizations. Galanti informs us that generalization is the gateway from which to begin the process of patient assessment, whereby stereotyping is the endpoint, the closed door, after which no more information is sought (Galanti, 1997). The goal here is to use generalizations as a framework from which to build an understanding of the diversity in refugees and immigrants.

Of course, culture does change, and while some may argue that those refugees and immigrants who have come to the West should, indeed must, adapt to the new ways of life, these changes can take years or even generations. Furthermore, while practices may appear to change on the outside, underlying worldviews may not. For example, it is not uncommon for refugee and immigrant patients to apply traditional hot–cold humoral theory to new medicines and treatments now available to them. We in no way consider this work to be an absolute compendium of cultural characteristics but rather an introduction to the richness in cultural diversity that is particularly pronounced in the intersection of refugees and immigrants with Western health care.

Decision-making and help-seeking

Health-related decision-making and help-seeking are underlying themes in the chapters on populations. What is provided in the chapters (family structure, age and gender roles, and health beliefs and practices) is best used as part of a matrix of understanding that includes all the determinants of decision-making and help-seeking. Among the determinants of decision-making and help-seeking related to illness, disease prevention, and health promotion (Bruce & McKane, 2000; Kemp, 2003; Uehara, 2003) are:

- attitudes, beliefs, and personal characteristics (including socioeconomic status) of the individual;
- attitudes, beliefs, and personal characteristics of the individual's culture and social networks, especially the family;
- past and present personal and social network experience in health or illness;
- past and present experience in seeking help, especially related to health and illness;
- characteristics and competencies of healthcare systems and individuals within the systems – the "community of solution" – as they interact with individuals and populations.

Anthropologists have demonstrated that all human cultures embrace a system of beliefs relating to the maintenance of health and illness causation, and concomitant therapeutic and preventive practices relating to these beliefs. In fact, most cultures have numerous and diverse therapeutic options. In this medical plurality, which option or options chosen are determined by a complex "hierarchy of resort," depending on such factors as cost, self-diagnosis, time, physical as well as cultural accessibility, and the like.

Clearly, the preceding is a brief summary of an extraordinarily complex and dynamic process. Yet maintaining awareness of these factors while interacting with individuals, families, and populations leads to a more complete understanding of people than simply characterization as a member of a particular culture.

Complementary and alternative medicine

As mentioned, in approaching an understanding of refugee and immigrant health, we must attempt to understand, or at least recognize, the wealth of medical systems across the globe that differ from those we experience in the West. In anthropology, this body of knowledge in the nonindustrialized world, from where many immigrants and refugees originate, is collectively known as ethnomedicine: "those beliefs and practices relating to disease which are the products of indigenous cultural development and are not explicitly derived from the conceptual framework of modern medicine" (Hughes, 1978, p. 151). Western medical researchers are beginning to refer to this body as Complementary and Alternative Medicine (CAM).

The National Center for Complementary and Alternative Medicine (NCCAM) classifies CAM therapies into five major categories (NCCAM, 2002).

Alternative medical systems

Alternative medical systems are built upon complete systems of theory and practice. Often, these systems have evolved apart from, and earlier than, the conventional medical approach used in the USA. Examples of alternative medical systems that have developed in Western cultures include homeopathic medicine and naturopathic medicine. Alternative medical systems that have developed in non-Western cultures include traditional Chinese medicine and the (East) Indian system of *Ayurveda*.

Mind–body interventions

Mind–body medicine uses a variety of techniques designed to enhance the mind's capacity to affect bodily function and symptoms. Some techniques that were considered CAM in the past are now mainstream Western approaches (for example, patient support groups and cognitive-behavioral therapy). Other mind–body techniques are still considered CAM, including meditation, prayer, mental healing, and therapies that use creative outlets such as art, music, or dance.

Biologically based therapies

Biologically based therapies in CAM use substances found in nature, such as herbs, foods, and vitamins. Some examples include dietary supplements, herbal products, and the use of other so-called "natural" but as yet scientifically unproven therapies (for example, using shark cartilage to treat cancer).

Manipulative and body-based methods

Manipulative and body-based methods in CAM are based on manipulation and/or movement of one or more parts of the body. Some examples include chiropractic or osteopathic manipulation, and massage.

Energy therapies

Energy therapies involve the use of what are known as "energy fields" of the body that are manipulated by the practitioner.

While embracing CAM as a means of better understanding health and illness, we are in no way endorsing the use of all CAM practices, particularly those that have not been analyzed to any degree by scientific inquiry and methodology. However, because CAM takes a different path than biomedicine, we do emphasize the many positive "complements" that CAM brings to the Western setting.

- Prevalent throughout much of traditional medicine is the emphasis on treating illness, the causes of the sickness as understood by the patient, in addition to treating disease, the etiology of the illness as defined by Western medicine. Similarly, CAM usually emphasizes addressing proximal, immediate causes of illness, such as infection, as well as the more distal causation, such as societal stressors.
- Prevention of disease is the cornerstone of much of CAM, through such avenues as nutrition, exercise, and stress reduction.

- CAM emphasizes holism or dealing with all aspects of the patient's life, including relationships with other people, and relationships with the natural and spiritual environment, in addition to physical or emotional symptoms.
- CAM principles in general get us closer to the World Health Organization (WHO) definition of health: "a state of complete physical, mental and social well-being and not merely the absence of disease or infirmity" (WHO, 1948).
- Practitioners and specialists of CAM, trusted individuals within their cultural group, can frequently serve as "gatekeepers" for public health interventions.

Culture-bound syndromes

The fourth edition of the *Diagnostic and Statistical Manual of Mental Disorders* (*DSM-IV*) (American Psychiatric Association (APA), 2000) included, for the first time, a Glossary of Culture-Bound Syndromes (CBS). Based on medical anthropological and cultural psychiatric research, the term CBS "denotes recurrent, locality-specific patterns of aberrant behavior and troubling experience that may, or may not, be linked to a particular DSM-IV diagnostic category. Many of these patterns are indigenously considered to be 'illnesses,' or at least afflictions, and most have local names" (APA, 2000, p. 898).

The understanding of CBS is very much in flux. For example, depression, once considered by some as specific to technologically advanced Western cultures, is now recognized as a global health problem, whose burden by the year 2020 will be second only to ischemic heart disease (Institute of Medicine, 1997; Lee, 2002). Similarly, *amok*, once considered specific to Malaysia has now been identified in Laos, Philippines, Polynesia, Papua New Guinea, and Puerto Rico. Moreover, analysis of multiple sudden mass assault(s) by a single individual (SMASI) in the West leads to the conclusion that, in most important respects, there are so many similarities between *amok* and SMASI that neither should be considered as a CBS (Hempel *et al.*, 2000). Finally, it should be understood that there is regional variation in descriptions of some CBS (Weller *et al.*, 2002). Despite disagreements among scholars, there *are* disorders or syndromes that are identified with certain cultures and recognized by those cultures. CBS are included in the discussions of specific cultures under health practices and beliefs.

Culture and the life cycle

In this book we utilize a medical anthropological framework as a tool to embrace this diversity and approach an understanding of immigrants and refugees within the Western medical system. We not only describe, but when possible explain, medical beliefs and practices within the cultural context. Medical anthropology draws upon both the biological and the social sciences in explaining health systems in this complex arena of cultural contact and change throughout the immigration experience. Consequently, medical anthropology offers paths to ultimately improve provider/patient rapport and medical compliance in these populations.

The life cycle course provides an excellent template from which to view health and illness cross-culturally. Anthropology focuses particularly on the social transitions that occur throughout the life cycle, including those linked to physiological changes (Helman, 2000). While culture defines the beginning and endpoints of age-grades, such as adolescence or old age, the events of childbirth, menarche, menopause and death are of course universal and are frequently surrounded by increased attention to the realm of health care. In fact, much has been said of the "medicalization" of the birth, menopause, and dying processes in Western cultures. Hence it is a useful to analyze medical beliefs and practices against the backdrop of the life cycle in order to gain insights into the medical systems of that particular culture.

Pregnancy and childbirth

Culture can have a profound effect on the health of the unborn child. For example, prescriptions and proscriptions on foods, medicine, and work can affect the size of the fetus and hence the healthful outcome of the pregnancy. Age at marriage and ultimately age at conception, in addition to access and use of birth control, are also largely cultural determinants which can impact the health of the mother and baby. Western prenatal care is largely absent from the developing world, not just because of cost, but moreover, because pregnancy is viewed as a natural physiological state. Also, time orientation is a common factor here, where more traditional societies are more focused on the daily living rather than on the future, in this case, on the outcome of the pregnancy (Galanti, 1997).

Childbirth is considered a life-affirming event, but many cultures the world over also recognize the health risks to mother and baby, entailing "a multitude of beliefs and rituals meant to help both mother and child and sometimes the entire family or community pass unharmed through this period of danger" (Jordan, 1993, pp. 3–4). These beliefs and rituals can be seen as helping to prepare the woman in her role transition from wife to mother. Most cultures have a specialized birth attendant of some sort. This specialist may assist in the prenatal and postpartum periods as well, such as providing social support for breastfeeding and a healthful diet, assistance with household tasks, and the like. Some cultures dictate rigid segregation between the sexes at all times, even more so during the peripartum stage, where it may be strictly forbidden for any male, including the husband, to have any contact with the birthing mother, for a specified period of time.

As mentioned, childbirth in Western cultures is frequently approached as a medical event requiring medical intervention rather than a natural human process. Beyond the use of midwifes, many immigrants and refugees from the third world are unaccustomed to this "medicalization" and possibly even uncomfortable with the concept of hospital-based birth. The (Western) idea of the father being present during delivery may also create discomfort.

Infancy and childhood

A common concept to many cultures from the Third World, where infant mortality is high, but with vestiges even in the Western world, is the ceremonial marking of "social birth" at some interval after biological birth, when membership in the society is formalized. For example, in many cultures a child is named only after days or weeks from birth, when there is relative certainty the newborn will survive, or perhaps even to discourage malevolent spirits from "calling" the baby during the critical early days of life. Circumcision, especially male circumcision in the West, is a similar ritual. Western providers may misinterpret cultural practices during this period of vulnerability as a lack of appropriate bonding (Galanti, 1997).

The feeding of infants is a significant concern to all cultures, but there is great variability cross-culturally in the techniques of feeding from birth. Colostrum is frequently perceived in the third world as "spoiled" or otherwise unsuitable and discarded. Breastfeeding incidence and duration has declined dramatically in most countries, especially in urban, industrialized societies or in non-Western societies undergoing modernization and urbanization (Helman, 2000). This transition from the breastfeeding norm to bottle feeding is multifactorial and well beyond the scope of this introduction, but in developing nations bottle feeding is associated with increased infection, malnutrition, and other health problems. For example, we found that recently arrived Cambodian refugee women, with no prior experience with bottle feeding, used the bottle inappropriately, as a pacifier, leading to deleterious health effects (Rasbridge and Kulig, 1995).

However, it should be noted that bottle feeding need not be inherently unhealthy, provided it is adequately explained to the inexperienced mother. All cultures have beliefs about what consists of appropriate weaning foods and when they can first be introduced. These foods are frequently simple enough, such as rice gruel, to be available in the new environments in which immigrants and refugees reside.

Care for the newborn and children in general is also culturally prescribed to a great extent. Although an extreme generalization, family size is frequently large and birth spacing short in the Third World, especially in agricultural areas, where labor needs are high. Hence childcare is sometimes entrusted to the barely older sibling, or in other cases to members of the extended family. Corporal punishment of children is not unusual cross-culturally, and many new immigrants may find themselves at odds with Western laws on the notion of acceptable child discipline. However, many cultural practices, such as the medical treatment known as "coining" practiced by many Asian societies, should be viewed within the larger cultural context for that group.

Childhood and adolescence are not necessarily periods of carefree bliss. Access to education is far from universal, especially for girls (Human Rights Watch (HRW), 2003a). Reams of evidence shows the shockingly high rates of forced child soldiering, sexual exploitation, and forced labor in many countries, especially those likely to be producing refugees (HRW, 2003b). Lifelong emotional as well as physical scars seem inevitable in these cases.

All cultures have some way in demarcating the social transition from childhood to adulthood, albeit not necessarily coincidental with biological puberty. These "rites of passage" surrounding puberty (as well as other stages of the life cycle) have been classically defined as occurring in the three stages of separation, transition, and finally, incorporation. While some stages may be less ritualized or emphasized, or even absent in certain cultures, the overall role transition during adolescence has universally profound implications in terms of increased responsibilities as well as rights. Often, this event signifies eligibility for marriage, especially for young women.

Menstruation and menopause

Menstruation in many traditional societies may be viewed as a state of physical impurity, which in some cases may lead to segregation of menstruating women, from their families, conjugal partners, and from religious and political institutions. However, it should be noted that women in non-Western societies, especially without physical or cultural access to birth control, spend far less time in the menstruating state than their Western counterparts, due to frequent pregnancies and lengthy breastfeeding (and the associated lactational ammenorhea). Menstruation can also frequently be interpreted as a necessary purging or cleansing of the female body of "pollutants," in which case menopause will be anticipated with some trepidation.

Like most other life events, menopause is a gradual process. Social conditions frequently affect the health and nutritional statuses of women, which in turn influences the timing as well as the degree of menstrual changes. Menopause may be viewed as consisting of a social transition as well as a biological one. The role and status of a post-menopausal woman frequently changes; in many societies post-menopausal women have more rights, as their expected role to produce children ceases. Menopause in Western society is frequently "medicalized," a pathological state that is seen to require therapeutic intervention.

End of life

Like all other points along the life cycle, dying and death are marked by significant cultural variation but consist of both biological death, the death of the human organism, and social death, which marks the conclusion of the deceased personal identity (Helman, 2000). The rituals surrounding dying and death are important, perhaps essential mechanisms for human societies to deal with loss and need to be respected by the host institutions to which refugees and immigrants interact.

In Western society, where death can sometimes be viewed as the failure of modern medicine, the dying process can be particularly medicalized. For example, institutionalization of dying patients and life-saving interventions are commonplace. In contrast, the dying person in non-Western societies is frequently surrounded by family members in the home setting. Western emphasis on autonomy and patient's "right to know" may conflict with cultural traditions to shield the patient from unfavorable prognoses (Galanti, 1997).

In most societies, death is seen not as a singular event in time but more as a process "where the deceased is slowly transferred from the land of the living to the land of the dead" (Helman, 2000, p. 161). During this process the "soul" or "spirit" is still in a state of limbo and can inflict harm on the living in the absence of prescribed rituals and activities. For example, in many cultures a widowed woman cannot remarry for a specified period because she is still married to the soul of the deceased until social death is realized.

Care and ultimate disposal of the corpse show tremendous variation cross-culturally. Many religions forbid the mutilation of the body in any way, such as with autopsy. In some societies, the body is prepared for burial or cremation by close family members, in others by religious officials, or even "traditional death attendants," specialists designated by the community. Immigrants to the West from areas where family or traditional death attendants care for the deceased may find the impersonal or practiced approach of professional morticians disconcerting (Helman, 2000).

Bereavement too is significantly culturally patterned. As Helman notes, "Cultures that believe in reincarnation – who see time as circular or spiral, and expect the souls of the dead eventually to be 'recycled' back onto Earth – are likely to have very different attitudes to mourning to those without such a belief, who see death as a final, permanent event" (Helman, 2000, p. 162). Similarly, in many traditions, the spirit of the deceased remains forever among the living, capable of protecting (as well as inflicting harm on) the living through the observance (or nonobservance) of propitiation rituals, such as offerings at shrines dedicated to the deceased, and other forms of ancestor worship.

REFERENCES

American Psychiatric Association (APA) (2000). *Diagnostic and Statistical Manual of Mental Disorders*: 4th edn, text revision. Washington, DC: Author.

Bruce, T. A. & McKane, S. U. (2000). *Community-based Public Health: A Partnership Model*. Washington, DC: American Public Health Association.

Dunn, A. M. (2002). Cultural competence and the primary care provider. *Journal of Pediatric Health Care*, **16**, 105–11.

Galanti, G.-A. (1997). *Caring for Patients from Different Cultures*, 2nd edn. Philadelphia, PA: University of Pennsylvania Press.

Helman, C. G. (2000). *Culture, Health and Illness*. Oxford: Butterworth Heinemann.

Hempel A. G., Levine R. E., Meloy, J. R., & Westermeyer, J. (2000). A cross-cultural review of sudden mass assault by a single individual in the oriental and occidental cultures. *Journal of Forensic Sciences*, **45**, 582–8.

Human Rights Watch (HRW) (2003a). *Women's Rights*. Retrieved August 9, 2003 from http://www.hrw.org/women/index.php.

  (2003b). *Children*. Retrieved August 9, 2003 from http://www.hrw.org/children/.

Hughes, C. (1978). Medical care: ethnomedicine. In *Health and the Human Condition*, ed. M. H. Logan & E. E. Hunt, North Scituate, MA.: Duxbury Press.

Institute of Medicine (1997). *America's Vital Interest in Global Health*. Washington, DC: National Academy Press.

Jordan, B. (1993). *Birth in Four Cultures: A Crosscultural Investigation of Childbirth in Yucatan, Holland, Sweden, and the United States*, 4th edn. Prospect Heights, IL: Waveland Press.

Kemp, C. E. (2003). Community health nursing education: where we are going and how to get there. *Nursing Education Perspectives*, **24**, 144–50.

Lee, S. (2002). Socio-cultural and global health perspectives for the development of future psychiatric diagnostic systems. *Psychopathology*, **35**, 152–7.

Lo, H.-T. & Fung, K. P. (2003). Culturally competent psychotherapy. *Canadian Journal of Psychiatry*, **48**, 161–70.

National Center for Complementary and Alternative Medicine (NCCAM) (2002). *What is Complementary and Alternative Medicine?* Retrieved August 8, 2003 from http://nccam.nih.gov.

Rasbridge, L. & Kulig. J. (1995). Infant feeding among Cambodian refugees. *Maternal Child Nursing*, **20**, 213–18.

Shaw-Taylor, Y. (2002). Culturally and linguistically appropriate health care for racial and ethnic minorities: analysis of the US Office of Minority Health's recommended standards. *Health Policy*, **62**, 211–21.

Uehara, E. S. (2003). Understanding the dynamics of illness and health-seeking: event-structure analysis and a Cambodian–American narrative of "Spirit Invasion." *Social Science and Medicine*, **52**, 519–36.

Weller, S. C., Baer, R. D., Garcia de Alba Garcia, J. *et al.* (2002). Regional variation in Latino descriptions of *susto. Culture, Medicine, and Psychiatry*, **26**, 449–72.

World Health Organization (WHO) (1948). *Definition of Health.* Geneva: Author. Retrieved August 12, 2003 from http://www.who.int/about/definition/en/.

2

Refugees and immigrants: concepts

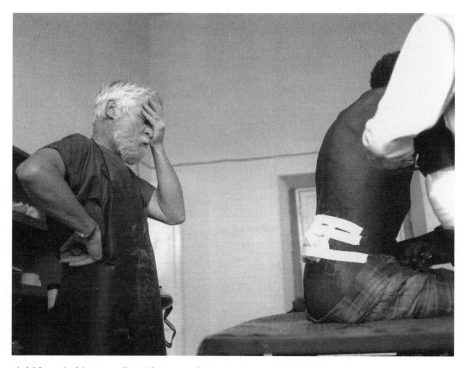

Field hospital in Somalia. (Photograph by courtesy of Judy Walgren.)

Refugee and Immigrant Health: A Handbook for Health Professionals, Charles Kemp and Lance A. Rasbridge.
Published by Cambridge University Press. © C. Kemp and L. A. Rasbridge 2004.

Introduction

Immigration and the control of peoples of foreign cultures crossing international borders, while always a contentious topic throughout modern history, has become a highly charged issue in the post-September 11th era. Across the world, refugees and immigrants affect, and are affected by, the cultures and nations they enter. In the modern West, policies toward immigrants and refugees range from the pragmatic to the humanitarian, and in all cases are under government, popular, and cultural scrutiny.

The purpose of this chapter is to explore briefly the different means of immigration by which peoples from foreign cultures ultimately come into contact with Western-based medical care providers. Immigration history often has a direct bearing on an individual's, or even an ethnic population's, health profile. Here, the categories of immigrants to be considered include economic migrants, refugees, asylees, asylum-seekers, and victims of trafficking (VOTs).

Immigrant types

Economic migrants

Economic migrants are those who enter a host country to pursue a better economic opportunity, or at least to ensure a better income for their offspring, either through legal immigration procedures (see below), or illegally, by surreptitiously crossing a border, with or without the help of smugglers, or otherwise violating the terms of a legal permit for entry, such as overstaying a tourist visa.

Legal immigration to the West is governed by diverse country policies, all of which have the goal of encouraging economic growth while restricting a drain on social resources, and of course some policies are more liberal than others. In the USA there are a myriad different types of visas for entry, broken down primarily into immigrant and nonimmigrant visas. Immigrant visas are solely for temporary residence, for example, tourist, student, or certain types of work visas. Nonimmigrant visas allow for permanent residency ("green card" admissions) and are of several types: family based, employment based, and specialty visas, the latter including entrepreneur, lottery/diversity and refugee/asylee visas (see below). All these categories are limited by government quotas.

Even in an era of increased border surveillance and heightened penalties, illegal immigration for purposes of financial gain remains a fact of life in all Western countries. There are always some migrants "able and willing to surmount legal and procedural barriers if opportunities on the other side are markedly better than those at home" (Collinson, 1994, p. 16). Policies in the West sometimes change from mass deportations to large-scale amnesties, in a pattern frequently related to economic cycles. Of course, the undocumented person's rights or abilities to access social services like health care vary from country to country but are more restricted than for the legal immigrant.

Refugees

It is difficult to read a newspaper today and not find a story on refugees somewhere in the world. Nonetheless, public perception of refugees can be misinformed, especially when refugees are lumped together with other types of migrants and immigrants. The 1951 United Nations (UN) Convention on the Status of Refugees, to which most Western countries are signatories, considers a refugee "any person who is outside any country of such person's nationality . . . and who is unwilling or unable to return . . . because of persecution or a well-founded fear of persecution on account of race, religion, nationality, membership in a particular social group, or political opinion" (UN High Commissioner for Refugees (UNHCR), 2003).

Herein lies the critical difference that sets refugees apart from other migrants: refugees flee persecution, sometimes for their lives, with little if any prior planning. Hence they can best be viewed as "pushed" from their country of origin rather than "pulled" to a new land for economic or social benefit. In reality, these distinctions are seldom clear-cut; many cases fall more accurately on a continuum between these two poles, and so the refugee definition, and the concomitant claim to asylum, is very difficult to adjudicate. On the whole, however, there are an estimated 20 million persons in the world today outside their country of origin and meeting this definition of a refugee (UNHCR, 2003).

In the classic scenario, once the refugee flees, three different "durable solutions" can ensue. For one, the refugee in some circumstances integrates into the community to which she or he fled, referred to as the first asylum country. This is a rare event as few countries, particularly those of the third world, where most refugees are found, can accommodate displaced neighbors either financially or socially. However, in a few specific cases like Cubans floating on rafts to US shores, Bosnians smuggled into Germany, or Vietnamese arriving on boats to Australia, fleeing refugees may be in a position to petition the host government for asylum directly.

More often, when displaced numbers reach a sufficiently large quantity to attract world attention, humanitarian relief organizations, typically led by the UNHCR, with the assistance of other nongovernmental organizations (NGOs) and host-country programs, provide the basic necessities like food, shelter, clothing, and medical care, together with protection, through the establishment of a refugee camp.

Conditions in refugee camps vary greatly around the world, dependent on both local and global political factors, but typically only the basic needs of refugees are met, and this may have a devastating psychological toll, as camp life, described as "halfway to nowhere," can endure for generations, as for example, with Palestinians.

Secondly, the more preferred "durable solution" is to repatriate refugees, returning them to their homelands to rebuild their lives, *when conditions change*. However, the United Nations has a strong mandate against "refoulement," or forcible repatriation against the will of the refugee. The repatriation option, accordingly, is controversial, as seen, for example with the mass protests by Vietnamese returning from Hong Kong. However, several more successful and large-scale efforts, when properly governed by world institutions, such as with the return of over one million Mozambicans from Angola, and to a lesser extent Cambodians from Thailand, demonstrate that this solution can work.

The third possibility, resettlement to a third country, or "secondary asylum," is by far the least likely to be undertaken: only a fraction of 1% of the World's 20 million or so refugees are ever resettled in third countries. Ideally, this should be the solution of last resort, as the costs are greatest, not just fiscally but in terms of discontinuity of culture and assimilation issues. In the final analysis, third country resettlement is equally a product of geopolitical politics and domestic lobbying as well as humanitarianism in the country of secondary asylum.

Resettlement

The USA, Canada, Australia, New Zealand, and the countries of the European Union are the chief providers of permanent refugee resettlement. Each country has its own resettlement policy but all have the same goal: the encouragement of assimilation and economic self-sufficiency. Since about two-thirds of all refugee resettlement in recent years occurs in the USA, the following discussion focuses on that country's program. Nevertheless, the same general issues surface in resettlement in all other Western countries as well.

The US program is best described as a government–private sector partnership. The government entities, at the federal level, include Congress, which in conjunction with the President approves overall refugee admission numbers for each fiscal year. Under those guidelines, the Justice Department conducts overseas interviews, most frequently in refugee camps, ostensibly to evaluate the "well-founded fear" basis. The State Department provides for overseas cultural orientation for those refugees approved for resettlement. Next, the US Public Health Service conducts the overseas medical examination (see Chapter 3).

Once the refugee is approved for resettlement, the linchpin of the resettlement process, the voluntary agencies (volags), assure the case. Through memoranda of agreement with the State Department, from whom they receive partial funding, these secular and church-based humanitarian organizations provide for, or arrange for, the requisite core services of resettlement like housing, medical attention, job training and procurement, social security and school enrolment, etc., for a finite period of time. The exact specifications of financial assistance and responsibility vary according to factors such as a direct sponsorship by the agency vs a sub-sponsorship, like a church group, a family reunion case vs a "free case," and inclusion in more specific programs such as the Cuban–Haitian program or the "Guam Kurd" program. Nevertheless, all refugees are entitled to certain social benefits, including limited government medical insurance.

Another federal entity, the Office of Refugee Resettlement, is charged with over-seeing the resettlement of refugees, and providing additional support and services, often through State offices for refugee assimilation. This office is also involved in encouraging and sponsoring mutual assistance associations, organizations com-posed of previously resettled refugees who aid newer arrivals in their assimilation, as well as other refugee assistance organizations.

In reality, the volag monies and programs are typically not sufficient to ensure full assimilation for refugees, and when additional funding is not forthcoming, adaptation may be negatively affected. Also, misplaced expectations loom large in the resettlement picture. Frequently, refugees hear rumors from friends, relatives, or even from television or videos about "the good life" in countries of second asy-lum. Overseas orientation prior to arrival is not always sufficient to fully inform refugees of the situation in countries of second asylum, and this may account for some adjustment difficulties upon arrival. Alternatively, many refugees are tremen-dously resourceful and surprisingly savvy to the resettlement process. Refugees are survivors, by virtual definition, and can and will manipulate systems to their best advantage when possible.

There is tremendous diversity both between resettled groups, and among indi-vidual ethnic groups. Within a group, there are sometimes different waves of arrivals over time, where the socioeconomic status is typically higher for the earlier refugees, those with the means or connections to flee first. It is often from these initial popu-lations that refugee service agencies hire translators and caseworkers. It is common for there to be significant class and other socioeconomic differences between these personnel and the later (usually larger) refugee population, thus creating tension between workers and clients.

Asylum-seekers and asylees

The asylum-seeker is an individual already in a Western country who is in the process of petitioning for permission to remain permanently because of a claim of persecution in the country of origin. This legal process can take several months or even years during which period the asylum-seeker is "out-of-status" and hence in a sort of legal limbo. In some European countries and in certain circumstances in the USA, the asylum-seeker may be detained or jailed, practices at the center of great political controversy (European Council on Refugees and Exiles (ECRE), 2003; Ladika, 2000; McMaster, 2001). Germany has by far the greatest number of asylum cases in Europe (Bloch, 2002).

The asylum-seeker may have originally entered the country through legal means and in time violated the terms of the legal permit for entry, e.g. overstaying a visa, or may have entered through illegal means such as falsified papers or have simply entered the country through various smuggling routes. Smuggling as the mode of entry is especially common in Europe, at 15–30% of all asylum petitioners overall, and as high as 50% in asylum cases in Germany and 60–70% in the Netherlands (ECRE, 2003).

Whatever the means of entry, asylum seekers in general come from the same countries as other refugees, typically from the Third World, and because of past histories and the subsequent flight from persecution, they have health profiles similar to other refugees. In some cases, their public health issues are even greater than those of refugees because of the lack of screening overseas. When asylum (and appeal) is denied by the courts, the asylum-seeker is deportable. When asylum is awarded, the individual is designated an asylee and is thenceforth eligible for the same benefits as refugees in most Western countries. There is presently legislation within the European union to "harmonize" asylum procedure throughout the region (Bloch, 2002).

Victims of trafficking (VOT)

Trafficking of humans is a worldwide humanitarian crisis, with the UN estimating the number of persons moved across borders through such schemes as indentured servitude, coercion and deception, and unlawful payment to be in the millions per year globally. The Trafficking Victims Protection Act of 2000 was enacted to protect the thousands of people, primarily women and children, who are lured into forced labor, prostitution and sometimes slavery in the USA. The Act enhances prosecution and penalties against those found guilty, but furthermore grants asylum, with full refugee benefits, to victims who agree to aid in the prosecution of the perpetrators. Similar protocols against human trafficking and smuggling were adopted by the UN in 2002 and ratified by the European Union to assist victims there.

Human rights

In conclusion, the cornerstone from which sound immigration policy is built, and in fact the driving force behind the publication of this present volume, lies with a basic respect for human rights and dignity. In 1948, the UN adopted the Universal Declaration of Human Rights (see Appendix B), a visionary document that detailed the fundamental rights of all humans. While other documents have followed, and in some cases refined or elaborated on, this document, the Universal Declaration stands today as a means of defining human rights and thus a means of defining humanity. Universally recognized human rights that are directly applicable to refugees include the rights to life, asylum, protection from torture and ill-treatment, and freedom of movement.

The right to life is the most fundamental right. Wherever there are refugees there is significant risk to life, whether through war, persecution, famine, or other dangers. The 20th century saw at least 167 million people – most civilians – slaughtered in war, concentration camps, wholesale murder, and so on (Brzezinski, 1996). No change is in sight in the 21st century.

Protection from torture and ill-treatment is also a basic and fundamental human right. The 20th and now 21st centuries show no decrease in this most grotesque of human rights violations. From video-taped torture of political prisoners in Liberia, to stoning of women in the Middle East, to institutionalized rape in Europe, torture and ill-treatment are not past barbarisms, but current political, cultural, or religious activities.

Freedom of movement encompasses the freedom to flee persecution and central to refugee rights, freedom from refoulement. This principle of non-refoulement is not specifically noted in the Universal Declaration, but is explicated in later human rights documents. Freedom of movement also includes the freedom to return to one's homeland.

Certainly other human rights violations or protections come to bear on refugees, and to a lesser extent, immigrants. In certain circumstances, other human rights may come to the forefront, for example, the right to education, to work, or to enter into a fully consenting marriage.

The future of refugee resettlement

Refugee resettlement, like so much else, is in a state of change in the post-9/11 era. Security concerns and international politics mean the following.

- Fewer refugees are arriving legally in the West as screening is much more rigorous and time-consuming than in the past.
- Fewer refugees or immigrants are arriving illegally in the West as border security is more rigorous than in the past. Still, large numbers of illegal refugees and immigrants do cross into Western countries to join large numbers already present.
- Vast numbers of refugees continue to flee war, persecution, famine, and other man-made and natural disasters.

Quite frankly, we expect the situation to deteriorate in the early 21st century. We expect there to be more need, less refuge, and fewer resources. We are saddened, but committed to continue the effort to offer refuge.

REFERENCES

Bloch, A. (2002). *The Migration and Settlement of Refugees in Britain.* New York: Plagrave MacMillan.

Brzezinski, Z. K. (1996). *Out of Control.* New York: Simon & Schuster.

Collinson, S. (1994). *Europe and International Migration.* London: Royal Institute for International Affairs.

European Council on Refugees and Exiles (2003). *Factfile.* Retrieved August 20, 2003 from http://www.ecre.org/factfile.

Ladika, S. (2000). Europe's unsettling immigrants. *The World and I Online Magazine.* Retrieved August 21, 2003 from http://www.worldandi.com/public/2000/may/immigs.html.

McMaster, D. (2001). *Asylum Seekers: Australia's Response to Refugees.* Victoria, Australia: Melbourne University Press.

United Nations (UN) (1948). *Universal Declaration of Human Rights.* Geneva: Author.

United Nations High Commissioner for Refugees (UNHCR) (2003). *Statistics.* Retrieved April 3, 2003 from http://www.unhcr.ch/cgi-bin/texis/vtx/statistics.

3

Health issues

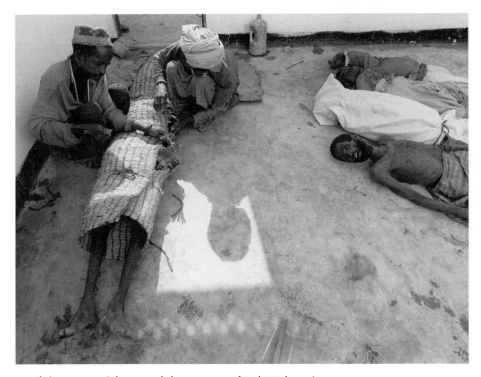

Death in a camp. (Photograph by courtesy of Judy Walgren.)

Refugee and Immigrant Health: A Handbook for Health Professionals, Charles Kemp and Lance A. Rasbridge.
Published by Cambridge University Press. © C. Kemp and L. A. Rasbridge 2004.

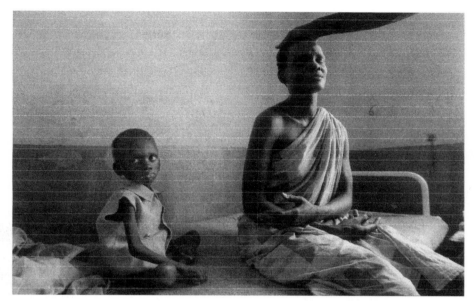

Hospital – where refugees share beds. (Photograph by courtesy of Judy Walgren.)

Introduction (refugees)

The first point of contact with health care for refugees is usually emergency care at a temporary border refugee camp in the country of first asylum, where primary care and hospital facilities treat injuries, severe malnutrition, acute (especially infectious) illness, and other pressing health problems (Hayes *et al.*, 2002). The border camp may be the only place of refuge in the country of first asylum, or there may be more permanent facilities located in a safer area away from the border. In either case, health problems of lesser acuity are addressed only after acute emergency health problems have been treated and after basic sanitation and safety needs have been met, which may be weeks to months after the refugee crisis begins. Hypertension, diabetes, and chronic parasitism, for example, are low priorities in many refugee camps. In relatively permanent refugee situations such as the Palestinian case, there may be a full range of health services similar to those in surrounding areas.

In most situations, services are provided by nongovernmental organizations (NGOs) that have private and/or government funding. Where there is active combat, military forces may, or may not, provide some basic services to refugees. NGOs play an enormous role worldwide in refugee health and welfare.

Unless there are pressing health problems on arrival in the country of second asylum, the first priorities for refugees and immigrants are usually shelter and employment. Only after these most basic needs have been met, do refugees and immigrants tend to seek health care. Seeking health care may also be delayed by concern that immigration status might be negatively affected by health problems, or in the case of illegal immigrants, that health providers may report them to immigration officials.

While there is no universal standard of care or screening procedure for newly arrived refugees in countries of second asylum, the most common first point of contact is the health department at the arrival site. Such contact may be through:

- refugee resettlement agencies that provide services through case workers and (usually) housing in rented apartments or houses are common in the USA.
- government refugee transit centers that provide 6–8 weeks of intensive orientation and other services, including health care, are typified in European resettlement.

Locales that utilize refugee transit centers probably realize better health outcomes than those that depend on a patchwork of refugee agencies and a variety of health providers.

The basis for screening and referral or treatment is to (a) identify communicable diseases that are public health risks and (b) eliminate health-related barriers to successful adaptation. Most countries require that all (documented) refugees and immigrants have a medical examination. Those applying for refugee or immigrant visas to the USA, for example, are screened before entry for communicable diseases of public health significance, documentation of immunizations, physical or mental disorders that may result in harm to self or others, and for drug addiction (American Public Health Association (APHA), 2002). These requirements are not significantly different from most other countries. Communicable diseases of public health significance in the USA (United States Centers for Disease Control and Prevention (CDC), 2002a) include:

- tuberculosis
- human immunodeficiency virus (HIV) infection
- syphilis
- chancroid
- gonorrhea
- granuloma inguinale
- lymphogranuloma venereum
- Hansen's disease

Vaccine-preventable diseases are listed below; vaccination for these is required prior to entry or by the time of adjustment to permanent residence:

- mumps
- measles

- rubella
- polio
- tetanus and diphtheria toxoids
- pertussis
- influenza type B
- hepatitis B

Depending on findings, a person may be granted entry, denied entry, or obtain a waiver for entry despite having significant health condition (CDC, 2002a). On arrival in the USA, refugees, but not most immigrants, are re-screened for health problems. Illegal immigrants are not screened, and because of deportation fears tend to delay contact with the healthcare system.

At its most basic level, domestic screening consists of a short history, vital signs, and testing for tuberculosis, sexually transmitted diseases, and gastrointestinal parasites. Treatment for tuberculosis and sexually transmitted diseases (STDs) is commonly through the local health department, while other health problems usually are referred to other facilities.

Referral procedures vary widely from locale to locale and except for tuberculosis and STDs, tracking of health status and treatment outcomes often does not occur. In countries without universal health coverage, refugees may have up to a year of government health insurance and then face paying full fee for services or obtaining private insurance.

The late 20th and early 21st centuries have seen an improvement in health status of refugees arriving in countries of second asylum. Previously, it was not uncommon to see entire families of refugees arrive in a state of malnourishment. The improvement in health status may be due to improved government and private agency services overseas, as well as to overall decreased numbers of refugees being admitted to countries of second asylum (Schlein, 2003). However, "health" is a relative concept, and in general, the health of newly arrived refugees is less than optimal, especially among those from countries with high disease prevalence rates and short life expectancies. In countries of second asylum, positive tuberculin skin tests are found in 42–53% of new arrivals, positive hepatitis B surface antigen in 5–15%, and gastrointestinal parasites in 19–36% (Benzeguir *et al.*, 1999; Hawn & Jung, 2003; Lifson *et al.*, 2002; Lopez-Velez *et al.*, 1997).

Refugee health issues and processes are quite complex, but may be best understood within the framework of a longitudinal model. The following discussion looks at refugee health at the level of a few representative ethnic groups, noting certain generalizations about their health pictures at the time of resettlement. Concordantly, the changing picture of health is examined longitudinally through the resettlement process, as each group explored can be viewed, on the whole, as representative of a different stage in the resettlement process.

The refugee health profile may be seen as changing along a hypothetical continuum from the acute phase, where illness is mostly a result of antecedent factors to resettlement, through to the chronic level, where the health picture is largely a consequence of long-term resettlement itself. The populations discussed here include Sudanese, Iraqis, Kurds from northern Iraq, and Cambodians.

Level I: acute phase

The acute phase is the level that attracts the most concern in the health arena, primarily because of the communicable nature of illnesses with which new arrivals present, and consequently the public health threat they represent. The groups discussed here, Sudanese and Iraqis after the Gulf War, were typical of new arrivals coming from poor healthcare backgrounds. For the Sudanese, the traumas of civil war, refugee flight and camp life were recent at the time of resettlement; for the Iraqis, war experiences, torture, and prison (in Saudi Arabia) are powerful past stressors. Parasitism abounded in both groups, as sanitation facilities were typically poor in the recent past for them (Peterson *et al.*, 2001). There are high prevalences of Mantoux skin test positivity and hepatitis (B, C, and D) markers (CDC, 2002B; Hobbs *et al.*, 2002; Lifson *et al.*, 2002).

New refugees attending domestic screening clinics frequently present with an extensive litany of complaints, as this may be their first access to Western medical care. For example, a Sudanese woman came to the clinic coordinated by one of the authors with a pre-translated page of complaints as follows,

severe headache always, fever, loss of weight, loss of appetite, emaciation, dizziness, weakness of the body, coughing, sometimes heart pain, unbalance of the body, and sometimes choking, the duration since we came from Africa.

With all new arrivals, in addition to the acute, there are chronic conditions that can be a function of events leading up to refugee flight, e.g. war-related trauma such as wounds and fractures left untreated. In many cases, no treatment is warranted for these old injuries, to the dismay of the patient.

As with other groups of refugees, many Sudanese and Iraqi refugees experienced an initial and brief period of optimism, followed quickly by a decline in health, especially mental health. Factors leading to psychological distress in this early phase include current circumstances such as poor social support, lack of meaningful activities, and long periods of waiting, and previous experiences, especially those related to war and persecution (Gorst-Unsworth & Goldenberg, 1998; Sondergaard *et al.*, 2001; Yaman *et al.*, 2002).

Level II: transition

Three to six years after arrival in 1991–92, the Kurdish community in the USA was representative of an intermediate stage of resettlement. Many believed that they were in the USA only temporarily and would return to their homeland in the eventuality that Saddam Hussein would be defeated in the next uprising. In the first several years of resettlement, many Kurdish children were viewed as future *peshmerga*, freedom fighters. Although talk of returning to fight continued for several years, the emphasis gradually shifted to assimilation and success in the new home.

Initially, health concerns were focused primarily on children's health and on the acute problems of adults. It was only after the children's needs had been largely met, that adults began coming forward in greater numbers seeking care. Even with these cases, frequently the initial access was to ask for prescription drugs needed by family members still in Kurdistan. Although the authors have not systematically inquired into this sensitive topic, it seems certain that some of the medications prescribed for patients in the USA find their way back to Kurdistan. Doctor shopping is common, as increasing numbers learn to maneuver through the complicated US healthcare system.

As with most groups, communicable diseases were prevalent in the first stages of resettlement, but later hypertension, diabetes, and goiter emerged as significant problems. Although there is a tendency to deny psychological distress, depression and post-traumatic stress disorder are common among Kurdish refugees (Silove *et al.*, 1997; Sondergaard *et al.*, 2001). Despite the presence of physical and psychological stressors, most of the younger Kurdish refugee men and even some women are now well integrated into the workforce.

Level III: chronic

Refugees who are assimilated, educated, adequately employed, and living in socially supportive circumstances are unlikely to enter this chronic phase. At this theoretical stage, 10 or more years after resettlement, refugees may suffer from a variety of chronic physical and psychological conditions. In this chronic stage, refugees are likely to live in isolated enclaves, have little access to health and social services, be unable to speak or write (more than rudimentarily) the language of the host country, have poor health, and have poor socioeconomic status (Kemp & Rasbridge, 2000).

Although many are well assimilated in the West, significant numbers of Cambodian refugees – even 20 years post-resettlement – are in a chronic state of poor health (D'Avanzo & Barab, 1998; Mollica *et al.*, 2002). Several factors are known to contribute to Cambodians and others being mired in this chronic state:

- high and often sustained levels of trauma such as torture, rape, beatings, forced labor, and the like prior to resettlement (Mollica *et al.*, 1998). As discussed in the chapter on Cambodians and the chapter on mental health, nearly the entire Cambodian *population* endured extraordinary trauma on an ongoing basis – such as not seen since the Holocaust.
- greater number of resettlement stressors (Blair, 2000). Conditions on the Thai–Cambodia border were brutal during the years of refugee influx (1979–1985) and in many cases resettlement in the West was poorly done. Cambodians were the first major group of severely traumatized refugees to be resettled in the West, and many agencies were ill prepared to address their needs.
- financial stress (Becker *et al.*, 2000; Blair, 2000; Uba & Chung, 1991). The relationship between poverty and poor health is clear and strong, with negative effects on all aspects of health and illness. With some exceptions, Cambodians have tended to have more financial difficulties than most other refugee populations. Lower levels of education, the liquidation of leadership by the ultra-Maoist regime, and higher levels of trauma have all played roles in the ongoing financial difficulties of Cambodian refugees.

This chronic state of refugee status and poor health is lived out or expressed in several ways.

- Traditional family structures break down, with age-related roles reversing as children take on power over parents as the children acculturate to a far greater extent than the parents; gender roles change and even reverse as women work outside the home and sometimes earn more than husbands; and people holding formerly respected roles (e.g., traditional healers, monks, scholars) find their roles have no value in the new land.
- Segments of the population gain a level of assimilation and move into middle or working-class communities while others withdraw into the "neither here nor there" world of the ethnic ghetto. The latter group then becomes isolated even from the upwardly mobile members of the culture.
- Untreated chronic health problems accumulate and long-term sequelae such as end-organ damage begin taking a toll.

When Cambodians first arrived in the West, mostly acute health issues such as tuberculosis, parasitism, prenatal care, and nutrition were, in most cases, the only health issues addressed (Erickson & Hoang, 1980). Now, 10–20 years later, chronic conditions such as coronary artery disease, hypertension, diabetes, depression, and alcoholism are the most frequently seen disorders among Cambodians accessing primary care. While the causes of these chronic conditions may in part be idiopathic, lifestyle changes in coming from an agrarian world to an urban environment surely play an important role, coupled with other aspects like dietary changes.

A recent case involved a 40-year-old Cambodian male who suffered a myocardial infarction and eventually died in the hospital after a week of "heroic" life-saving measures, including the amputation of a leg (secondary to use of vasopressor medication). While he had a known recent history of hypertension, he went relatively unmedicated by choice, claiming, naturally, that he was young and felt fine. Ironically, after his death, and after several other similar examples, rumors were rampant in the community that it was the hospitalization itself that caused this patient to die. Who could explain how a young man in visibly good health could die from this Western disease? The fear of hospitalization remains among a portion of the community.

Another case illustrates the complexities of cultural isolation and barriers to healthcare access. A middle-aged Cambodian woman died from heart failure, after missing several follow-up appointments and failing to obtain refills for her antihypertensives. She was initially connected to the healthcare system by community health workers who discovered her hypertension through routine screening. However, an all-too-familiar scenario played out when the outreach workers eventually became involved elsewhere and the patient either did not seek further care for lack of concern or could not due to accessibility barriers. While the compassion fatigue is marked within the medical community, so too is the weariness of battling an often-insurmountable medical system on the part of refugees.

Another sure indicator of acculturative stress, the wear and tear of material and spiritual poverty, on the health of resettled Cambodians is the increase in prevalence of self-abusive behaviors and the concomitant health sequelae. Notable here is the widespread use and abuse of alcohol. At the risk of overstatement, one of the most frequent pastimes for women in the inner-city enclave, those widowed or having husbands working, is the day-long card game, gambling, complete with the continuous consumption of betel nut and cigarettes, and the slow but steady intake of beer. Not surprisingly, there are anecdotal reports of high rates of cirrhosis, and other concomitants to heavy alcohol consumption in this population, especially among women, with several dying in recent months of end-stage kidney and liver disease.

Mental health issues loom large in this population. Post-traumatic stress disorder (PTSD) and depression are common (Blair, 2000; Mollica *et al.*, 2002; Silove *et al.*, 1997). The response to such distress is often withdrawal and heavy alcohol use (Kemp & Rasbridge, 2000). Premigration distress predictors of high-dose trauma bear heavily on the acculturation outcomes of Cambodian and other refugee populations. Mental health is discussed in Chapter 4.

Immigrants

Immigrants do not usually present with the same dramatic backgrounds of war and persecution as refugees. In some cases, immigrants come from privileged backgrounds and are able to maintain prestige and lifestyles comparable or even exceeding the past. In other cases, however, immigrants come from desperate backgrounds and live desperate lifestyles in their new homes. From Paris to San Francisco, there are ethnic immigrant enclaves with many inhabitants living in abject poverty and often outside the law because of illegal immigration status.

While the health status of illegal immigrants varies from locale to locale, in most cases, health status is poorer than the general population and access to care is limited (Gailly, n.d.; Ku & Freilich, 1991; Matteelli *et al.*, 2001). Gaining a complete understanding of the health status of illegal immigrants is challenging to researchers.

The previous discussion of phases in the refugee process may also be applied, at least to some extent, to poorer or illegal immigrants. Health status varies significantly with circumstances of immigration. Chinese immigrants, for example, who have traveled in crowded ships for lengthy periods of time may arrive with both acute and chronic illnesses. Persons who arrive via air are less likely to present with illness (though illnesses with lengthy incubation periods may manifest after arrival). Like refugees, immigrants tend to arrive in their new country with great optimism – especially about expected employment.

In the second or transition phase, immigrant health concerns – like the concerns of refugees – are focused primarily on children's health and on the acute problems of adults. Usually, it is only after those priorities are met that adults come forward in greater numbers seeking care for chronic conditions such as hypertension or diabetes. Unless overwhelming, psychological distress is seldom addressed by immigrants (except through self-medication with, for example, alcohol consumption). Immigrants who make the transition from "other" and migrant status to full-time employment with benefits (as opposed to day labor jobs paid with cash), leave this negative cycle to become to a large extent, members of their community. Those who remain on the margins of society, enter a third or chronic stage.

This chronic immigrant state is marked by a chronic state of "other" status and poor health lived out or expressed in several ways, including:
• traditional family structures break down, with age, family, and gender-related roles reversing;
• withdrawal into the isolated "neither here nor there" world of the ethnic ghetto;
• accumulation of untreated chronic health problems and the beginning of long-term sequelae such as end-organ damage.

Unquestionably, there are many exceptions and countless variations on these phases of assimilation. However, on a broad or macro level, they hold relatively true.

Regardless of resolution, immigrants often experience a "sadness from losing their sense of place" (Skidmore, 2002, p. 92).

Conclusions

In the refugee, illness from the refugee experience and morbidity as a consequence of resettlement are two distinct entities. For long-term resettled refugees like Cambodians and other Southeast Asians, some having been in the West for 20 years or more, there is a general dearth of long-term care. It is often difficult to find support for outreach efforts in this community, particularly in the light of the more acute, and more public health-threatening illnesses of more recent arrivals.

There are various layers to refugee and immigrant health and illness. To address these complex problems, culturally competent care from outreach to tertiary care should be broadly based. Clearly, public health agencies must continue to focus on identifying and treating acute diseases, and primary care providers need to do more outreach into addressing health risk behaviors, e.g., alcohol abuse, before the chronic problems develop. The development of cultural competence among health providers is enormously important. Integral to this situation is a discussion of definition – when does one stop being a refugee or an immigrant? While there is no simple answer, it is clear (to the authors, at least) that the legal and political definitions drawn of "refugee" are frequently far too limited and unrealistic.

Health risks and screening parameters

The following are general and specific guidelines for health screening of refugees and immigrants. Note that these are not completely inclusive. Clinical and other judgments are essential in determining health risks and screening requirements of groups and individuals. Conditions in regions of the world change and problems not noted here may arise (Ackerman, 1997; CDC, 2002a; Gavagan & Brodyaga, 1998; Kemp, 2002; Minnesota Department of Health, 2001).

Health risks: global
- Malnutrition
- Intestinal parasites (especially amebiasis, giardiasis, ascariasis, strongyloidiasis, hookworm, trichuriasis, enterobiasis)
- Hepatitis B
- Tuberculosis
- Low immunization rate (risk for measles, mumps, rubella, diphtheria, pertussis, tetanus)

- Dental caries
- Malaria
- Sexually transmitted infections, including cervical cancer, HIV/AIDS, chancroid, chlamydia, gonorrhea, granuloma inguinale, lymphogranuloma venereum, syphilis
- Diarrheal illnesses
- Long-term effects of trauma, rape, torture (PTSD)
- Neonatal tetanus
- Rheumatic heart disease
- *Among children, high lead levels are increasingly seen worldwide.*

Screening and laboratory recommendations (global)

- Tuberculosis (PPD)
- Intestinal parasites (stool for O and P ×3)
- Hepatitis (including hepatitis surface antigen (HBsAg), hepatitis B surface antibody (anti-HBs), and hepatitis B core antibody (anti-HBc))
- HIV (ELISA and western blot)
- VDRL/RPR for syphilis
- CBC with differential
- Urine analysis (UA) (if abnormal, consider UC, urine AFB, or urine O and P)
- Other sexually transmitted infections (chancroid, gonorrhea, granuloma inguinale, lymphogranuloma venereum)
- Hansen's disease
- Immunization status
- Nutritional status

Consider the following, based on history and findings

- Malaria (thick and thin blood smears)
- Pregnancy test
- Varicella titer

REFERENCES

Ackerman, L. K. (1997). Health problems of refugees. *Journal of the American Board of Family Practice*, **10**, 337–48.

American Public Health Association (APHA) (2002). *Understanding the Health Culture of Recent Immigrants to the United States: A Cross-cultural Maternal Health Information Catalog.* Retrieved November 5, 2002 from http://www.apha.org/ppp/red/index.htm.

Becker, G., Beyene, Y. & Ken, P. (2000). Health, welfare reform, and narratives of uncertainty among Cambodian refugees. *Culture, Medicine, and Psychiatry*, **24**, 139–63.

Benzeguir, A. K., Capraru, T., Aust-Kettis, A. & Bjorkman, A. (1999). High frequency of gastrointestinal parasites in refugees and asylum seekers upon arrival in Sweden. *Scandinavian Journal of Infectious Disease*, **31**, 79–82.

Blair, R. G. (2000). Risk factors associated with PTSD and major depression among Cambodian refugees in Utah. *Health and Social Work*, **25**, 23–30.

Centers for Disease Control and Prevention (CDC) (2002a). *Medical Examinations of Aliens (Refugees and Immigrants)*. Retrieved November 11, 2002 from http://www.cdc.gov/ncidod/dq/health.htm.

(2002b). Increase in African immigrants and refugees with tuberculosis – Seattle-King County, Washington, 1998–2001. *Morbidity and Mortality Weekly Report*, **39**, 882–3.

D'Avanzo, C. E. & Barab, S. A. (1998). Depression and anxiety among Cambodian refugee women in France and the United States. *Issues in Mental Health Nursing*, **19**, 541–56.

Erickson, R. V. & Hoang, G. N. (1980). Health problems among Indochinese refugees. *American Journal of Public Health*, **70**, 1003–6.

Gailly, A. (n.d.). *The Access of Immigrants to Healthcare in Belgium: Perceptions and Good Practices*. Retrieved May 14, 2003 from http://www.salutepertutti.org/.

Gavagan, T. & Brodyaga, L. (1998). Medical care for immigrants and refugees. *American Family Physician*, **57**, 1061–8.

Gorst-Unsworth, C. & Goldenberg, E. (1998). Psychological sequelae of torture and organized violence suffered by refugees from Iraq. *British Journal of Psychiatry*, **172**, 90–4.

Hawn, T. R. & Jung, E. C. (2003). Health screening in immigrants, refugees, and internationally adopted orphans. In *The Travel and Tropical Medicine Manual*, 3rd edn., ed. E. C. Jong and R. McMullen, pp. 255–65. Philadelphia, PA: W. B. Saunders.

Hayes, M., Sheik, M., Wilson, H. G., & Spiegel, P. (2002). Reproductive health indicators and outcomes among refugees and internally displaced persons in postemergency phase camps. *Journal of the American Medical Association*, **288**, 595–603.

Hobbs, M., Moor, C., Wansbrough, T., & Calder, L. (2002). The health status of asylum seekers screened by Auckland Public Health in 1999 and 2000. *New Zealand Medical Journal*, **115**, 152.

Kemp, C. (2002). *Infectious Diseases: Bioterrorism and Infectious Diseases of Refugees and Immigrants*. Retrieved November 20, 2002 from http://www3.baylor.edu/~Charles_Kemp/Infectious_Disease.htm.

Kemp, C. & Rasbridge, L. A. (2000). *Cambodian Refugees and Health Care in the Inner-city*. Retrieved November 30, 2002 from http://www3.baylor.edu/~Charles_Kemp/cambodian_health.html.

Ku, L. & Freilich, A. (1991). Caring for immigrants: health care safety nets in Los Angeles, New York, Miami, and Houston. *Kaiser Commission on Medicaid and the Uninsured*. Retrieved June 1, 2003 from http://aspe.hhs.gov/hsp/immigration/caring01/report.pdf.

Lifson, A. R., Thai, D., O'Fallon, A., Mills, W. A., & Hang, K. (2002). Prevalence of tuberculosis, hepatitis B virus, and intestinal parasitic infections among refugees to Minnesota. *Public Health Reports*, **117**, 69–77.

Lopez-Velez, R., Turrientes C., Gutierrez, C., & Mateos, M. (1997). Prevalence of hepatitis B, C, and D markers in Sub-Saharan African immigrants. *Journal of Clinical Gastroenterology*, **25**, 650–2.

Matteelli, A., Volonterio, A., Gulletta, M. *et al.* (2001). Malaria in illegal Chinese immigrants, Italy. *Emerging Infectious Diseases*, **7**, Retrieved June 20, 2003 from http://www.cdc.gov/ncidod/eid/vol7no6/matteelli.htm.

Minnesota Department of Health, (2001). *Minnesota Refugee Health Provider Guide.* Author: Minneapolis.

Mollica, R. F., McInnes, K., Poole, C., & Tor, S. (1998). Dose–effect relationships of trauma to symptoms of depression and post-traumatic stress disorder among Cambodian survivors of mass violence. *British Journal of Psychiatry*, **173**, 482–8.

Mollica, R. F., Henderson, D. C., & Tor, S. (2002). Psychiatric effects of traumatic brain injury events in Cambodian survivors of mass violence. *British Journal of Psychiatry*, **181**, 339–47.

Peterson, M. H., Konczyk, M. R., Ambrosino, K., Carpenter, D. F., Wilhelm, J. & Kocka, F. E. (2001). Parasitic screening of a refugee population in Illinois. *Diagnostic Microbiology and Infectious Disease*, **40**, 75–6.

Schlein, L. (2003). Refugees continue to be unwelcome says UNHCR. *Voice of America News.* Retrieved June 21, 2003 from http://www.voanews.com/.

Silove, D., Sinnerbrink, I. Field, A., Manicavasagar, V., & Steel, Z. (1997). Anxiety, depression, and PTSD in asylum-seekers: associations with pre-migration trauma and post-migration stressors. *British Journal of Psychiatry*, **70**, 351–7.

Skidmore, M. (2002). Menstrual madness: Women's health and well-being in urban Burma. *Women and Health*, **35**, 81–99.

Sondergaard, H. P., Ekblad, S., & Theorell, T. (2001). Self-reported life event patterns and their relation to health among recently resettled Iraqi and Kurdish refugees in Sweden. *The Journal of Nervous and Mental Disease*, **189**, 838–45.

Uba, L. & Chung, R. C.-Y. (1991). The relationship between trauma and financial and physical well-being among Cambodians in the United States. *The Journal of General Psychology*, **118**, 215–25.

Yaman, H., Kut, A., Yaman, A., & Ungan, M. (2002). Health problems among UN refugees at a family medical centre in Ankara, Turkey. *Scandinavian Journal of Primary Health Care*, **20**, 85–7.

4

Mental health

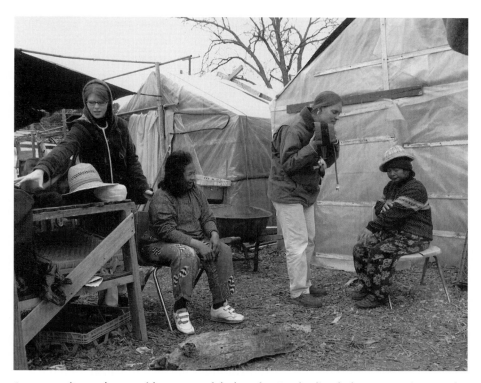

A community garden provides a peaceful place for Cambodian holocaust survivors and a place for nursing students to learn community health. (Photograph by courtesy of Charles Kemp.)

Refugee and Immigrant Health: A Handbook for Health Professionals, Charles Kemp and Lance A. Rasbridge. Published by Cambridge University Press. © C. Kemp and L. A. Rasbridge 2004.

Introduction

Many refugees are at high risk for mental health problems as a direct result of the refugee experience, especially war/trauma experience and displacement (Fazel & Stein, 2002; Kivling-Boden & Sundbom, 2002; Lie, 2002; Mollica, 2001; Silove, 1999). Many also experience psychosocial and environmental problems in the host country that negatively affect mental health. Refugees are also subject to the same mental health problems as any other population.

Some immigrants, especially those who have a difficult or dangerous journey to the host country or who live in poverty or isolated in the host country, are also at risk for mental health problems as sequelae to the immigration experience. Immigrants whose journey is risk free and who do not have daily struggles in the host country are at less risk for mental health problems. However, even this group still may live as "other" and thus have ongoing negative life experiences and be at risk for mental illness.

In this chapter we will first examine mental health issues specific to refugees, and then look briefly at mental health issues of immigrants. Readers should note that many of the concepts discussed under refugees may also be applied to nonrefugee immigrants.

War/trauma experience

War is brutal. Caught in the middle and burdened by family and possessions, refugees often experience far greater brutality than combatants. Common to all such experiences are shattered illusions of safety and a penetrating awareness of vulnerability. Traumatic experiences of refugees (Blair, 2000; Cunningham & Cunningham, 1997; Mollica et al., 2002; Silove, 1999; Weinstein et al., 2001) may include experiencing or witnessing the following.

- Imprisonment is common and being held in isolation tends to be more traumatic. In contrast to imprisonment in lawful circumstances, imprisonment for refugees seldom includes visitors.
- Rape and other assaults are common and torture is also common. Physical torture may include beating, electric shock (increasingly used because no signs are left), burning, asphyxiation, stretching, genital trauma, and rape. Psychological torture may include threats, isolation, mock execution, forced witnessing of torture or execution, and sleep deprivation. In some cases, rape is an institutionalized weapon of war.
- Combat atrocities, including bombing, explosions, and other means of mass killing are very common. Refugees may witness multiple killings extending over time.

- Home and possessions are destroyed or left behind. The majority of refugees come to countries of second asylum with nothing but clothes and perhaps one or two momentos of their former life.
- Family members are often separated, wounded, or killed. This is a source of chronic unresolved grief for many survivors.

How I Came to America (anonymous elementary school essay)

It was very difficult to leave Cambodia. There was very little food, even though people were made to work very hard. Pol Pot's soldiers killed many people. The Vietnamese came and fought with Pol Pot's army.

I remember being happy in Cambodia when I was little. I remember helping my Grandfather and Grandmother make clothes to sell. They let me fold and help cut material. Then they would sew the material to make clothes.

I remember playing games, fresh coconuts, and the temple Angkor Wat.

I remember many things that make me very sad. I will tell you about them.

We rode the train from Phnom Penh to Battambang. From Battambang we started walking to Thailand. We had to leave. My father, my mother, brother, sister, grandfather and grandmother all went together. We were walking through the forest. The trees bent back and forth, the leaves fell to the ground like raindrops, but there were no clouds in the sky. The Vietnamese and Pol Pot's soldiers captured us. They did some terrible things I will never forget.

They tied my mother and father to trees. My mother was going to have a baby but she was very skinny. They took a sword and cut her stomach opened and cut the baby out and killed it and cut her again. She screamed and screamed! Many days I put my head on my desk and still hear her screaming. They shot my father in the head. They dug a big hole and put my grandfather and grandmother in it and other people too. They threw grenades into it and blew all the bodies apart. This soldier helped us try to get away with my aunt. They shot at us. They threw a grenade. They shot my toes and part of the grenade hit me in the back. I almost died.

The Vietnamese came and made Pol Pot's soldiers leave. The Vietnamese doctor came and gave me a shot and took me to a hospital in a tent. I got better. My aunt carried me to Thailand.

I went to school 4 days in Thailand. I came to America on June 25, 1981.

- Hunger is widespread. Food (or its lack) is a classic and effective weapon of war, and civilians, of course, are the last priority for receiving food and the first to have it taken away.
- Health is compromised. Risk factors include nutritional deficiencies, shortages of medicine, shortages of health personnel, and lack of facilities.
- Life in refugee camps, especially in countries of first asylum, is usually difficult. Conditions in most camps are primitive and dangerous, with some camps similar to third-world prisons.

These and other factors lead to a high incidence of (a) anxiety disorders, especially post-traumatic stress disorder (PTSD) or combat stress reaction (CSR) and to a lesser extent (b) depressive disorders (Fazel & Stein, 2002; Lie, 2002; Sack *et al.*, 1997). Grief is a major factor in the lives of many refugees and grief therapy is a helpful model in counseling refugees with PTSD and other distress (Kemp, 2000).

Displacement

"*When we came to America we were so scared. Somehow we just lost. Maybe our souls. We don't know.*" (Anonymous)

Refugees leave their homeland and culture with little hope of return. "Culture shock" is thus overwhelming and for older generations with less ability to adapt, unrelenting. A lifetime of memories, familiarity, and accomplishment is abandoned and a completely new and often incomprehensible and hostile world is entered. Language, customs, and values of the new world are not only different from those of the refugee, but also are perceived by some refugees and some people in the country of refuge as superior to the language, customs, and values of the refugee. Adjustment to the culture in the new home is often more difficult for refugees than for immigrants and is often most difficult for older refugees.

Constructs such as "social displacement syndrome" and "survivor syndrome" applied to refugees give a relatively consistent picture of responses to displacement. Although presented as "stages" here, these are better thought of as a process of common states of mind/response(s) often experienced by refugees, especially those who have had traumatic displacement experiences. These phases, especially the latter ones, coincide with the stages discussed in Chapter 3 (Fazel & Stein, 2002; Kemp, 2000; Phillips *et al.*, 1982).

The first phase of displacement

This is the wartime and/or repression that led to the necessity of leaving. This is discussed earlier in the section on war/trauma experience.

The barbed wire phase (a term from Holocaust literature)

This represents time spent in hostile circumstances such as under a totalitarian government or in refugee, austerity, or even concentration camps. This phase is characterized by suppression or repression of feelings and normal responses to circumstances. For example, Rule 6 of the "Security Regulations" at Tuol Sleng Prison in Cambodia stated, "WHILE GETTING LASHES OR ELECTRIFICATION YOU MUST NOT CRY AT ALL" The genesis of *chronic* PTSD may be found in this and other phases, when normal responses to stress are not allowed or experienced.

The liberation and following year phase

This may begin with life in the country of first asylum if living and other conditions there are positive. If living conditions in the country of first asylum are difficult, liberation may not be felt to begin until the country of second asylum is reached. This phase is characterized by some euphoria, and a degree of cognitive or emotional disorganization related in some cases to separation of family members.

The early after-effects phase

This occurs when a refugee reaches stable and relatively safe refuge, such as the country of second asylum. Ambivalence in thought and behavior are characteristic of this phase as the refugee reorganizes patterns of living and perception to deal with life in the new land. New and effective behaviors may be in conflict with old and more deeply held values. It is at this time that the refugee may begin to confront behaviors that resulted in survival but conflict with the ego ideal, e.g., fleeing for survival while others may have stayed to fight. Chronic anxiety, flattened emotions, loss of self-esteem, depression, and recurrent nightmares are features of this stage.

The delayed after-effects phase

This is characterized by withdrawal and exacerbation of the above problems masked in many cases by frequent alcohol or other drug use. Family conflict may worsen and be exacerbated by young people's embrace of new cultural values and rejection of the past.

The recovery phase

With some degree of assimilation and acceptance of the new circumstances this is, hopefully, the last phase.

The consequences of war/trauma experience and displacement

The most common negative outcome of war/trauma experience and displacement is PTSD or some variation on PTSD. These and other mental health problems are compounded by great difficulty in accessing and obtaining, on a consistent basis, any sort of effective health care; an inability to access mental health services existing in the host country; and separation from traditional sources of care for mental distress.

The Diagnostic and Statistical Manual of Mental Disorders, 4th edn (DSM IV) identifies "psychosocial and environmental problems that may affect the diagnosis, treatment, and prognosis of mental disorders" (American Psychiatric Association

(APA), 2000, page 29). These problems fit – to a startling extent – the circumstances of many refugees. They include:

- problems with the primary support group, such as the death of a family member, family disruption, and abuse;
- problems related to the social environment, such as death or loss of a friend, inadequate social support, acculturation problems, and discrimination;
- educational problems, including illiteracy and academic problems;
- occupational problems, including unemployment and stress at work;
- housing problems, such as inadequate housing, unsafe neighborhoods, or problems with neighbors;
- economic problems;
- problems with access to health services;
- problems related to the legal system;
- other psychosocial and environmental problems.

All these (except problems related to the legal system – usually) fit the circumstances of virtually all refugees, especially early in the refugee process. Most of these problems also fit the circumstances of many immigrants. The cumulative negative effects of these factors contribute to the development or exacerbation of mental and other health problems.

Post-traumatic stress disorder

Anxiety disorders such as PTSD and/or combat stress reaction (CSR) are common responses to war and related or similar trauma (Fazel & Stein, 2002; Lie, 2002; Solomon, 1993). Symptoms of PTSD or PTSD-like disorders are often accompanied by depressive symptoms (Lie, 2002). The focus here is on PTSD because most studies on refugees have identified PTSD as a primary problem rather than CSR (e.g., Kivling-Boden & Sundbom, 2002; Lie, 2002). Diagnostic criteria (or assessment parameters) of PTSD as defined in the DSM IV include:

- exposure to a traumatic event involving (a) actual or threatened death or serious injury to self or others and (b) a response of intense fear, helplessness, or horror.
- persistent and distressing re-experiencing of the traumatic event in one or more of the following ways: (a) intrusive recollections, (b) dreams of the event, (c) reliving the event such as in flashbacks, (d) intense psychological distress from exposure to external or internal cues to the event, (e) physiological activity (increased heart rate, chest pain, difficulty breathing, diaphoresis, etc.) from exposure to external or internal cues to the event.
- persistent avoidance of stimuli related to the trauma and "numbing of general responsiveness (not present before the trauma)" such as (a) attempts to avoid stimuli such as thoughts, feelings, places, or people related to the trauma,

(b) inability to remember key aspects of the trauma, (c) decreased interest or participation in activities, (d) feeling detached or estranged from others, (e) decreased affect such as inability to feel love, and/or (f) decreased sense of future.

- persistent "increased arousal (not present before the trauma)" such as (a) difficulty sleeping, (b) irritability or anger, (c) difficulty concentrating, (d) hypervigilance, and/or (e) increased startle response.
- symptoms lasting more than 1 month.
- distress resulting in significant symptoms or impairment.

PTSD is classified as acute if symptoms last less than 3 months, chronic if symptoms last more than 3 months, and delayed onset if onset is at least 6 months after the traumatic event. Most refugees with PTSD in countries of second asylum would thus have chronic (and often delayed onset and chronic) PTSD.

The incidence of PTSD as defined by the DSM IV among adult and child refugees from war zones ranges from 25–94% (Goldstein *et al.*, 1997; Holtz, 1998; Lie; 2002; Sack *et al.*, 1997). The incidence and severity of PTSD are related to several factors (Basoglu *et al.*, 1997; Kemp, 2000; Mollica *et al.*, 2002), including:

- the frequency and severity of trauma;
- preparedness for trauma;
- the existence or absence of spirituality and other protective factors in the person experiencing trauma.

In the case of refugees, a common exacerbating factor in developing PTSD or a confounding factor in treating it is that there is neither time nor resources available after the trauma(s) for dealing with or integrating the trauma. War-time presents little opportunity for dealing with anxiety, and some totalitarian regimes do not allow expression of feelings. Living as an asylum-seeker in the country of first asylum adds to the uncertainty and stress, and living in the country of second asylum may mean an absence of culturally, linguistically, and/or spiritually appropriate means of addressing psychological/emotional pain. In countries of second asylum many refugees also work extraordinarily hard, hence have little energy for dealing with problems. Conversely, many refugees are unemployed and unable to mobilize themselves for life itself, much less, addressing psychological problems.

The incidence or severity of PTSD or PTSD-related disorders tends to decrease with time after the stressful event(s). Although healing is slower in more traumatized persons and groups, there is an overall reduction in symptoms and decline in distress. A common pattern is alternating responses of intrusion and avoidance that changes as an individual works through or adapts to the trauma. Intrusion gradually shifts more into avoidance as time passes (Solomon, 1993). Yet, regardless of patterns, severe trauma has a life-long negative effect among many (Shmotkin *et al.*, 2003).

Grief

Grief is the normal response to loss and must be considered in an attempt to understand the mental health of refugees and immigrants (Kemp, in press). Responses to trauma and loss often resemble or can be described in terms of grief reaction or delayed grief reaction. Through displacement and war, refugees lose their home, possessions, and often, loved ones or sense of self. Immigrants lose – at a minimum – their sense of place and comfort. Any one of these might result in severe grief. Other losses that may be less obvious:

- The unconditional loss of a war, i.e., complete dominance by a hostile force, may be a shattering blow to individual and community esteem.
- Decisions made during war or flight from war may come to haunt refugees as they shift from circumstances of war to those of peace. What seemed necessary, if not right, at one time may be later perceived as wrong or unnecessary.
- Old ways of life are seldom valued in the new life. The respected family or village elder becomes irrelevant, impotent, or even an object of ridicule. Relations within families or groups undergo irrevocable change. Rituals, ceremonies, and perhaps religions do not fit with the mainstream culture and may thus lose at least some of their power. Adjustment to the new culture, for which many refugees and immigrants strive, means losing the old while never quite gaining the new.
- Loss of future is a subtle and little-understood phenomenon. For many refugees the future seems at best uncertain. Once safety is reached, there is a sense of great relief. However, the relief is often followed by persistent and well-founded uncertainty and anxiety about the future.
- As is true with PTSD, grief may affect individuals, their families, communities, or even be seen in terms of cultural grief and bereavement.

Dysfunctional or complicated grief is grief that lasts longer and is characterized by greater disability or dysfunctional patterns than is usual among persons of a particular culture (Kemp, in press; Silverman *et al.*, 2001; Tomita & Kitamura, 2002). Assessment parameters include (a) the loss of something important (see above) and (b) responses including prolonged, disabling changes in life patterns, e.g., changes in sleep, dreams, libido, concentration; excessive anger, crying, sadness, guilt; difficulty expressing or denial of the loss; repetitive reliving of experiences related to the loss and/or ineffective attempts to address the loss or replace the lost object; and verbal expression of lasting distress over the loss.

Immigrants

The immigration experience ranges from desperate and sometimes lethal journeys through desert or jungle where some die from exposure or dehydration, and encounters with bandits are routine and terrible, to first-class flights where the greatest trauma is immigration delays. In the first case, previous discussions of trauma, PTSD, and grief experienced by refugees apply to immigrants. In the latter case, there is no apparent trauma, yet there still remains stress. The stress translates both to mental *and* physical health problems. Stressors specific to immigrants (Fossion *et al.*, 2002; Jaber *et al.*, 2003; Pernice & Brook, 1994; Ritsner & Ponizovsky, 2003; Yeh, 2003) include the following:

- Culture change (or "culture shock") is inevitable, even for the most Westernized immigrants. The degree of stress and subsequent distress is greater among the less Westernized who also are more likely to be at a lower socioeconomic status.
- Language change is a problem for nearly all immigrants, even for most of those who speak the language of the host country. Idioms and regional variations and references may confound even the best-educated immigrant, thus causing anxiety.
- Family disruption is universal. There may be little stress in separation of a few weeks' or months' duration, but for most immigrants, separation is long-lasting and when illness or crisis strikes, there may not be an opportunity to return home where social support is available.
- Lack of social support is an ongoing problem for many immigrants. Coping with this isolation includes living in ethnic enclaves, adopting fictive older kin, sending home for relatives or a spouse, spending large amounts of time at ethnic "hang-outs," watching videos or cable television from the home country, and so on – in all cases, maintaining links to the familiar.
- Family role changes affect all ages and genders. Children, with their ability to more quickly learn the new language may be called upon to translate or serve as the family interface with the outside world. Elders may be perceived first by the outside world, and then within the family, as less valuable due to their inability to interact with the host culture. In male-dominated cultures, women having an easier time finding and keeping work, or in some cases being paid at higher rates than men is enormously stressful to both men and women.
- Poor, non-affirming, or superficial relations with people native to the host country are common. This creates a sense of ongoing devaluation of the immigrant's self and culture.

Often, when thinking of immigrants and psychological distress, the focus is on poor or otherwise marginalized people. However, contrary to popular conceptions, even privileged and educated immigrants, especially the younger and older (vs middle-aged), experience significant distress *and* the distress continues over time *and* on return to the home country (Furukawa, 1997; Ritsner & Ponizovsky, 2003).

The tasks of bereavement applied to refugees

The tasks of bereavement (Carpenito, 2002; Cooley, 1992; Kemp, 1999) include all or most of the below. These may be applied to refugees or immigrants according to circumstances of individuals.

Telling the story of the loss or trauma

The story usually needs to be told repeatedly, with details emerging over time (Mollica, 2001). The client may need help in sequencing events, clarifying details, and separating what is real from what is not. The story of the loss or trauma may also include reflection and discussion of the "good times" in the life before the trauma.

Expressing and accepting the sadness and pain (catharsis of the expected emotions/responses)

Many people fear an emotional catastrophe if the sadness and related feelings are expressed and thus re-experienced. There also are cultural, gender, and other issues in expressing or controlling feelings.

Expressing and accepting guilt, anger, and other negatively perceived feelings (contrast to expected responses above)

Denied or hidden guilt and/or anger are common defenses. As with addressing sadness and pain, there are cultural, gender, and other issues related to guilt, anger, and other feelings. Catharsis is a powerful and sometimes frightening process in this step. Group work may be especially helpful here. Because guilt is almost universal, it should be directly addressed, including working with the client to help her or him reach the conclusion that neither the trauma nor the response is the victim's fault. Forgiveness of self can be a powerful experience.

Reviewing the relationship with what was lost, e.g., loved ones, culture, sense of self, trust, dignity, and so on

This step is obviously valuable when grief is the primary issue, but is also part of dealing with the losses related to trauma, including torture – when the loss is trust in self or sense of self.

Understanding common processes and problems in responses to trauma

Although the pain is not lessened, it is highly beneficial to know that responses (such as described earlier) are normal and even common. Like other people in distress, refugees often feel that nobody else has experienced what they have experienced nor responded as they have responded. Some feel that their responses indicate mental illness. Understanding common processes helps decrease the sense of shame and isolation. Therapeutic/information groups are a helpful means of increasing understanding and decreasing isolation.

Being understood or accepted by others

Isolation is common and functions to exacerbate problems among refugees. Understanding and acceptance are healing factors.

Exploring possibilities in the new life

From the ashes of pain and destruction may rise a new and sometimes stronger life. Some things or aspects of self are never regained and some wounds are never healed. Even so, through a process of grieving for the old life, setting achievable goals for the new, and successfully solving problems; and with the social and spiritual support discussed throughout this chapter, the client can go forward.

Working on, and to some extent, through these tasks decreases distress and moves the client toward healing. However, recovery from the trauma of torture and some war experiences is a long process and periods of regression may occur, manifested by depression or alcohol and/or other drug abuse; or by crisis situations involving violence toward others or self. Intermittent emergency and/or long-term support is often required.

Much of the Western literature on trauma focuses on the use of psychotherapeutic or professional counseling intervention in the treatment of persons who have been tortured or otherwise traumatized. Clearly, trauma such as torture inflicts spiritual as well as physical and psychological injury. Consideration should thus also be given to the spiritual component in the response to or treatment of trauma. Traditional treatments and ceremonies often have a spiritual component and may be an effective recourse for traumatized and/or grieving clients. If clients are referred to a source of spiritual care, the referring party should ensure that the source of care is aware of the realities and consequences of war-related trauma.

REFERENCES

American Psychiatric Association (APA) (2000). *Diagnostic and Statistical Manual of Mental Disorders*, 4th edn, text revision. Washington, DC: Author.

Basoglu, M., Mineka, S., Paker, M., Aker, T., Livanou, M., & Gok, S. (1997). Psychological preparedness for trauma as a protective factor in survivors of torture. *Psychological Medicine*, **27**, 1421–33.

Blair, R. G. (2000). Risk factors associated with PTSD and major depression among Cambodian refugees in Utah. *Health and Social Work*, **25**, 23–30.

Carpenito, L. J. (2002). *Nursing Diagnosis: Application to Clinical Practice*. Philadelphia, PA: J. B. Lippincott.

Cooley, M. E. (1992). Bereavement care: a role for nurses. *Cancer Nursing*, **15**, 125–9.

Cunningham, M. & Cunningham, J. D. (1997). Patterns of symptomatology and patterns of torture and trauma experiences in resettled refugees. *Australian and New Zealand Journal of Psychiatry*, **31**, 555–65.

Fazel, M. & Stein, A. (2002). The mental health of refugee children. *Archives of Disease in Childhood*, **87**, 366–70.

Fossion, P., Ledoux, Y., Valente, F. *et al.* (2002). Psychiatric disorders and social characteristics among second-generation Moroccan migrants in Belgium: an age-and gender-controlled study conducted in a psychiatric emergency department. *European Psychiatry*, **17**, 443–50.

Furukawa, T. (1997). Sojourner readjustment: Mental health of international students after one year's foreign sojourn and its psychosocial correlates. *Journal of Nervous and Mental Disease*, **185**, 263–8.

Goldstein, R. D., Wampler, N. S., & Wise, P. H. (1997). War experiences and distress symptoms of Bosnian children. *Pediatrics*, **100**, 873–8.

Holtz, T. H. (1998). Refugee trauma versus torture trauma: A retrospective controlled cohort study of Tibetan refugees. *Journal of Nervous and Mental Disease*, **186**, 24–34.

Jaber, L. A., Brown, M. B., Hammad, A., Zhu, Q., & Herman, W. H. (2003). Lack of acculturation is a risk factor for diabetes in Arab immigrants in the US. *Diabetes Care*, **26**, 2010–14.

Kemp, C. (1999). *Terminal Illness: A Guide to Nursing Care*, 2nd edn. Philadelphia, PA: J. B. Lippincott.

  (2000). *Refugee Mental Health*. Accessed 2/25/2003 from http://www3.baylor.edu/~Charles_Kemp/refugee_mental_health.htm.

Kemp, C. (in press). Grief and loss. In *Psychiatric Mental Health Nursing*, 3rd edn., ed. K. M. Fortinash & P. A. Holoday-Worret St. Louis: Mosby.

Kivling-Boden, G. & Sundbom, E. (2002). The relationship between post-traumatic symptoms and life in exile in a clinical group of refugees from the former Yugoslavia. *Acta Psychiatrica Scandanavia*, **105**, 461–8.

Lie, B. (2002). A 3-year follow-up study of psychosocial functioning and general symptoms in settled refugees. *Acta Psychiatrica Scandanavia*, **106**, 415–25.

Mollica, R. F. (2001). The trauma story: a phenomenological approach to the traumatic life experiences of refugee survivors. *Psychiatry*, **64**, 60–3.

Mollica, R. F., Henderson, D. C., & Tor, S. (2002). Psychiatric effects of traumatic brain injury events in Cambodian survivors of mass violence. *British Journal of Psychiatry*, **181**, 339–47.

Pernice, R., & Brook, J. (1994). Relationship of migrant status (refugee or immigrant) to mental health. *International Journal of Social Psychiatry*, **40**, 177–88.

Phillips, S., Baker, R., & Pearson, R. (1982). A critical review of terminology and psychosocial issues related to the survival of refugees who have experience the threat of genocide. *Proceedings of the International Conference on the Holocaust and Genocide*. Tel Aviv.

Ritsner, M. & Ponizovsky, A. (2003). Age differences in stress process of recent immigrants. *Comprehensive Psychiatry*, **44**, 135–41.

Sack, W. H., Seeley, J. R., & Clarke, G. N. (1997). Does PTSD transcend cultural barriers? A study from the Khmer adolescent refugee project. *Journal of the American Academy of Child and Adolescent Psychiatry*, **36**, 49–54.

Shmotkin, D., Blumstein, T., & Modan, B. (2003). Tracing long-term effects of early trauma: a broad-scope view of Holocaust survivors in late life. *Journal of Consulting and Clinical Psychology*, **71**, 223–34.

Silove, D. (1999). The psychosocial effects of torture, mass human rights violations, and refugee trauma. *The Journal of Nervous and Mental Disease*, **187**, 200–7.

Silverman, G. K., Johnson, J. G., & Prigerson, H. G. (2001). Preliminary explorations of the effects of prior trauma and loss on risk for psychiatric disorders in recently widowed people, *Israel Journal of Psychiatry and Related Sciences*, **38**, 202–15.

Solomon, Z. (1993). *Combat Stress Reaction: The Enduring Toll of War*. New York: Plenum Press.

Tomita, T. & Kitamura, T. (2002). Clinical and research measures of grief: a reconsideration. *Comprehensive Psychiatry*, **43**, 95–102.

Weinstein, C. S., Fucetola, R., & Mollica, R. (2001). Neuropsychological issues in the assessment of refugees and victims of mass violence. *Neuropsychology Review*, **11**, 131–41.

Yeh, C. J. (2003). Age, acculturation, cultural adjustment, and mental health symptoms of Chinese, Korean, and Japanese immigrant youths. *Cultural Diversity and Ethnic Minor Psychology*, **9**, 34–48.

5

Religions

Sonal Bhungalia and Charles Kemp

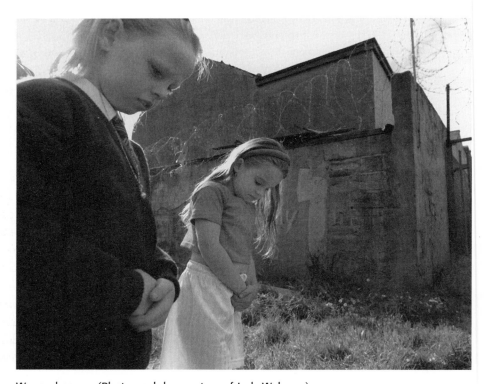

War and peace. (Photograph by courtesy of Judy Walgren.)

Refugee and Immigrant Health: A Handbook for Health Professionals, Charles Kemp and Lance A. Rasbridge.
Published by Cambridge University Press. © C. Kemp and L. A. Rasbridge 2004.

Introduction

Refugees and immigrants bring a variety of religions and faith traditions to their new homes. Like other people, refugees and immigrants cannot easily be categorized as Muslim or Christian or Buddhist and then be expected to follow a particular set of behaviors based on that religion. Within all religions there are differences of opinion about even some of the most basic tenets of the religion and other doctrinal issues. Here we seek only to acquaint readers with some basics about world religions and how they sometimes influence health care beliefs and practices.

Being a stranger in a new land, along with the suffering from war, loss of home, loss of culture, loss of identity, and the challenges (and sometimes failures) of life in the new country, is sometimes experienced as a spiritual crisis. Most or all the basic spiritual needs (hope, meaning, relatedness, forgiveness or acceptance, and transcendence) are threatened and often unmet when people have no place of their own. Although meeting spiritual needs is not the focus of this work, we do want to state as clearly as possible that unmet spiritual needs are a threat to health and that supporting faith *per se* is important in improving health.

This chapter addresses only the major world religions (Hinduism, Buddhism, Judaism, Christianity, and Islam). They are discussed in approximate order of age, with the oldest coming first and the newest last.

Hinduism

The earliest records of Hinduism date back to about the time that Moses was said to have received the Ten Commandments, around 1000 to 1500 BC (Grun, 1982; Roberts, 1993). The major Hindu scriptures are the *Vedas*, the *Upanishads*, and the most recent, the *Bhagavad-Gita* (often referred to as the *Gita*). The early Hindu scriptures are a collection of writings by seers or prophets, while the *Bhagavad-Gita* is a dialogue between Lord Krishna and Prince Arjuna.

The goal of Hinduism is freedom (of the soul or *Atman*) from endless re-incarnations and the suffering inherent in existence. In popular usage, re-incarnation and transmigration (rebirth) of the soul are viewed similarly. The endless re-incarnations are the result of *karma*, the actions of the individual in this present life and also the accumulation of actions from past lives.

"Free us from sins committed by our fathers; from those through which we ourselves offended" (from a hymn to Varuna in the *Rigveda*)

Except for Western devotees of the Krishna Consciousness cult, Hindus are almost exclusively Indian. There is little interest in proselytizing as there is no call to convert others: one either is or is not Hindu. Indeed, some Hindus would say that Hinduism is less a belief than a statement of universal law – under which all beings are governed.

The caste system is an integral part of Hinduism. Caste divides society into four social classes, with the highest class being the priest class, or the *Brahmans* and the lowest class being the laborer class, or *Sudras*. Caste is inherited at birth and is based on *karma*. Aspects of Hinduism that commonly affect health decisions and communications between patient, family, and provider are as follows.

- *Karma* is a law of behavior and consequences in which actions in past live(s) affect the circumstances in which one is born and lives in this life. Thus a person may feel that his or her circumstances or illness is caused by *karma*, even though there may be a concurrent complete understanding of biological causes of illness.
- Belief in one God (*Brahma* the Creator or ultimate reality), many gods (such as *Brahma*, *Shiva*, *Vishnu*, *Krishna*, and others), in no gods, or in all the preceding with a focus on a particular deity or deities. How can this be, the Western mind may ask? "*Atman* is *Brahman*, *Brahman* is *Atman*. You yourself are the ultimate reality, but you are not what you seem" (Kaufman, 1976, p. 218). In other words, this faith is understood through the experience of enlightenment, and not through linear logic.
- Meditation and prayer are used by many Hindus. Some meditate silently, while others chant "*Aum*" and other prayers aloud.
- Vegetarianism is universal among devout Hindus and is based on belief in reincarnation, the idea that the soul of a person enters back into creation as a living being. Hindus pray a specific prayer before eating, in which one asks forgiveness for eating a plant or vegetable in which a soul could dwell.

Health beliefs and practices

The traditional Indian (and thus Hindu) system of medicine is known as *Ayurveda*, which means "knowledge of life." Diagnosis according to *Ayruveda* is based on determining the root cause of a disease, which is not always inside the body. When curing disease, it is important not to cause new symptoms by suppressing the presenting symptoms.

In the *Ayurveda* system, the body is composed of three primary forces, termed *dosha*. The three *dosha* (or tridosha) are called *Vata*, *Pitta*, and *Kapha*. Each *dosha* represents characteristics derived from the five elements of space, air, fire, water, and earth. Equilibrium among the *dosha* is perceived as a state of health and imbalance is disease. Once the aggravated or unbalanced *dosha* is known, it is brought into balance by using different kinds of therapies. Space represents the ears and is responsible for hearing, speech, and sound. Air represents skin, which is responsible for touch, pressure, and the feeling of cold to dry sensation. Fire represents the eyes, which are responsible for sight, heat, and light. Water represents the tongue, which is responsible for taste, liquids, and hot or cold. Earth represents the nose, hence is responsible for smelling and odor.

There are approximately 1400 plants used in *Ayurvedic* medicine, none of which is synonymous with instant pain relievers or antibiotics. The herbs used in *Ayurvedic* remedies are thought to gradually metabolize and have few side effects on the body. There is increasing availability of these herbs in the West, especially in large urban areas.

Most educated Hindus are fully conversant with modern scientific explanations of illness and Western or cosmopolitan medicine. As noted earlier, this does not preclude complete belief in karma as a cause of illness, nor does it, in some case, preclude the use of *Ayurvedic* and other traditional practices.

End of life

Many Hindu patients prefer to die at home, and some will go back to India – especially to the sacred city of Varanasi, to die. Consistent with the Western idea of resolving unfinished business, a Hindu who is elderly or terminally ill may put significant effort into resolving relationships and other such personal matters. Dying full of anger or fear leads to a lower level of rebirth than dying full of love and acceptance. It is important to understand that a devout Hindu believes that she or he has already been born and died many times in the past, and this contributes to increased acceptance of death.

The idea that suffering is inevitable and the result of *karma* may result in difficulty with reporting symptoms and with symptom control. Many will seek a conscious dying process and death, and hence will choose discomfort over clouded sensorium. Difficulties between hospice staff and family or the patient may arise when therapeutic measures are refused, especially when it seems that the patient may want or need the therapy, but the family influences her or him to refuse.

A person near death may be placed with her or his head facing east and a lamp placed near the head. Family members are likely to be present in large numbers as death nears. Chanting and prayer, incense, and various rituals are part of the process. These may include application of sacred ash or paste to the person's forehead and placing a few drops of milk or water from the sacred Ganges River (*Ganga Ma*) in the dying person's mouth. Ideally, the person who is dying will chant her or his mantra (a personal sacred phrase) as death occurs. If this is not possible, a family member may softly chant the mantra in the person's right ear. If there is not a chosen mantra, then the mantra *Aum Namo Narayana* or *Aum Nama Sivaya* may be used.

The moment of death is seen by some as similar to falling asleep, with the difference being that, in sleep, the silver cord that is thought to connect the body to the soul stays intact, but in death, the cord breaks.

After death, the family should be the only ones to touch the body, hence healthcare staff should touch the body as little as possible. Ideally, a family member should clean the body and this person should be of the same sex as the deceased. After cleaning, a cloth is tied under the chin and over the top of the head, the thumbs and great toes tied together, and the body is wrapped in a red cloth and placed with the head facing south. Embalming and organ donation are prohibited.

When a person dies in a hospital, the family may want the death certificate signed as soon as possible and then transport the body home rather than to a funeral home. At the home, religious pictures are turned to the wall and mirrors may also be covered. The ceremony at the home includes prayer, incense, chanting, and singing sacred songs.

The preference is for cremation and ideally, the ashes are spread over the holy river, *Ganga Ma*. The men and boys of the family may shave their hair as a symbol of mourning for the dead. The mourning family may wear all white and wish to have a *Brahman* at the funeral to perform a prayer and blessing.

Judaism

Judaism dates back to the Prophet Abraham around 1500–1000 BC. The central belief in Judaism is in the one God. "*Hear O Israel: the LORD our God is one LORD*" (the *Shema*, from Deuteronomy 6). The practice of this belief includes following the Law, living according to the ethics derived from the Law, following ritual, and supporting "the people, Israel." The sacred books of Judaism are:

- the *Torah* (Genesis–Deuteronomy).
- the *TaNaK* or the Hebrew Bible (*Torah*; *Neviim* or prophets such as Joshua, Samuel, Isaiah; and *K'tuvim* or sacred writings such as those of King David, Jeremiah and Eichah).
- the Talmud, consisting of a legal code written in Hebrew called the *Mishnah* and an Aramaic commentary on the *Mishnah* called the *Gemara*.

From the *Torah*, from millennia of pogroms, and from the Holocaust, have come Zionism and the modern state of Israel. "*The LORD said to Abram, 'Go from your country and your kindred and your father's house to the land that I will show you*" (Genesis 12: 1).

There are three main branches or movements (Rich, 2002) in Judaism:

- Orthodox Jews (7% of American Jews) practice strict observance of *halakhah* or Jewish Law, and believe that God (written as G-d to avoid defacing the name of the Lord) gave Moses the entire *Torah* as well as the oral tradition of the *Torah*. Within the Orthodox movement are modern Orthodox who tend to blend into society as a whole and the *Chasidim* (sometimes erroneously termed "ultra-Orthodox"), who live separately and dress distinctively.
- Conservative Jews (38% of American Jews) view the *Torah* and other sacred writings as coming from God, but transmitted by humans and thus possessing a human component. Conservative Jews follow *halakhah*, but with the belief that

the Law can remain true to Judaism's values while changing in accordance with the dominant culture.

- Reform Jews (42% of American Jews) are the most liberal and do not believe that the *Torah* was written by God. While not following the strict interpretation of the Law, Reform Jews hold to the values and ethics of the faith.

There are other movements, such as Reconstructionism, but these have significantly fewer followers than those discussed above.

The Sabbath or *Shabbat* begins on Friday, 18 minutes before sunset and ends on Saturday, about 40 minutes after sunset, when three stars can be seen. *Shabbat* should not be confused with the Christian Sabbath. *Shabbat* is primarily a time of rest and spiritual enrichment, and is composed of two main components:

- to remember the significance of *Shabbat* as a commemoration of creation and as a commemoration of Jewish freedom from slavery in Egypt;
- to observe *Shabbat* by following ritual and prohibitions. Note that what is normally prohibited on *Shabbat* (see below) is permitted to preserve life. The original prohibitions were based on work necessary to build the sanctuary and the modern prohibitions are derived from these.

There are a number of religious holidays, celebrated to various extents according to movement and personal inclination. These include *Yom Kippur* or the Day of Atonement (fall), *Pesach* or Passover (early spring), and *Rosh Hashana* or the Jewish New Year (fall).

Health beliefs and practices

Judaism has a long tradition of scientific and intellectual inquiry, and Jews, in general, tend to ascribe to modern medical and health practices. The care of Orthodox, and to a lesser extent, Conservative Jews, is most likely to be influenced by religious beliefs. Among the religious issues that may influence health care are the following.

- The observation of Sabbath and holy days includes proscriptions against using electricity, riding in a car, handling money, writing, and cooking. The exception to these restrictions is when life is in danger. For example, an ambulance and/or elevator may be used to save a person's life, but not for the convenience of family members or physicians.
- Dietary law includes consuming only kosher foods, i.e., those prepared or slaughtered according to kosher guidelines. Pork, shellfish, and raw meats or blood are forbidden, as is mixing meat and dairy at meals or in the preparation of food. Utensils that have been used to prepare or serve forbidden foods are also forbidden.
- Fasting is done for 24 hours during Yom Kippur. Medical needs for food or medicine take precedence over the religious observation in most cases. There is

a 24-hour fast during the summer on *Tisha b'av*. During Passover, no leavened bread or related products are eaten.

- Circumcision (*brit milah*) is performed on all males 8 days after birth by a *mohel*, a Jew with training in the procedure.
- Prayer is encouraged during illness. There are specific prayers for the sick, as well as personal intercessory prayers. Spiritual care is provided by a rabbi and/or family and friends.
- Organ transplants and amputations are accepted by most Jews, but some are opposed. In these and other ethical issues, a rabbi may be consulted.

End of life

Jewish patients in developed countries do not seem to have a strong preference for place of death. The issue more critical than place may be the availability of spiritual support and freedom to practice ritual. Spiritual care is best provided by a rabbi, but a person of any faith may appropriately read to the patient from the *Torah*, Psalms, or other Jewish holy books. Family involvement is likely to be considerable, especially among Orthodox Jews.

Withholding or withdrawing treatment in terminal illness is a matter of personal preference. Treatment with double-effect (palliation of symptoms at the cost of life) is not proscribed, but euthanasia and assisted suicide are clearly forbidden. Autopsy is acceptable if required by law, but no parts should be removed. Organ transplants are permitted with consultation from a rabbi (Andrews & Hanson, 1999).

Deathbed confession and repentance are traditional, as are blessings and ethical instruction to loved ones. There is not, however, a corollary to last rites as seen among Catholics.

After death, the body's eyes should be closed, preferably by a relative, but there are no proscriptions against non-Jewish persons touching the body. The body should then be straightened and covered. Ideally, a family member stays with the body until burial. Cremation, embalming, and what funeral homes often term "restoration" (applying make-up and the like) of the body are prohibited, as is public viewing and the use of an ornate coffin. Most synagogues have a *chevra kaddisha* or burial society that prepares the body according to Jewish practice. Burial should occur within 24 hours of death, except that burial should not take place on the Sabbath.

The *Kaddish* is an ancient Jewish prayer associated with the end of life. Observant Jews only recite the *Kaddish* in the presence of ten males, and even liberal Jews say the prayer in Aramaic.

There is a prescribed period and ritual of mourning. The first period is called *shivah* and is divided into an initial period between death and burial in which the mourner is exempt from certain religious obligations. The mourner is said to be between life and death and is called a *goses*. The 7-day period of mourning between burial and the end of the *shivah* has special stringencies such as sitting only on a low bench or on the floor. During that period it is improper for friends to exchange greetings with the mourner. One simply comes into the mourner's presence, except that it is permitted to use this phrase in Hebrew: "May you be comforted among the mourners of Zion and Jerusalem."

The 30 days following *shivah* (*shloshim*) have fewer restrictions than the first 7. For example, mourners can sit on regular chairs and exchange greetings. But until the end of the mourning period, mourners are prohibited from attending parties or other such occasions. The *Kaddish Yatom* (orphan's Kaddish) is said regularly until the conclusion of the mourning period.

After 1 year, there is for some, a modern convention of a ceremony in which the name of the deceased is placed in a memorial room in the synagogue. Another modern convention is the practice of unveiling a grave stone on the first anniversary of death and saying *Kaddish* with friends and family at the graveside.

Buddhism

Buddhism began in the 6th century BC, both as a reform of Hinduism and as a response to the suffering inherent in the human condition, epitomized by illness, aging, and death. The founder of Buddhism was Gautama Siddharta (also spelled Siddhartha), the Buddha (in Sanskrit, "The Awakened," "The Enlightened").

There are two main branches in Buddhism:
- Theravada Buddhism, or the "lesser vehicle," is practiced most often by people from Cambodia, Laos, Thailand, Burma, and Sri Lanka.
- Mahayana Buddhism, or the "greater vehicle," is practiced most often by people from Vietnam, China, and Japan.

There also are other aspects of Buddhism, such as the Zen Buddhism of Japan and the Lamaism of Tibet. In the Western world, there are differences based on nationality or ethnicity, so that in a particular location, there may be one or more each of a Laotian temple, a Cambodian temple, a Chinese temple, and so on. One Buddhist group that reaches out to other ethnicities, especially in works of charity, is the Buddhist Compassion Relief Tzu Chi Foundation.

In Theravada Buddhism, nirvana is achievable only through complete renunciation (non-attachment) and through living as a monk. The Buddha is "revered, not as a god but as one who has shown the way" (Bradley, 1963, p. 116). In practice, among the laity and many monks, the reverence shown to the Buddha and images of the Buddha is like that shown to a god. In some branches of Mahayana Buddhism, nirvana is possible for nonmonks, and among lay persons there appears to be a greater belief in (often multiple) deities, in heaven, and in hell. More sophisticated monks are apt to view these as states of mind.

The earliest Buddhist scripture is the Theravada *Tipitika* or Three Baskets. The *Tipitika* is written in *Pali*, the liturgical language of Theravada Buddhism and is very lengthy and along with later scripture comprises an immense body of work. The essence of Buddhism is found in the Four Noble Truths, the realization of which resulted in Gautama becoming the Buddha. The Four Noble Truths are as follows.

- All sentient beings suffer. Birth, illness, death, and other separations are inescapably part of life.
- The cause of suffering is desire (*tanha*). Desire is manifested by attachment to life, to security, to others, and most specifically, the desire "to be" (Carse, 1980).
- The way to end suffering is to cease to desire.
- The way to cease to desire is to follow the Eightfold Path: (1) right belief, (2) right intent, (3) right speech, (4) right conduct or action, (5) right endeavor or livelihood, (6) right effort, (7) right mindfulness, and (8) right meditation.

Following the Eightfold Path leads to cessation of desire and to nirvana, or emancipation from rebirth. Note that this is not a path of complete renunciation; Buddhism advocates a Middle Way between extreme asceticism and self-indulgence. Following the Middle Way includes living life with kindness, compassion, respect, and moderation. To achieve this it is necessary to understand that the material world is transient and ever-changing. Other concepts in Buddhism include the following.

- Nirvana is a state of "nothingness" that occurs when enlightenment is reached and there is no more suffering. Nirvana is the ultimate goal of the Buddhist.
- The Five Precepts are a moral code of avoidance, including destroying life, taking what is not given, wrong-doing in sexual desires, false speech, and consumption of distilled and fermented intoxicants causing carelessness.
- The principle of karma (or *kamma*) is basic to the practice of Buddhism. Karma is popularly interpreted as a moral precept: do right and one will be reborn into a higher state; do wrong and rebirth will be to a lower state. A more accurate understanding is that Karma is neither reward nor punishment, but simply cause and effect.

Although Buddhist scripture has nothing to say about magic, belief in magic is common among some Buddhists, especially people from the Theravada countries of Thailand, Cambodia, and Laos, and also among Tibetans. Magico-religious practices include use of amulets, spells, and the presence and power of spirits.

Health beliefs and practices

Buddhist scripture does not speak directly to health and related matters. However, Buddhist philosophy has clear application to health and health practices in several respects, including following the middle way, proscriptions against taking life, and acceptance of life and suffering. Buddhism explicitly seeks "the middle way" to enlightenment and in all aspects of life. Thus, following or practicing Buddhism should entail moderation in lifestyle. Proscriptions against taking life extend to prohibition of killing or eating animals. Though not as pervasive as the vegetarianism among Hindus, vegetarianism is widely practiced by Buddhists.

The acceptance of life and suffering in Buddhist philosophy begins with the premise that to live is to suffer (the first Noble Truth). Much has been made by Westerners of the Buddhist (and by extension, Asian) propensity to fatalism. This fatalism or more accurately, *acceptance* of what cannot be changed – especially suffering – is central to Buddhism. The direct application to health-related matters of this acceptance of life and suffering is as follows.

- There is a common reluctance to complain or express pain. Suffering or discomfort may thus be accepted to a greater extent by Buddhists than by people of other faiths.
- Acceptance of suffering as a reality of life leads some to accept spiritual or social problems or conflicts of life. For example, many Buddhists see no conflict between the fundamental precepts of Buddhism and other religions: syncretism in religion, medicine, and other matters makes perfect sense.
- How one lives/dies may be as important as whether one dies.

These points do not mean that Buddhists should be expected to suffer silently and gracefully, full of acceptance for all aspects of life and death. To the contrary, Buddhists may show as much fear of illness, suffering and death as others. Truly devout Buddhists, like other truly devout people experience less fear of suffering and death.

End of life

The Buddha did not give specific answers to the questions of dying, death, and afterlife – except that they are inevitable. On the question of immortality, the Buddha gave the "fourfold denial".

"A saint is after death. A saint is not after death. A saint is and is not after death. A saint neither is nor is not after death" (quoted by Carse, 1980).

Buddhist scholars thus see four possibilities regarding life after death; the less scholarly, i.e., the majority of Buddhists, are likely to believe in rebirth according to deeds, i.e., karma.

A key issue in dying for many Buddhist patients and families is to maintain consciousness so that patients can go through the process of dying with equanimity and "wholesome thoughts." Wholesome thoughts include awareness of the transient nature of existence, reflection on past "good efforts," and letting go of life "without clinging and grasping" (Ratanakul, 1991, p. 396). A quiet place for dying is preferred to a noisy or busy unit. A monk or lay religious leader may chant or lead chants to help promote a peaceful or insightful state of mind at death. Incense may be burned and amulets, including images of the Buddha, may be placed near the person who is dying.

Organ transplant, autopsy, and touching the body are nonissues for most Buddhists. The question of burial or cremation is more cultural than religious. Among some Southeast Asians, the family will wash the body and place the hands in a prayerful position. In many cases, if possible, the body should be kept at the home so that ceremonies may be conducted. White is usually the color of mourning and some close relatives may shave their heads as a sign of mourning. The temple is also the site of ceremonies, both soon after the death, at 100 days, and at other times, e.g., when there is enough money for a proper ceremony.

"Thus shall ye think of all this fleeting world:
A star at dawn, a bubble in a stream;
A flash of lightening in a summer cloud,
A flickering lamp, a phantom, and a dream."
　　　　From the *Diamond Sutra* (of the Buddha)

Christianity

Christianity includes the doctrines and religious groups based on the teachings of Jesus Christ. Jesus is the proper name and Christ refers to his position as Messiah, i.e., chosen by God as "the anointed one." As Christianity grew, Jesus was increasingly presented as the risen Lord.

There are, of course, many branches of Christianity. The divisions best known by laypersons in the Western world are Protestant and Catholic. There are also innumerable divisions according to variations on the basic beliefs and the great division between those who take the Bible as the literal Word of God and those who take the Bible as the inspired word of God. The earliest division was in 1054 between the Western Church or Church of Rome (Catholic) and the Eastern Church or Greek Church when Pope Leo IX condemned the Patriarch of Constantinople.

The Catholic Church

Late in the life of Christ and during the missions of the Apostles, the term catholic referred to the universal beliefs and practices of the church at the time. Over time and in general use, the term evolved into the more specific Roman Catholic Church. Catholicism is based on the Bible and also on declarations of the Pope and papal councils. The authority of the Catholic Church is thus the Pope and clergy as opposed to individual or denominational interpretation of the Bible. There are seven sacraments in Catholicism:
• baptism
• reconciliation (more commonly known as Penance or Confession)

- the Eucharist or Holy Communion
- confirmation
- matrimony
- Holy orders (of clergy)
- anointing of the Sick (Formerly known as Last Rites or Extreme Unction)

There are several Catholic beliefs or practices that directly relate to health care, including prohibition of family planning other than what is based on the ovulatory cycle. Oral contraceptives, condoms, vasectomy, and the like are thus prohibited. In actual practice, large numbers of Catholics do, in fact, use these latter means of family planning. Abortion is prohibited and there is recent tradition of the Pope and other clergy working actively to abolish abortion.

Baptism is ideally performed by a priest, but in emergencies when life is in danger, can be performed by a parent, nurse, physician, or other lay (and non-Catholic) person. The Sacrament of the Sick is provided to Catholics who are ill – including when recovery is expected. The Sacrament of the Sick includes anointing and prayer, and, like the Sacrament of Reconciliation, is provided only by a priest.

The Eastern Church

The Eastern Church includes the Orthodox Church, the Greek (Orthodox) Church, the Russian Orthodox Church and others, including The Ethiopian, Coptic, Armenian, Syrian and Indian Churches. Although the term Greek Orthodox is often used as a name for the Eastern Church, it is used most accurately for the Church of Greece and related churches that use the Byzantine rite. In the Eastern Church, in general, there is a sacramental view of life with the spiritual and physical worlds perceived as sacred. Thus there is widespread use of icons of Jesus, Mary, and apostles. Worship includes a greater degree of ritual that in most Protestant churches and the liturgy is always sung.

The clergy of the Eastern Church includes bishops or Patriarchs (whose authority is said to go back to the Apostle Mark) and priests. Parish priests are allowed to marry, but bishops and monks are not. The jurisdiction of the Pope is denied. There are seven Sacraments in the Eastern Church, with the first four expected of every believer and the last three not expected of all:

- baptism (by triple immersion)
- penance
- unction of the sick (as grace for recovery)
- matrimony
- confirmation (anointing)
- Holy communion
- Holy orders

Although there have been a number of unsuccessful attempts at reunion between the Catholic and Eastern Churches, there has been increasing progress toward an improved relationship.

Protestantism

Protestantism began with Martin Luther's questioning the authority of the Catholic Pope over Scripture. The Protestant Reformation followed and Protestantism spread across Europe in the 16th century. The basic beliefs of Protestantism are as follows.
- Salvation is through faith alone rather than through works.
- Religious authority lies in the Word of God as revealed in the Bible.
- The church is the entire community of believers rather than only the clergy.
- Individuals serve God according to their individual calling and all vocations have equal merit.

There are seemingly infinite variations on these themes and hundreds of denominations and subdivisions of denominations and sects that are considered to be Protestant denominations.

End of life

Except as described above, Christian practices related to the end of life are relatively similar. Repentance, whether formal as among Catholics, or less ritualistic as among Protestants, is common. Protestants do not believe that forgiveness is granted or mediated by humans, but still, many find comfort in companionship as they repent. Comfort is also found through prayer and reading the Bible. Ideally, the patient's pastor provides much of the spiritual care, but there is a long Christian tradition of spiritual care provided by lay persons. There are no specific Sacraments at the end of life, but those who receive Holy communion usually find great comfort in the ritual. In terminal situations, prayers tend to be focused on comfort in what is to come and the hope for resurrection. Most Christians have no religious objection to autopsy. There is enormous variation in funeral and bereavement practices.

Islam

Islam is based on what is considered by Muslims to be the Word of God as revealed to the Prophet Muhammad by (primarily) the Angel Gabriel beginning in the year AD 610. The word Islam, in Arabic, means surrender, specifically to God; a Muslim is one who surrenders to God. The foundation and unifying belief or *tawhid* of all Islam is the belief in One God (Allah). "God! There is no God but Him, the Living, the Ever-existent one." *Qur'an*, The *Imrans* 3:1

The scripture of Islam is the Koran or *Qur'an*, the direct and infallible revelation of God to The Prophet Muhammad. The *Qur'an* is divided by chapters or *Surahs*, which are arranged according to revelation. Except for the first *Surah*, arrangement is from longest to shortest. The *Qur'an* gives explicit rules or "legislation" for Muslims, with *halal* describing what is lawful and *haram* what is unlawful. Although the *Qur'an* has received little scholarly inquiry or analysis, examination of the earliest known copies of the *Qur'an* show significant differences between early and more recent editions, and between history and dogma (Stille, 2002). In addition to the *Qur'an* there is the Tradition or *Hadith*, "the Sayings and Doings of the Prophet Muhammad." The *Hadith* is the body of traditions upon which much of the life and traditions of the Muslim community is based. The *Hadith* is a vast work that evolved from texts appearing from 130–300 years after Muhammad's death and may, in some respects modify or contradict the *Qur'an* (Rahman, 1987; Stille, 2002).

As with other religions, there are divisions within Islam, including between fundamentalists and secularists, between *Sunni* and *Shi'a* (or Shiite), and the various schools or sects within the larger divisions.

The difference between Sunni (90% of Muslims) and Shi'a (10% of Muslims) has its basis in a split among Muhammad's followers after his death with no male heir. Those who became Sunni appointed a spiritual leader (the Caliph) while those who became Shi'a believed that Ali, the husband of Muhammad's favorite daughter, was the legitimate heir to Muhammad's role as the spiritual leader of Islam.

After belief in God there is belief in angels, Satan, spirits (*jinn*), the Day of Reckoning, Heaven and Hell, and in the Prophets and Messengers (including Abraham, Moses, Joseph, and Jesus). Muhammad is considered to be God's (Allah's) final Prophet and Messenger. There are also "five pillars of faith." These are:

- faith in the one God, explicated by daily recitation of the testimony or *shahada*: "There is no God but Allah, and Muhammad is His Prophet;"
- daily prayer or *salat* at least five times daily;
- alms-giving or *zahat* (or *zakat*);
- fasting or *sawm* (sunrise through sundown), principally during Ramadan;
- pilgrimage or *hajj* to Mecca at least once, if possible.

Friday is the most important day of worship. Regular worship takes place in mosques and in non-Muslim countries, major holidays or celebrations of religious ceremonies may be held at public places to accommodate large crowds.

Health beliefs and practices

While The *Qur'an* seldom speaks directly to issues of sickness or physical health, related issues are addressed. There are also religious obligations and customs associated with Islam that affect healthcare practices and beliefs. Common health-related issues among Muslims include the following.

- Cleanliness is a requirement for Muslims, with mouth, hands, and feet washed at least five times each day before the required prayers.
- Menstruation is regarded as "an illness" and women are required to remain separate during this time (*Qur'an*, The Cow 2:222).
- Modesty is important, especially among adults who have "carnal knowledge," i.e., sexual awareness (*Qur'an*, Light 24:31). Women and men (but women more than men) are expected to dress and behave conservatively. Health and personal care or assessments from different-gender persons usually are distressing to more conservative or less cosmopolitan Muslims, and complaints or responses to questions may be edited on the basis of the gender of the health care provider and/or translator.
- Dietary restrictions include pork and meat from animals killed outside of Muslim custom, and eating from dishes or with utensils that have had contact with proscribed foods (*Qur'an*, The Table 5:3). Hospitalized patients may restrict their diet to only food brought by the family, a vegetarian diet, or kosher foods. During Ramadan, adult Muslims fast from dawn to sun-down. The month of Ramadan is in the ninth month of the Islamic (Julian) calendar – which is ten days shorter than the Gregorian calendar or solar year. This means that Ramadan moves seasonally by ten days each year, and in the course of a full lifespan, a person will fast in all seasons. Fasting for some includes all food, water, and medicine, while others allow water and/or medicine during the day. Patients who need to take medicine or eat to survive may fast at a time other than Ramadan. The *Qur'an* allows people who are ill or traveling to defer fasting (*Qur'an*, The Cow 2: 185).
- Some descriptions of Islam focus on the tendency of Muslims to be fatalistic, citing belief in and surrender to the Will of Allah, or *inshallah*. Illness or tragedy may be explained and accepted through *inshallah*. On the other hand, Islam is an increasingly activist religion in which change or action are readily accepted or sought when possible.

While Islam demands acceptance of Allah and thus supersedes allegiance to clan and family (Hiro, 1989), the family remains the major unit of social organization among Muslims. In all health decisions, family concerns take precedence over individual concerns. Healthcare decisions usually include discussion among family members, with the oldest man having the final say.

In some cases, the death of a husband results in the widow marrying her husband's brother, even if he is already married. Thus in this and some other circumstances, a man may have more than one wife.

". . . you may marry other women who seem good to you: two, three, or four of them." *Qur'an*, Women 4:3

Islam gives women the right to inherit property (one-half as much as men), remarry, and not be forced into sex or marriage. Islam also gives specific rules prohibiting incest.

Ritual female genital cutting (FGC) is practiced in some Muslim cultures in Africa and the Middle East, but is not based on the *Qur'an* or Islamic tradition. See Chapter 6 on women and chapters on specific cultures.

Marriage for women may occur at a young age, shortly after puberty. For men and women, marriage is often arranged. Marriage is generally arranged for the purpose of developing or strengthening ties between families. In some situations, the sister of a man's wife is expected to marry her sister's husband's brother.

End of life

Among Muslims from the Middle East, quick pain/symptom relief is expected, but the expression of pain, except during labor and delivery, is often private. It is seldom desirable for a non-Muslim to read from the *Qur'an* as a means of spiritual care, and seldom practical, as the *Qur'an* is generally read in Arabic. Rituals related to dying include the patient facing Mecca, confession of sins, prayer, and reading or recitation of verses from the *Qur'an* (especially the 36th surah, *Ya Sin*) into the ear of the person who is dying by the eldest man present.

"Lo! those who merit Paradise this day are happily employed, They and their wives, in pleasant shade, on thrones reclining; Theirs the fruit (of their good deeds) and theirs (all) that they ask; The word from a Merciful Lord (for them) is: Peace! But avaunt ye, O ye guilty, this day!" *Qur'an*, *Ya Sin* 55–59

After death, non-Muslims should not touch the body. The family or a designated person from the community is responsible for washing and preparing the body. Most Muslim scholars have the opinion (*fatwa*) that autopsies are not allowed (Sheikh, 1998) except when required by civil law and that organ donation may be allowed when necessary (Al-Mousawi *et al.*, 1997). The funeral should take place as quickly as possible and the body buried in a Muslim cemetery when available. Mourning is a family and public community process, with men and women separate.

REFERENCES

Al-Mousawi, M., Hamed, T., & Al-Matouk, H. (1997). Views of Muslim scholars on organ donation and brain death. *Transplantation Proceedings*, **29**, 3217.

Andrews, M. M. & Hanson, P. A. (1999). Religion, culture, and nursing. In *Transcultural Concepts in Nursing Care*, 3rd edn., ed. M. M. Andrews and J. S. Boyle, pp. 378–443. Philadelphia, PA: Lippincott.

Bradley, D. G. (1963). *A Guide to the World's Religions*. Englewood Cliffs, NJ: Prentice-Hall.

Carse, J. P. (1980). *Death and Existence: A Conceptual History of Human Mortality*. New York: John Wiley & Sons.

Grun, B. (1982). *The Timetables of History*. New York: Touchstone.

Hiro, D. (1989). *Holy Wars: The Rise of Islamic Fundamentalism*. New York: Routledge.

Kaufman, W. (1976). *Religions in Four Dimensions*. New York: Readers Digest Press.

Rahman, F. (1987). *Health and Medicine in the Islamic Tradition*. New York: Crossroad.

Ratanakul, P. (1991). Buddhism: discussion of dying with dignity. In *Dying with Dignity*, Facilitator M. Abivan, pp. 395–7. *World Health Forum*, **12**, 375–99.

Rich, T. R. (2002). *Judaism 101*. Retrieved January 1, 2003 from http://www.jewfaq.org/.

Roberts, J. M. (1993). *History of the World*. New York: Oxford University Press.

Sheikh, A. (1998). Death and dying – a Muslim perspective. *Journal of the Royal Society of Medicine*, **91**, 138–140.

Stille, A. (2002, March 2). Scholars are quietly offering new theories of the Koran. *New York Times*. Section A, page 1, 19.

FURTHER READING

Holy Bible, Revised standard version. Cleveland, OH: Collins.

The Koran. Translation by N. J. Dawood (1990). New York: Penguin Books.

The Koran. Translation by M. Pickthall (1992). New York: Alfred A. Knopf.

6

Women

Jennifer Foster, Brenda Newell, and Charles Kemp

"Millions of women throughout the world live in conditions of abject deprivation of, and attacks against, their fundamental human rights for no other reason than that they are women."

(Human Rights Watch (HRW), 2003)

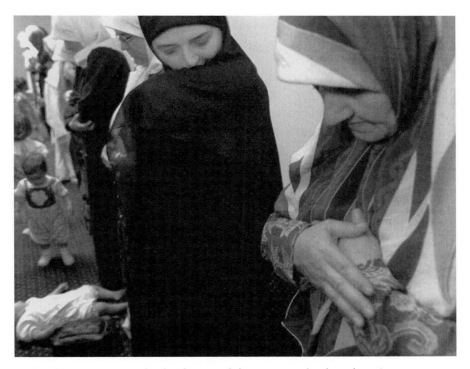

Finding her way in a new land. (Photograph by courtesy of Judy Walgren.)

Refugee and Immigrant Health: A Handbook for Health Professionals, Charles Kemp and Lance A. Rasbridge. Published by Cambridge University Press. © C. Kemp and L. A. Rasbridge 2004.

Introduction

Among immigrants and refugees from the developing world, women are a highly vulnerable population primarily because of traditional cultural roles and perspectives that place them inferior and subservient to men. Women tend to have lower educational levels, more health problems, less treatment for health problems, and once in the new country, tend to be more isolated than men (Aroian, 2001; Cohen, 1998; HRW, 2003; Meadows *et al.*, 2001; United Nations High Commissioner for Refugees (UNHCR), 1998). Although women and children comprise fully 80% of refugees, even the most fundamental health services for women – reproductive health care – are a low priority before arrival in the new country, and a challenge to access once in the new country (United States Committee for Refugees (USCR), 1999).

Access to health care

Refugees are required to have a screening examination before or shortly after arrival in the country of second asylum. However, this may be the only form of health care provided to many during this time period, and for women, may not include a pelvic examination. Immigrants may have no screening or health care on arrival. Language barriers, limited transportation, social service agency ignorance of health needs, and the refugee's or immigrant's limited knowledge of healthcare sources all inhibit the woman's access to primary and specialty health care (USCR, 1999).

Personal and cultural issues may also cause a woman to hesitate seeking health care. Many refugee and immigrant women come from cultures that place little or no value on women's health, or may have cultural values that preclude obstetric or gynecological examinations or even histories. Others have always relied on traditional methods of treating illness, and may distrust Western medicine techniques (Downs *et al.*, 1997).

Diet and nutrition

Malnourishment is common to refugees in general, but is especially common to women, and particularly so in war conditions or refugee camps in countries of first asylum. Often there is a period of weeks to months of insufficient food prior to and after arrival in first asylum camps. In other cases, food distribution may be prioritized with food going first to male family members who work outside the home to support the family. In addition, through menstruation, pregnancy, or breastfeeding, women lose nutrients. All this results in women living for varying lengths of time with less than optimal nutritional intake (or absorption) of calories and nutrients. Inadequate intake is less a problem among immigrant women and in Western countries of second asylum. However, poor nutrition leading to obesity may become a problem.

Shelter

A factor that may greatly increase or decrease the refugee woman's vulnerability is her source of shelter. In many countries of first asylum, refugee women live in crowded refugee camps where exposure, violence, and illness are common. Some women may live in brothels or sweatshops to survive. Although there may be different options for refugee women in countries of second asylum or for immigrant women – especially those who are single heads of households – shelter that is safe, clean, and affordable may still be difficult to find.

Reproductive health

Refugee women tend to have greater parity, delayed prenatal care, and lower hematocrits than their host country counterparts. Refugee women are also more likely to have complications during labor and delivery and to deliver low birth weight babies (Kang *et al.*, 1998). Financial implications of having children may also increase the physical and emotional strains on refugee women.

Rape and sexual abuse

Refugee and immigrant women are extremely vulnerable to sexual abuse and rape. Women of many cultures tend to be dependent upon men for the essentials of daily survival; in some cultures, women are viewed as property and are expected to submit to men. This, coupled with the fact that men are generally physically stronger than women, opens the door to sexual and physical abuse outside and inside marriage. In most Third World countries, abuse is not even reported due to the social status of women. Refugee and immigrant women bring this background to their countries of asylum. Major sources of rape and sexual abuse include the following:

- Soldiers and paramilitaries sometimes torture and rape prisoners of war and residents of the towns and villages they invade. The "ethnic cleansing" practiced by Serbian soldiers against Bosnians and Iraqi pogroms against Kurds and Shiite Muslims are examples of institutional abuse where rape is used as a weapon of war. Individual acts of rape on the part of the military are also common in wartime.

- Spouses and family members may also commit rape and abuse. In India, for example, in-laws may participate in wife abuse and "bride burning." Traditional gender roles in many cultures allow men to abuse their wives, along with having full control of the sexual aspects of the relationship.
- Criminals in countries of second asylum may take advantage of unsuspecting and frightened immigrant or refugee women and by deceptive means lure them into situations they are unprepared to handle.
- Trafficking (discussed in Chapter 2) is the importation of people for sexual and/or other exploitation. Trafficked women present with the devastating issues of sexual and/or other exploitation, as well as the problems common to immigrants and refugees (Orhant, 2001).

Determination of whether sexual abuse is occurring or has occurred is challenging in many cases for health or social service staff, with deep shame, anger, and a sense of enormous vulnerability complicating assessment. Some women, constrained by cultural values and practices, will doubt that anything can be done to stop abuse. Female providers or, at the very least, female interpreters, are essential to uncover and address problems of abuse.

Female genital cutting

Until just a few years ago, few in the West were aware of the practice of female genital cutting (FGC) or female genital mutilation (FGM). FGC has also been called female circumcision (FC), but this promotes a comparison with male circumcision, which in many cases is misleading (as male circumcision does not cause discomfort other than the procedure, is not related to control over the circumcised person, and does not decrease sexual response). In this work we use the term FGC.

FGC involves the removal or, in some cases, ritual scarring of genital tissue. There are four types of FGC classified by the World Health Organization (WHO).

- Type I is the removal of the prepuce and/or part or all of the clitoris. "Sunna circumcision" is a non-WHO classification that consists of the removal of the prepuce and/or the tip of the clitoris.
- Type II is the removal of the prepuce and clitoris together with the partial or complete excision of the labia minora. Clitoridectomy consists of the removal of the entire clitoris (both prepuce and the glans) and the removal of the adjacent labia.
- Type III (or infibulation) is the most extreme form of FGC and consists of the removal of the clitoris, the adjacent labia (majora and minora), followed by the pulling of the scraped sides of the vulva across the vagina. The sides are then

secured with thorns or sewn with catgut or thread. A small opening to allow passage of urine and menstrual fluid is left. An infibulated woman must be cut open to allow for intercourse on her wedding night, and the opening may then be closed again afterwards to secure fidelity to her husband.

- Type IV Unclassified refers to any of several practices, including pricking, piercing, or excision of the clitoris or labia; stretching of the clitoris or labia; regional cauterization; scraping the vaginal orifice (angurya cuts) or cutting the vagina (gishiri cuts); introducing caustic substances into the vagina to cause narrowing; and other practices that damage female genitalia.

Prevalence rates and types of FGC by country*

Prevalence	Country	Type(s) most commonly practiced
50%	Benin	Type II
70%	Burkina Faso	Type II
20%	Cameroon	Types I and II
43%	Central African Republic	Types I and II
60%	Chad	(Type III only in eastern parts of the country bordering Sudan)
5%	Democratic Republic of Congo (formerly Zaire)	Type II
43%	Cote d'Ivoire (Ivory Coast)	Type II
98%	Djibouti	Types II and III
97%	Egypt	Types II (72%), I (17%), and III (9%)
95%	Eritrea	Types I (64%), III (34%), and II (4%)
90%	Ethiopia	(Type III is practiced only in regions bordering Sudan and Somalia)
80%	Gambia	Type II Type I practiced only in some parts
30%	Ghana	Type II
50%	Guinea	Type II
50%	Guinea Bissau	Type I and II
50%	Kenya	(Type III practice in eastern regions bordering Somalia)
60%	Liberia	Type II Types I (52%) and II (47%)
94%	Mali	(Type III practiced in the southern part of the country (1%))
25%	Mauritania	Types I and II
20%	Niger	Type II

60%	Nigeria	(II is predominant in the South and Type III practiced only in the North)
20%	Senegal	Type II
90%	Sierra Leone	Type II
98%	Somalia	Type III
89%	Sudan-North	Type III (82%), I (15%), and II (3%)
18%	Tanzania	Types II and III
50%	Togo	Types II
5%	Uganda	Types I and II

* From the book, *Caring for Women With Circumcision*, by Nahid Toubia, MD. Used with permission from Rainbo Publications.

Worldwide, about 2 000 000 girls are subjected to FGC each year. The age at which the cutting is done is usually between 4 and 12 years, but it may also be done at other ages, from infancy to first pregnancy, based on the type of cutting to be done and the customs of the area in which the procedure is to be performed (US Department of Health and Human services [DHHS], 2001).

A major concern about FGC, beyond the pain and deleterious long-term effects it causes, are the circumstances in which it is done. Frequently, conditions are unsanitary, and the procedure is done by a "midwife" using a non-sterile sharp instrument such as a razor blade, scissors, kitchen knife, or a piece of glass. These instruments may be used on several girls in succession and are rarely cleaned beyond wiping. This greatly increases the risk and incidence of infection, and in some cases results in the transmission of HIV. Primary fatalities result from shock, hemorrhage, and septicemia (DHHS, 2001).

Other long-term complications may occur as well. Dyspareunia, aversion to sex, genital malformation, delayed menarche, and chronic pelvic complications are common results. Menstruation, which may last 10 days or longer, causes pain and often is malodorous. A woman who has been tightly infibulated urinates drop by drop and may need 15 minutes to void. This often results in urinary retention and causes recurrent urinary tract infection (DHHS, 2001; Toubia, 1999).

The rationales given for FGC are varied, complex, often poorly understood, and in most cases, deeply imbedded in the practicing cultures. From a human rights perspective, FGC is a form of violence against girls and women, a means of controlling women, and a clear human rights violation (DHHS, 2001). Culture-based rationales given for FGC include the following:

- necessary rite of passage to womanhood;
- prerequisite for qualifying for wifehood;
- means of enhancing male sexuality;
- means of curbing female sexual desire, thus preventing promiscuity and preserving virginity;
- aesthetic, purifying or hygienic benefits (the clitoris is seen by some as an unhealthy, unattractive and/or lethal organ);

Because FGC is practiced by many Muslims, it is seen as some as a religion-based practice. However, neither the Qur'an nor Hadiths make any mention of the practice (DHHS, 2001; Toubia, 1999).

Disease

Many refugee women come from countries where tropical and infectious diseases uncommon to the USA are endemic. While in their homes or in refugee camps, where infection spreads rapidly, refugee women may have contracted diseases such as malaria, intestinal parasites, filariasis, schistosomiasis, and other disorders (please see the section on health for risks specific to various areas of the world).

Along with these are diseases more commonly seen in the USA, such as hepatitis, tuberculosis, and sexually transmitted diseases (STDs). STDs occurring in refugee women include those common in Western countries (gonorrhea, syphilis, chlamydia, HIV) and those less common in the West (trachoma, lymphogranuloma venereum, granuloma inguinale). Women are especially at risk for STDs because of the sexual violence that may have occurred, choices made by some (e.g., sex for food), and because women contract STDs at a greater rate than men due to differences in female and male anatomy (Aroian, 2001; Bello, 1995).

Post-traumatic stress disorder

Mental health problems are present in every group of people and among immigrants and refugees, especially women, are significantly over-represented (Aroian, 2001). Some women may have had pre-existing conditions that were triggered or worsened by the stress of immigration and related events. Other women experience new onset conditions as a result of the stress of the homeland situation, trauma, flight, or relocation. Depression and anxiety disorders are seen in approximately 58% and 24% of refugee women, respectively (Kang et al., 1998). The most common diagnosis among refugee women, however, is post-traumatic stress disorder (PTSD). In one study of Yugoslavian refugee women, 65% developed PTSD (Kang *et al.*, 1998). In refugee women who have experienced physical or sexual torture, even more develop the disorder. In addition to traumatic occurrences, many women develop high levels of anxiety upon being separated from their families, which increases the chances of developing or exacerbating PTSD.

Relocation stress

Some studies have shown that the period of the greatest psychological strain for immigrant and refugee women is just after their arrival in the new home (Aroian, 2001). The role changes a refugee woman undergoes and the lack of under-standing she may have of the system contribute to this. However, there is no time in the life of an immigrant or refugee when there is no risk of stress. Immigrant and refugee women come from many different backgrounds and may find themselves in a setting completely unlike that which they are used to, e.g., after a lifetime in the rural developing world, a woman may find herself living in a large, metropolitan area. This would be a major stressor even to a woman who spoke the language and was used to the customs of the new land. For the immigrant or refugee woman, it can be overwhelming. Major psychosocial issues in immigration and resettlement are as follows.

Housing

Finding housing that is safe, comfortable, and affordable is a major challenge in resettlement. Housing in countries of second asylum is usually very different from the country of origin. Women may not be used to having hot and cold water, flush toilets, and other such devices, hence may need instructions on related safety issues.

Transportation

Immigrants and refugees may live in proximity to some, but never all, essential resources. A major reason for noncompliance with health care is lack of trans-portation to the clinics – especially after the first few months of intensive services from social service agencies.

Language

Difficulty learning a new language creates a great deal of the stress associated with relocation. Most communities offer ESL (English as a Second Language – or French or whatever the language of the new country) classes, and others provide translator services in some settings. However, learning a new culture, means of livelihood, and all the other new experiences in the life of an immigrant or refugee, make learning the language very difficult for many. Older people in particular have great difficulty with language. If the refugee woman attempts to learn the new language, she may face the stress of trying to maintain the cultural traditions of the family without being criticized for giving up the old language (which always involves some loss of culture as well). Using a refugee's children or other young person to translate also creates stress for all concerned.

Customs and protocols

Everything in the host country is new, from obtaining food, to registering in school, to childbirth, to the money. Further, immigrant or refugee women may have no concept of what insurance or benefits are, even up through the time they become citizens.

Technology

The technology in most Western countries of asylum is far more advanced than that of many countries around the world, including most of the ones from which these women have fled. Items taken for granted in the host country, such as washing machines, televisions, VCRs, telephones, microwaves, and computers may be rare in the countries of origin. Immigrants and refugees must learn quickly to use at least some of these machines to succeed in their new homes.

Perhaps the key to understanding relocation stress is recognition of the overwhelming unknown variables in the woman's life. She may see her present and future as utterly uncertain, even down to the smallest detail.

Role strain and changes

Role strain occurs when one's normal pattern of behavior developed in response to the demands and expectations of others changes abruptly, resulting in feelings of stress. This frequently occurs when women from one part of the world come to another part of the world – where foreign ways are seldom valued by the larger society. In addition to the changes in the woman's role, the stresses on the family's roles and structure may lead to role strain in each of its members. Role strain is common among immigrant and refugee women as they try to adjust to life in their host countries, while attempting to maintain the traditions and cultures of their homelands (as concurrently, their children embrace the new culture). Pressure is frequently put upon the woman to create a haven or to recreate the "old home," which when coupled with society's expectations of the woman to become somewhat Westernized, may lead to significant stress and role strain.

The role of women in many countries worldwide is subservient, especially concerning matters outside of the household. Upon arrival in the West, they may gain much freedom. However, it may be difficult and uncomfortable for the woman to reconcile this new freedom to her traditional views on the role of the woman. It usually is even more difficult for the men to reconcile these changes. In addition, married women may find a job before their husbands, which adds the new stressors of work to their load (while not decreasing women's domestic responsibilities). An immigrant or refugee woman may have mixed feelings about her new role as the person financially supporting the family. The husband may feel guilt that he is not the one supporting the family and may resent his wife's contribution to the family, creating conflict and additional stress for the woman.

Early marriage

In some cultures, it is common for girls to marry at an early age. When these women come to the USA as refugees, they may be only 14–17 years old. The difference of age in married women here, may cause the woman to feel further isolated in the larger society and she may have a more difficult time making friends, since she may feel she does not "belong" with girls her own age or with older married women. Due to their young age, these women generally have fewer personal resources to deal with the strain of being a wife in the new culture, as well as to deal with stress created by relocation in general.

Children

Immigrant and refugee children generally are the first in their families to adjust to the major changes of relocation and resettlement. They usually learn the language far more quickly and completely than their parents and become adept at the living in the new system. However, this may raise some issues within the family and create new concerns for the refugee mothers.

Respect for elders, parents, and tradition is considered important in most traditional families. However, usually the average level of respect shown to parents by their children is lower in the Western world than in the developing world/woman's place of origin. The woman may not know how to maintain family structure as her children act in a way that would have been considered inappropriate and disrespectful in the old land, but is "normal" in her new location. This also can create a great deal of stress as the woman feels she is losing control of her family and losing her influence and the influence of her culture and traditions in her children.

Discipline becomes an issue as parents try to deal with respect and simple disobedience problems. However, this, in itself, may become a problem. In many cultures slaps and hits with sticks are viewed as acceptable methods of punishment. In the West, this can lead to accusations and convictions of child abuse.

Children may be hurt by environmental hazards in a new place as well. Mothers may not know the hazards present in their own home. Traffic, electrical outlets, gas outlets, and cleaning supplies are just a few sources of danger that may be new to the women. In addition, the weather in the new residence may be significantly warmer or cooler than in the nation of origin, requiring teaching about clothing, air conditioning, and gas heater safety.

Finally, education may be a major issue in immigrant and refugee families. Many cultures do not give any importance to the education of girls, beyond household skills. This mentality may either cause refugee women to avoid education and to discourage the education of their daughters, or it may encourage them to take advantage of the new opportunities open to them. In turn, this may lead to conflict between the refugee woman and her husband and culture. Most refugee women try to ensure that their children obtain a higher level of education than they themselves achieved.

Family separation

It is common for immigrant and refugee women to have lived in close proximity to their extended family for their entire life, and it is thus difficult to live in different country and without access to family support. The separation may be stressful to the woman and may make it difficult for her to build confidence in herself in a new setting.

Ownership issues

Many immigrants and refugees come from regions where women have no, or unequal, property or inheritance rights. This may become an issue immediately for widowed, divorced, or single women, or may arise at a later time in families.

Religion

Religion is a key part of life for many women. In a few cultures, religious practice affects all aspects of life, while in others, there is separation of faith and daily life. In some cases religious beliefs will reinforce the previously noted sense of powerlessness, and in other cases, serve to empower women.

Conclusions

Immigrant and refugee women should be treated with special sensitivity and respect. Healthcare providers should watch carefully and take note of things that make the woman more or less uncomfortable. If possible, another woman should provide care, as many cultures and individuals view this as most appropriate.

Immigrant and refugee women have concerns and needs that vary from person to person and encompass every aspect of life. They may carry the heavy weight of a violent, frightening, and often tragic past, as well as the pressure of facing an unknown future. Yet they press on, daily fighting against the odds to survive.

The key to assisting immigrants and refugees is education and knowledge. The more one learns about cultures and the special needs and issues of immigrants and refugees, the better one can identify needs and serve in some way to help meet them.

A key characteristic of nations to which immigrants and refugees come, is freedom. With support and opportunity, some immigrant and refugee women will become contributing members of the community. As the UNHCR notes, women tend to be peace builders and may act to facilitate a greater sense of peace in the community, both at home and abroad (UNHCR, 1998).

REFERENCES

Aroian, K. J. (2001). Immigrant women and their health. In *Annual Review of Nursing Research*, Series ed. J. J. Fitzpatrick, Vol. 19: *Women's Health Research*, ed. D. Taylor and N. F. Woods. New York: Springer Publishing.

Bello, K. (1995). Vesicovaginal fistula (VVF): only to a woman accursed. In *The Female Client and the Health-care Provider*, ed. J. H. Roberts and C. Vlassof. Ottawa: International Development Research Centre. Retrieved 5/13/2003 from http://www.idrc.ca/books/focus/773/bello.html.

Cohen, S. A. (1998). The reproductive health needs of refugees: emerging consensus attracts predictable controversy. *The Guttmacher Report*, **1**, 10–12.

Downs, K., Bernstein, J., & Marchese, T. (1997). Providing culturally competent primary care for immigrant and refugee women. *Journal of Nurse-Midwifery*, **42**, 499–508.

Human Rights Watch (HRW) (2003). *Women's Rights*. Retrieved August 9, 2003 from http://www.hrw.org/women/index.php.

Kang, D. S., Kahler, L. R., & Tesar, C. M. (1998). Cultural aspects of caring for refugees. *American Family Physician*. Retrieved September 27, 1999 from http://www.aafp.org/afp/980315ap/medsoc.html.

Meadows, L. M., Thurston, W. E., & Melton, C. (2001). Immigrant women's health. *Social Science and Medicine*, **52**, 1451–8.

Orhant, M. (2001). *Trafficking in Persons: Myths, Methods, and Human Rights*. Population Reference Bureau. Retrieved 2/2/2003 from http://www.prb.org/Content/ContentGroups/Articles/011/ Trafficking_in_Persons_Myths,_Methods,_and_Human_Rights.htm.

Toubia, N. (1999). *Caring for Women with Circumcision*. New York: Rainbo Publications. www.rainbo.org.

United Nations High Commissioner of Refugees (UNHCR) (May, 1998). *Progress Report on Refugee Women.* (Report No. SC/1998/INF.1). Retrieved October 8, 1999 from http://www.unhcr.ch/refworld/unhcr/excom/standcom/1998/ REFW.html.

US Committee for Refugees (USCR) (1999). *Refugee Women: The Forgotten Majority.* Worldwide Refugee Information. Retrieved September 16, 1999 from http://www.refugees.org/ world/articles/women_refugees.htm.

US Department of Health and Human Services (DHSS) (2001). *Female Genital Cutting: Frequently Asked Questions.* Retrieved July 30, 2003 from http://www.4woman.gov/faq/fgc.htm.

Part II

Cultural traditions and populations

7

Afghanistan

Introduction

Like many populations of immigrants and refugees in the West, Afghans show marked intraethnic and socioeconomic diversity. The population of Afghanistan is composed of diverse tribal groups who generally show allegiance primarily to the local tribe rather than to a centralized Afghan state (Robson & Lipson, 2002). The largest ethnic group is the Pashtuns, comprising about 38% of the population, with various subtribal divisions. Pashtuns speak *Pashto* and are predominantly Sunni Moslems. Most are small-scale agriculturalists, animal herders, or small-scale traders. The majority of the *mujahadeen*, the "holy warriors" who fought the Soviets and later the United States forces in Afghanistan were ethnic Pashtuns.

The second largest ethnic group in Afghanistan is the Tajiks, about one-quarter of the population. Their history, cultural characteristics and language, known as *Dari*, are all related to Persia (Iran). They are predominantly townspeople and sedentary farmers, mostly in the fertile eastern valleys north and south of the Hindu Kush mountains. Tajiks are virtually all Sunni Moslem but, on the whole, are less conservative in their practice than the Pashtuns.

The third largest ethnic group is the Hazaras, about 19% of the population, a nomadic people of Mongol origin. Like the Tajiks, they also speak *Dari*. The remainder of the population is divided among the more than 19 ethnic groups in Afghanistan, such as the Baluchis, Uzbeks, and Turkmens (Robson & Lipson, 2002).

History of immigration

The population of Afghanistan is difficult to assess, but most estimates place the total at over 27 million (CIA, 2003). However, due to the nearly constant civil strife of the last several decades, at least one of every five Afghans lives as a refugee in

Refugee and Immigrant Health: A Handbook for Health Professionals, Charles Kemp and Lance A. Rasbridge.
Published by Cambridge University Press. © C. Kemp and L. A. Rasbridge 2004.

the teeming camps along the borders and in neighboring Pakistan and Iran. These numbers represent the largest group of refugees in the world, although millions of Afghans have begun to return since the recent US-backed overthrow of the Taliban.

The first wave of resettled refugees to the West from Afghanistan were primarily well-educated urbanites fleeing the Soviet invasion in 1979. These were followed by larger numbers of less-affluent, more traditional Afghans from the growing refugee camps or directly from countries like Pakistan and India. Then, in 1989, in the wake of the Soviet withdrawal from Afghanistan, factional infighting destroyed much of the country and led to even greater numbers fleeing the country, especially professionals. And in 1996 the Pashtun-dominated Taliban regime came to power and instituted a fanatical brand of Islam on the country, causing millions more Afghans to flee, especially Tajiks and other minorities.

Through 2002, about 15 000 Afghans were resettled to the United States (Immigration and Refugee Services of America (IRSA), 2002), with the largest populations in the San Francisco Bay Area, northern Virginia, and Los Angeles. In Europe, Germany, the Netherlands, and Great Britain have resettled sizeable groups as well (United Nations High Commissioner for Refugees (UNHCR), 2003). Most resettled Afghans are Pashtun and Tajik, but smaller, and sometimes separate, ethnic minority communities like Hazaras also are found (Robson & Lipson, 2002). Over the years, many resettled Afghans have become citizens and have reached levels of economic self-sufficiency, while other families remain marginalized and welfare dependent, a decade or more after their initial resettlement.

Culture and social relations

"In Afghanistan, life doesn't belong to just one person. . . . Every decision is connected to the family – we are all tied together" (An Afghan man quoted in Robson and Lipson, 2002)

One cannot overemphasize the importance Afghans place on allegiance to the family, with strict obedience to the father's authority and elders in general. Traditionally, life's activities were focused within a walled compound consisting of the landowner and his extended family. Even in more modern families the "wall" still remains symbolically. Robson and Lipson (2002) note that "an Afghan's family is sacrosanct and a matter of great privacy."

In general, in this patrilineal society, women are subservient to men, and there is great concern for the chastity of unmarried women and the sequestering of women in general. Until the Taliban were overthrown, *all* women were fully veiled in their infrequent trips outside the household compound. Typically, women of the household of all ages form a single work group in the care of children and other household duties. There is little emphasis on education for girls, who marry at a young age.

Although many resettled women are finding the necessity to go to work in order to help support the family, the idealized adult female role remains that of care-taker for children and the household in general. While women resettled in the West undoubtedly have more freedoms in general and may have a voice in the marriage proposal contract, arranged marriages, usually between extended family members, are the norm both in countries of resettlement and in Afghanistan. There are some parents and single men themselves who return temporarily to Afghanistan or Pakistan to visit relatives and seek out marriage prospects, thus ensuring the continuity of family ties and even Afghan culture itself (Lipson & Omidian, 1997).

There is some polygamy in Afghanistan, as Islam allows up to four wives. However, only wealthy men or large landholders can afford such an arrangement. Divorce is possible, under both Islamic law and traditional Afghan culture, but stigma, family pressures, and a complete lack of options for divorced women discourage most women from divorcing, except in extreme cases (D'Avanzo & Geissler, 2003; Lipson & Omidian, 1997).

Not surprisingly, Afghans resettled as refugees face great stress when confronted with the openness and freedoms of the West. While traditional Afghan family values may slowly change, many challenges will remain for at least a generation. For example, even the more liberal women are very reluctant to see a male physician, especially for gynecological issues, and in general both men and women are reluctant to discuss health and other personal concerns with anyone outside of the extended family. Furthermore, Robson and Lipson note,

"In the United States, Afghans perceive school and social service agency intervention as under-mining parental authority, responsibility and control, even demeaning marriage, the purpose of which is to bear and raise children" (2002).

Communication

Pashto and *Dari* are the two national languages of Afghanistan. Both are written in a variant of the Persian (*Farsi*) script, which itself is based on Arabic. Spoken *Pashto* has two major dialects, but typically speakers of each can readily understand the other. *Dari*, spoken by the Tajiks in the north and west, also has internal dialect differences. On the whole, it is related to spoken Persian (*Farsi*). However, a native-born Iranian speaker of *Farsi* describes *Dari* as a rather distant dialect, so that interpretation by *Farsi*-speakers for *Dari*-speakers is somewhat inexact.

Dari is considered the more prestigious language and is the language of business and higher education. However, because of the political power of the Pashtuns, *Pashto* is the language of government, and is a required school subject even in *Dari*-speaking Tajik areas. *Pashto* speakers are frequently bilingual in *Dari*, but older *Dari*-speakers may not be conversant in *Pashto*. The rate of illiteracy in

Afghanistan is substantial, estimated by the US Central Intelligence Agency (CIA) (2003) as 49% for men and 79% for women.

Religion

Despite the considerable ethnic diversity in Afghanistan, the practice of Islam is nearly universal. The vast majority of Afghans follow the Sunni sect, but there is a Shiite minority, as well as less formalized "folk" practitioners. Virtually all Afghans adhere to the more fundamental aspects of Islam pertaining to morality, hygiene, and modesty, especially concerning women. However, adherence to all the rituals and dictums of Islam varies at the individual level as well as that of the ethnic group: on the whole, Tajiks are less strict in their interpretation and practice of Islam than the Pashtuns.

Health beliefs and practices

There is a deep history in Afghan culture on the observance and use of magico-religious rites in the prevention of and treatment of illness. For example, amulets and charms are frequently worn to ward off evil spirits. There is a folk belief that these spirits have the potential to cause various afflictions to the nervous system. Also, written verses from the Koran, wrapped in stuffing, and worn on a string are believed to guard against "evil-eye" and other forms of jealousy. Written Arabic is believed to contain a mystical power in and of itself, especially by the older generation, even though or perhaps because few can read it.

The traditional medicine pharmacopoeia of Afghanistan is known as *atary* in *Dari* and consists of herbs, plants, leaves, and bark (but no animal parts, which an informant confided would be "disgusting"). These medicines were commonly available in Afghan marketplaces, where the aroma alone would attract buyers, and usually taken in powdered form or boiled into tea. Some examples are as follows: sore throats are commonly treated with a tonic of water and a seed from a pear-like fruit common to Afghanistan, boiled to a gelatin-like state and swallowed. Dental caries are treated with a cantaloupe seed mixture. Heart conditions are treated with Valaria root tea.

There are *atary* specialists in Afghanistan that are more knowledgeable about prescribing for particular ailments. This knowledge (and experimentation) has accumulated for at least 1000 years. Ibn Sina, an ancient Persian scientist, is credited as the founder of much of *atary* medicine (Islamic Affairs Department (IAD), 1999).

Some of the more common herbs are imported and are available in markets in the West, especially in Iranian stores. However, there appear to be few, if any, *atary* specialists among the resettled refugees.

There are also other types of traditional medicine practiced in Afghanistan, and undoubtedly some of these ideas are retained among the resettled refugee population, especially among the elderly. For example, in Afghanistan there exists a whole practice of massage therapy and body manipulation specialists, known as *dalal* in *Dari*, very similar to Western chiropractics, who also employ a sauna-like procedure.

Furthermore, there are some elements of humoral balance in Afghan illness etiology and treatment, known as *sard* or "coldness" and *garm* or "warmness." For example, a certain type of lamb stew consumed in excess is understood to create a "cold" state in the body, an imbalance which can cause illness. Alternatively, honey and crystallized sugar is understood to be humorally "hot."

It should be noted too that opium, ubiquitous to Afghanistan, is commonly used in folk medicine. Raw opium in a wrapped form, known as *bast*, is used to treat extreme pain, increase sexual stamina, and stimulate the appetite.

Pregnancy and childbirth

Children are greatly valued, especially male children, as an economic asset in adding their labor to the household compound. Births are usually assisted by a midwife, known as a *dais*, especially in the rural areas, where health services of any sort for women are rare. Breastfeeding is nearly universal and usually continues until subsequent conception. However, it is thought that many women introduce tea-soaked bread to infants' diets as early as 3 months. This early weaning, along with contaminated water, food shortages, and other factors contributes to high prevalences of diarrhea and malnutrition; two-thirds of children show signs of protein-energy malnutrition (D'Avanzo & Geissler, 2003).

Babies are frequently given only a first name, albeit sometimes a compound name, and surnames are typically not used, except sometimes for the wealthy or political elite. In Western society this represents a difficulty, such that many resettled refugees adopt a surname, frequently the name of their tribe (or have a surname somewhat arbitrarily assigned by immigration officials). Education of children frequently takes place in religious schools, at least for boys, as the Taliban had banned schools for all females. Physical punishment for discipline is the norm.

End of life

Rituals surrounding death follow the tenets of Islam. A mullah or other clergyman prays over the body and reads from the Koran, with friends and relatives gathered at the home. The body is washed by relatives of the same sex, wrapped in a white shroud, and placed in a coffin. Burial must be within 24 hours. Two days after burial, a ceremony and meal commemorating the deceased is held in the home or in the local mosque (D'Avanzo & Geissler, 2003).

Health problems and screening

The public health picture for Afghanistan over the last few decades has been abysmal due to the almost complete destruction of an already rudimentary health care infrastructure. Refugee flight and camp life took its toll on the health of Afghan refugees, with high rates of depression and hypertension, especially for women, who did not have access for female health care workers and were not permitted to be treated by male doctors (Lipson & Omidian, 1997).

The healthy life expectancy or HALE in Afghanistan is 33.4 years and the full life expectancy is 45 years (Population Reference Bureau (PRB), 2002; World Health Organization (WHO), 2002a). Infant mortality is high in Afghanistan (147 deaths/1000 live births), and infectious diseases the leading causes of death and disability (Central Intelligence Agency (CIA), 2003; WHO, 2002a). Afghanistan is one of 22 countries worldwide with a "high burden" of tuberculosis, one of nine countries in the world with indigenous transmission of polio (low transmission rate), and with a 35% immunization rate, one of 11 countries accounting for more than 66% of world deaths from measles (Stein *et al.*, 2003; WHO, 2002b; WHO, 2003). Afghanistan is also one of only three countries worldwide in which women die at a younger age than men (PRB, 2002).

The most frequent diagnoses among Afghans seen at the author's clinic are hypertension and diabetes, similar to other studies (Lipson *et al.*, 1995a,b; Lipson & Omidian, 1993), along with constipation, headaches, dental caries, and joint pain. In one interesting case, a woman first presented at the clinic with her head completely covered, in the heat of the Dallas summer, with hypertension and frequent headaches. Over a few months, her head covering was increasingly loosened every time she came in. One day, she came in nearly unrecognizable with her head covering completely removed, and perhaps coincidently, her headaches gone and her hypertension well controlled.

The concepts of health and wellness take on a psychosocial component for Afghans. As defined by an Afghan refugee in California: "Being healthy is having family members all here and together; it does not matter too much if physically they aren't doing too well" (quoted in Lipson and Omidian, 1996, p. 69). Afghans endured extreme and sustained psychological trauma over the last 25 years, with over 40% of the population either killed or driven out of their homeland by the incessant fighting (Lipson & Omidian, 1997). Many survivors were imprisoned and tortured and are otherwise witnesses to atrocities. Even those resettled to the West suffered extreme loss: loss of family members killed or left behind, loss of social status, and even wholesale loss of culture. Not unexpectedly, depression, somatization, and post-traumatic stress disorder are the most frequent mental health diagnoses among Afghans living in the United States (Lipson, 1993).

Even after years of resettlement in the West, the issues of depression and marginalization may not dissipate but in fact may worsen, especially among the elderly. Like other refugees, many Afghans fear dying in a country which is not their "home" and to which they did not choose to come. As Lipson points out, homebound elderly "are isolated and lonely when they speak insufficient English to talk with American neighbors or are culturally restrained from moving outside their family circle" (1993, p. 414).

Health risks in refugees and immigrants from Afghanistan (Kemp, 2002; Stein *et al.*, 2003; WHO, 2001, 2002a,b) include:

- amebiasis
- anthrax
- boutonneuse fever
- brucellosis or undulant fever
- cholera
- Crimean–Congo hemorrhagic fever
- cysticercosis (tapeworm)
- dracunculiasis (Guinea worm disease)
- echinococcosis (hydatid disease)
- giardia
- hepatitis
- hookworm
- leishmaniasis
- malaria
- measles
- plague
- schistosomiasis (bilharzia)
- toxocariasis
- trachoma
- trematodes
- trichinosis (trichinella)
- tuberculosis
- typhus
- post-traumatic stress disorder

REFERENCES

Central Intelligence Agency (CIA) (2003). *World Factbook.* Retrieved June 11, 2003 from http://www.cia.gov/cia/publications/factbook/geos/af.html.

D'Avanzo, C. E. & Geissler, E. M. (2003). Afghanistan. In *Cultural Health Assessment*, 3rd edn. St. Louis: Mosby.

Immigration and Refugee Services of America (IRSA) (2002). *Refugee Reports, 23*. Retrieved April 3, 2003 from http://www.refugees.org/.

Islamic Affairs Department (IAD) (1999). *The Medical Sciences*. Retrieved April 3, 2003 from http://www.iad.org/Islam/medicine.html.

Kemp, C. (2002). *Infectious Diseases*. Retrieved April 12, 2003 from http://www3.baylor.edu/ ~ Charles_Kemp/Infectious_Disease.htm.

Lipson, J. (1993). Afghan refugees in California: mental health issues. *Issues in Mental Health Nursing*, **14**, 411–23.

Lipson, J. & Omidian, P. (1993). Health among San Francisco Bay area Afghans: a community assessment. *The Afghanistan Studies Journal*, **4**, 71–86.

(1996). Afghans. In *Refugees in the 1990s*, ed. D. Haines, pp. 63–80. Westport, CT: Greenwood Press.

(1997). Afghan refugee issues in the U.S. social environment. *Western Journal of Nursing Research*, **19**, 110–26.

Lipson, J., Hosseini, T., Kabir, S., Omidian, P. & Edmonston, F. (1995a). Health issues among Afghan women in California. *Health Care for Women International*, **16**, 279–86.

Lipson, J., Omidian, P., & Paul, S. (1995b). Afghan health education project: A community survey. *Public Health Nursing*, **12**, 143–50.

Population Reference Bureau (PRB) (2002). *2002 World Population Data Sheet*. Retrieved May 12, 2003 from http://www.prb.org/pdf/WorldPopulationDS02_Eng.pdf.

Robson, B. & Lipson, J. (2002). *Afghans: Their History and Culture. Cultural Orientation Project*. Retrieved April 3, 2003 from http://www.culturalorientation.net.

Stein, C. E., Birmingham, M., Kurian, M., Duclos, P., & Strebel, P. (2003). The global burden of measles in the year 2000 – a model that uses country-specific indicators. *Journal of Infectious Diseases*. **187** (Suppl. 1), S8–S14.

United Nations High Commissioner for Refugees (UNHCR) (2003). *2002 Annual Statistical Report: Afghanistan*. Retrieved August 20, 2003 from http://www.unhcr.ch.

World Health Organization (WHO) (2001). *Communicable Disease Profile: Afghanistan and Neighboring Countries*. Geneva: World Health Organization.

(2002a). *World Health Report*. Retrieved June 5, 2003 from http://www.who.int/whr/2002/en/.

(2002b). *Global Polio Status 2002*. Retrieved May 9, 2003 from http://www.polioeradication. org/all/global/.

(2003). *Global TB Control Report 2003*. Retrieved June 1, 2003 from http://www.who.int/gtb/ publications/globrep/index.html.

8

Bosnia

Tracey Mackling and Charles Kemp

Note: Bosnia – now the Federation of Bosnia-Herzegovina is a joint Bosniak/Croat federation founded in 1994. Within the political borders of Bosnia-Herzegovina are two tiers of government: (1) the Bosniak/Croat Federation of Bosnia and Herzegovina and (2) the Bosnian Serb-led Republika Srpska (RS). To prevent an outbreak of violence such as occurred in the 1990s, the North Atlantic Treaty Organization maintains a Stabilization Force (SFOR) in Bosnia-Herzegovina. The term "Bosniak" refers to Bosnian Muslims (Central Intelligence Agency (CIA), 2002).

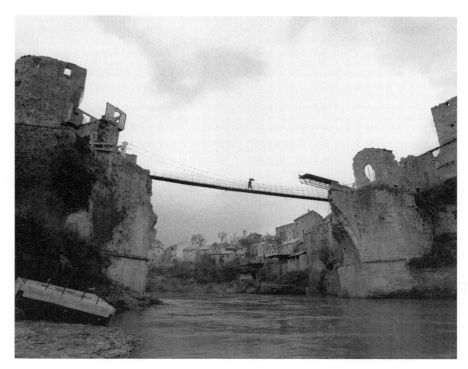

Destroyed bridge in Mostar. (Photograph by courtesy of Judy Walgren.)

Refugee and Immigrant Health: A Handbook for Health Professionals, Charles Kemp and Lance A. Rasbridge. Published by Cambridge University Press. © C. Kemp and L. A. Rasbridge 2004.

Introduction

The dissolution of the Soviet Union in 1990 led to the creation or re-creation of a number of Eastern European or Balkan states, including Bosnia-Herzegovina, Croatia, and Macedonia. Borders and populations changed, in some cases leading to, or renewing, conflict among ethnic and religious groups. Conflict was most pronounced between Serbia (the former Yugoslavia) and Bosnia (formerly part of Yugoslavia). The roots of the conflict lay in the past history of the areas (e.g., forced assimilation and different allegiances in World War II), in religious differences (Christian and Muslim), and in atavistic nationalism.

Conflict began in 1991, and in 1992, Bosnia (the Federation of Bosnia and Herzegovina) declared independence from Yugoslavia. The conflict included "ethnic cleansing" of Muslims in Bosnia by Serb military and police. This genocide was characterized by concentration camps, mass murders (especially of men), and a Serb policy of raping Muslim women. In 1995, for example, the Serbian army took a United Nations safe area (Srebenica) and in 5 days, systematically murdered more than 7000 men and boys, and raped an unknown number of women (Public Broadcasting System, 2000).

The vast majority of casualties in the war (approximately 250 000 killed) were civilian. An outflow of refugees resulted in approximately 2 000 000 Bosnians displaced to other countries and more than 200 000 coming to the United States (CNN, n.d.; Johnstone & Mandryk, 2001; Goldstein *et al.*, 1997).

Prior to the conflicts of the 1990s, Bosnia was seen by many as a model of religious and ethnic tolerance, with Christians, Muslims and different ethnic groups living in relative harmony. Currently, the Bosnia-Herzegovina population is 48% Bosniak, 37% Serb, and 14% Croatian (CIA, 2002). Most Bosniaks are Muslim, most Serbs are Greek Orthodox, and most Croats are Catholic, with Bosniaks tending to be more diverse with respect to religion than Serbs or Croats. The religious breakdown is Muslim 40%, Orthodox 31%, Roman Catholic 15%, Protestant 4%, and other 10% (CIA, 2002).

Culture and social relations

Bosniaks tend to be cosmopolitan and from urban backgrounds. Those from rural backgrounds generally had homes with electricity, appliances, and indoor plumbing, hence are not in any sense peasants. Nearly all are literate and most have completed at least the eighth grade. Except at festivals or among amateur folklore ensembles, men and women alike dress as do other cosmopolitan Europeans in jeans or slacks, dresses, and the like; older women often wear scarves as head coverings.

Although there are extended families living together in rural Bosnia, most Bosniaks live in a nuclear family. Many families have a history of both wife and husband employed outside the home. Men usually have greater authority than women, but there is not a tradition of extreme repression. Although polygamy is sanctioned in the *Qur'an* ("marry of the women, who seem good to you, two or three or four . . ." Women: 4), it is very rarely practiced among Bosniaks (Ranard, 1995).

Communications

The language of Bosnia is Serbo-Croatian (Bosniaks now refer to their language as Bosnian), and many people also speak German, English, or another second language. In most respects, Serbo-Croatian is similar enough to English that Bosnians are able to learn English without exceptional difficulty. A relatively high level of education (at least eighth grade) helps in learning English. Some have difficulty with question formation and recognition of gender-specific names (many Bosnian women have a name ending in "ica" or "a") (Ranard, 1995).

Religion

Virtually all Bosnian refugees are Muslim. Islamic influences on health care beliefs and practices are discussed in the chapter on religions. As discussed in that chapter, there are many factors that influence the extent to which a religion impacts health-related behavior. In the case of Bosniaks, generally a cosmopolitan group, Islam may have less of an impact on health beliefs and practices than among others from more fundamentalist backgrounds. Bosniak women, for example, tend to be less intent on maintaining extreme modesty and are more willing to report gynecological problems than women from some other groups. At most, Bosniak women, especially older women, wear a scarf over their head and dress conservatively.

Health beliefs and practices

Except that the healthcare system in Bosnia is socialized, basic health care is similar in many respects to that in most of the West. There is a strong emphasis on primary care and some sophisticated tests and procedures are generally unavailable. However, except for conflict and war-related shortages, primary care, at least, is similar. Nearly all Bosnians are familiar with Western conceptions of hypertension, coronary disease, diabetes, treatment of infections, and so on. Some arrive in the US or other countries of second asylum, with histories of treatment for thyroid deficiency, cancer surgery, and other sophisticated procedures.

Health problems and screening

Research and the authors' experience have uncovered no specific health problems or risks among Bosniaks other than those related to war experiences, i.e., risk for post-traumatic stress disorder (PTSD), combat stress disorder (CSR), depression, and other sequelae of psychological trauma including, despite Islamic prohibitions against alcohol, alcoholism. Reactions to war trauma are discussed in detail in the chapter on mental health. Readers are strongly encouraged to refer to that chapter, as many Bosniaks of all ages have lived through genocidal experiences and thus have a very high risk for delayed reactions. Readers should also note that these experiences are similar to holocaust experiences, hence reactions may continue through at least a second generation.

Like other refugees, Bosniak refugees tend to have a poorer "global health" status than other people in the host country. In Bosnia and Herzogovina, the healthy life expectancy (HALE) is 62.5 years and the full life expectancy is 68 years (Population Reference Bureau, 2002; World Health Organization (WHO), 2002). Chronic non-infectious diseases are the leading causes of death and disability; and health risks for new Bosniak immigrants are primarily cardiac disease and related, cancer, diabetes, and other chronic noninfectious diseases. Health risks (Kemp, 2002; WHO, 2002) include:

- babesiosis (rare)
- boutonneuse fever
- encephalitis (most likely to be tick-borne)
- hemorrhagic fevers (HFs) (HF with renal syndrome and tick-borne HFs)
- lyme disease
- trematode infection (opisthorchiasis)
- chronic non-infectious diseases and conditions such as cardiac disease and related, cancer, diabetes, and COPD.

REFERENCES

Central Intelligence Agency (2002). *World Factbook* (revised 2003). Retrieved December 23, 2002 from http://www.cia.gov/cia/publications/factbook/geos/bk.html.

CNN (n.d.). *The Balkan Tragedy*. Retrieved May, 12, 2003 from http://www.cnn.com/WORLD/Bosnia/history/index.html.

Goldstein, R. D., Wampler, N. S., & Wise, P. H. (1997). War experiences and distress symptoms of Bosnian children. *Pediatrics*, **100**, 873–8.

Johnstone, P. & Mandryk, J. (2001). *Operation World: 21st Century Edition*. Waynesboro, GA: Paternoster USA.

Kemp, C. (2002). *Infectious Diseases*. Retrieved April 12, 2003 from http://www3.baylor.edu/ ~Charles_Kemp/Infectious_Disease.htm.

Population Reference Bureau (2002). *2002 World Population Data Sheet*. Retrieved May 12, 2003 from http://www.prb.org/pdf/WorldPopulationDS02_Eng.pdf.

Public Broadcasting System (2000). *Srebrenica: A Cry from the Grave*. Retrieved April 22, 2002 from http://www.pbs.org/wnet/cryfromthegrave/about/about.html.

Ranard, D. A. (1995). *The Bosnians*. New York: Church World Service.

World Health Organization (2002). *World Health Report*. Retrieved June 5, 2003 from http://www.who.int/whr/2002/en/.

9

Burma

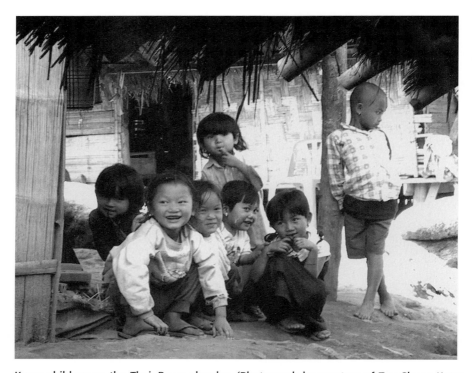

Karen children on the Thai–Burma border. (Photograph by courtesy of Tao Sheng Kwan-Gett.)

Refugee and Immigrant Health: A Handbook for Health Professionals, Charles Kemp and Lance A. Rasbridge.
Published by Cambridge University Press. © C. Kemp and L. A. Rasbridge 2004.

Introduction

Burma (called Myanmar by Burma's ruling military State Peace and Development Council or SPDC) is in mainland Southeast Asia and is bordered by Thailand and Laos on the East, India and Bangladesh on the West, and China on the North. The primary population centers are along the centrally located Irrawaddy river valley. Most of the rest of the country is mountainous and the climate throughout is tropical monsoonal.

There are more than 48 000 000 people in Burma. Ethnic groups include the Burmese or Burmans (68% of the population), followed by the Shan, Karen (original indigenous people), Rakhine, Chinese, Indian, Mon, and others (e.g., Kachin, Chin, Wa, and other indigenous peoples) (Central Intelligence Agency (CIA), 2002). Many of the ethnic minority groups or indigenous people are "hill tribes" who occupy the mountain jungle areas.

Although there is a legendary list of Kings of Arakan (in Burma) dating to 2666 BC, the first record of a Burmese capital was in 500 BC. For the next several millennia there were a number of Burmese kingdoms of various sizes. Burma became a province of British India in 1886 and gained independence in 1948. A military dictatorship took power in 1962 and in 1988 declared martial law, which continues as this is written.

History of immigration

There have long been Burmese immigrants to the West, especially Britain. The modern outflow of refugees began after the military took power, especially in the late 1980s when Burma's ruling generals annulled an election, declared martial law and crushed the democratically elected opposition led by Nobel Peace Prize winner Daw Aung San Suu Kyi. In addition to Burmese political refugees, there are more than 100 000 Karen, Shan, and other indigenous people who are refugees on the Thai–Burma border. Living conditions on the border, especially within ethnic hilltribe areas, are very difficult and there are frequent mass movements of internally displaced people (IDPs), as the SPDC army continues its military campaign to bring the entire country under its control. The Burmese term for refugee is *dukkha-the*, "one who has to bear *dukkha*, suffering" (Lang, 1995). Human rights violations in Burma are "massive" and include murder, rape, torture, forced relocation, and forced labor of dissidents and minorities (Petersen *et al.*, 1998; Skidmore, 2002).

Culture and social relations

Burma is primarily an agricultural country with little industry and almost no technology. At one time Burma was the largest rice producer in Southeast Asia.

However, economic development has been poor under SPDC rule due to corruption and mismanagement. Even the second largest city, Mandalay, has a distinctly rural or small-town atmosphere. The years of self-imposed isolation since 1962 have meant that, in many ways, this traditionally rural, non-industrial culture has remained so. At the same time, however, 40 years of repression has had significant negative impact on traditional Burmese culture.

Burmese culture is traditionally family and religion oriented. This holds true for ethnic minorities as well, though indigenous people such as the Karen may have family and community structures different from the Burmese. Traditionally, families are extended, but among refugees and immigrants, nuclear families are the norm. Parents are held to be sacred and one of the "five objects of worship" in Buddhism, hence disobedience to a parent is considered a sin (Way, 1985). Social class lines are strong and thus there is little opportunity for social mobility.

Marriage is often arranged and may involve consultation with the family astrologer to determine whether the two young people will be compatible. Initiation to adulthood begins at age nine with the *shin-pyu* ceremony for boys, which is followed by several weeks in a monastery; and the *nahtwin* ceremony for girls, which includes having the ears pierced. A distinctly Burmese cultural practice, carried over in some cases to new lands is the use of *thanaka*, a pale yellow paste applied to the cheeks, forehead, and sometimes arms of both genders but more frequently in girls and women.

Communications

As noted above, Burmese culture is very old. Interactions between social equals tend to be characterized by politeness and concern for the other person. The Burmese term, *a-nah-dah* expresses the Burmese cultural value of "an attitude of delicacy, expressive of a solicitousness for other people's feelings or convenience" (Way, p. 279, 1985). An example of the application of *a-nah-dah* is a tendency to try to convince another person that what cannot be given, e.g., an affirmative answer to a question, is not worth having (Cultural Profiles Project, n.d.).

The primary language of Burma is Burmese, one of the Tibeto-Burmese family of languages. Burmese is tonal and at least to the Western ear, does not have the musicality or softness of most other Southeast Asian languages. The indigenous people each have their own language, though most also speak at least some Burmese. Forms of Burmese address are usually couched in terms of relationship and include the following.

- *U* means uncle and is also a term of respect. *U* Thant, for example, was the Secretary General of the United Nations.

- *Daw* is the term for aunt and is the term of respect for women, e.g., *Daw* Aung San Suu Kyi.
- *Ko* is the term for older brother or friend.
- *Ma* means sister or young girl.
- *Maung* means a boy or young man.
- *Bo* means leader.
- *Saya* is the term for teacher or master, and also for traditional healer.

As is common throughout Buddhist Southeast Asia, the head of an adult *or* child is figuratively the highest part of the body and should not be touched by another person – although exception is made for medical examination. It also is impolite to sit in a seat higher or at the same level as an older or more respected person. Shoes are not worn in the home or pagoda. When sitting on the floor, such as in a pagoda or a formal situation, men and women sit with their legs flexed sideways so that their feet are pointed to the rear rather than at a Buddha image or other people. However, in informal situations, men may sit cross-legged. Pointing one's finger, hand, or foot at another person is considered rude, and calling another person with upraised index finger is insulting.

Religion

Almost 90% of Burmese are Theravada Buddhist, with most of the rest of Burmese equally divided between Christians and Muslims (CIA, 2002). Many ethnic "hilltribe" villagers are animist, or combine animist traditions with one of the three primary religions. Related to the animism that existed before Buddhism, *nat* (literally, lord) or spirit worship is pervasive among Burmese Buddhists. Readers are referred to the discussion of Theravada Buddhism in Chapter 5 on religions.

Based on tradition and the artifice that *nats* are themselves devotees of the Buddha, *nat* worship is very much blended with Buddhism. There are 37 inner *nats* who are allowed inside the pagoda and hundreds or perhaps thousands of outer *nats* who are not allowed in the pagoda. Some *nats* are basically protective, some capable of possessing humans, while others are associated with particular places or activities. The Little Lady of the Flute, for example, acts as a guardian and playmate of children, and makes children smile in their sleep. In general, *nats* require appeasement, such as maintaining a "house *nat*" shrine on the south side of the home (Courtauld, 1984).

Astrological computations are commonly used to predict the future and to guide many life decisions such as choosing a child's name, a wedding day, and when to travel. The Burmese astrological system is based upon the Hindu system, and representations of Hindu gods may be found in some Burmese Buddhist homes.

Health beliefs and practices

Traditionally, health is considered to be related to harmony in and between the body, mind, and soul and the universe, with the latter encompassing everyday life, socioeconomic conditions, as well as spiritual circumstances. The idea of harmony is most commonly expressed as a balance of "hot" and "cold" elements or states, e.g., illnesses or states of health may be seen as hot or cold so treatment should then be with opposite medicines or foods. The postpartum period, for example is a cold state, hence hot foods or medicines should be taken. Despite common assertions that hot and cold states are not related to temperature, most Burmese and other Southeast Asians avoid cold drinks for people in a cold state.

Changes in diet are commonly used to treat illness. Depending on the illness, an increase in or reduction of one or more of the six Burmese tastes (sweet, sour, hot, cold, salty, bitter) may be indicated. *Yesah* is a herbal cure-all substance used by many Burmese.

Culture bound illnesses among Burmese include spirit possession by a Nat or an ancestor and *Koro*. *Koro* is the intense fear that the genitalia will recede into the body and that, if the genitalia recede completely, death will occur (Way 1985). Among women, menstrual flow is critical to health and, depending on the flow, an indication of good or poor health – including mental health (Skidmore, 2002).

Pregnancy and childbirth

Traditionally prenatal and neonatal care is often provided by a midwife or *let-thare*. In cities, however, clinics and hospitals are commonly used, and as in the West, the value of prenatal and neonatal care is well recognized. Traditional dietary restrictions during pregnancy, especially among the hilltribe ethnic groups, make prenatal nutrition counseling essential. The risk of neonatal sepsis or tetanus is significant in some hilltribe villages, where midwives lacking proper equipment or training may cut the umbilical cord after delivery with a bamboo sliver and paint the umbilical stump with charcoal. The postpartum period (*me dwin*) is viewed as a time of susceptibility to illness as the mother's body is "cold" from blood loss. The body should be warmed with external heat as well as warm drinks and foods with "hot" properties. Sour and bitter foods are also taken postpartum as these are thought to reduce blood loss (Skidmore, 2002). Oral contraceptives are thought by many to cause menstrual irregularity, while Depo-Provera injections are thought to provide regularity (despite the common adverse reaction of irregular bleeding).

End of life

Buddhist philosophy and outlook are the greatest influences on how many Burmese approach dying and death. Equanimity and mindfulness are central to the process, and in some cases may be more valued than measures to manage symptoms. For example, patients or families may elect for a greater degree of alertness over complete pain control and accompanying clouded sensorium. It is thus important to counsel patients and families that with current standards of care, many patients are pain-free and alert.

Health problems and screening

Burma is an isolated, developing rural nation that has been in a state of civil war for much of the past half-century. These factors contribute to the Burmese having a healthy life expectancy 10 years less than the neighboring Thai (WHO, 2002a). Infectious diseases are the greatest health problem among the Burmese.

Accurate vital statistics are difficult to obtain because of Burma's ongoing civil war and disruption of the country's health services infrastructure. Life expectancy at birth is 54.6 years for males and 59.9 years for females. The healthy life expectancy (HALE) at birth for males is 46.5 years and 51.4 years for females. The infant mortality rate is 72/1000 and the child mortality per 1000 is 121 for males and 106 for females (CIA, 2002; Population Reference Bureau, 2002; World Health Organization (WHO) (2002a).

Health risks for new Burmese immigrants or refugees (Allden *et al.*, 1996; Cho-Min-Naing, 2000; Kemp, 2002; Okada *et al.*, 2000; Petersen *et al.*, 1998; WHO, 2002b; Win *et al.*, 2002; Wongsrichanalai *et al.*, 2001) include:

- amebiasis
- angiostrongyliasis
- anthrax
- capillariasis
- chikungunya
- cholera
- cryptococcosis
- cryptosporidiosis
- cysticercosis (tapeworm)
- dengue Fever (including dengue hemorrhagic fever)
- filariasis: (Bancroftian filariasis and Malayan filariasis)
- gnathostomiasis
- helminthiasis (ascariasis, echinococcosis/hydatid disease, schistosomiasis)

- hepatitis B (15% carriage rate)
- HIV/AIDS
- hookworm
- leishmaniasis
- leprosy
- leptospirosis
- malaria, including multidrug resistant (MDR) from *Plasmodium falciparum* resistant parasites and especially from malaria re-infection. MDR malaria is especially common on the Thai–Burma border, where most refugees are found. Other malaria-causing parasites in Burma include *P. Vivax*, and much less commonly *P. malariae*, and *P. ovale*.
- melioidosis
- mycetoma
- paragonimiasis
- sexually transmitted infections, including HIV/AIDS, cervical cancer, chancroid, gonorrhea, granuloma inguinale, lymphogranuloma venereum, syphilis)
- strongylodiasis
- thalassemias
- trematodes (liver-dwelling: clonorchiasis and opisthorchiasis; blood-dwelling: schistosomiasis or bilharzia; intestine-dwelling; and lung-dwelling)
- tropical sprue
- tuberculosis (Burma is one of 22 countries worldwide designated by WHO as "high burden" for tuberculosis)
- typhus, Scrub
- yaws (frambesia)
- post-traumatic stress disorder
- physical sequelae of torture
- injuries from landmines and unexploded ordinance
- malnutrition
- anemia
- thalassemia

Acknowledgement

Tao Sheng Kwan-Gett, M.D., M.P.H.

REFERENCES

Allden, K., Poole, C., Chantavanich, S., Ohmar, K., Aung, N. N., & Mollica, R. F. (1996). Burmese political dissidents in Thailand: trauma and survival among young adults in exile. *American Journal of Public Health*, **86**, 1561–9.

Central Intelligence Agency (2002). *World Factbook*. Author. Accessed 12/14/2002 http://www.cia.gov/cia/publications/factbook/geos/bm.html.

Cho-Min-Naing, (2000). Assessment of dengue hemorrhagic fever in Myanmar. *Southeast Asian Journal of Tropical Medicine and Public Health*, **31**, 636–41.

Courtauld, C. (1984). *In Search of Burma*. London: Frederick Muller Limited.

Cultural Profiles Project (n.d.). *Myanmar*. University of Toronto. Retrieved December 14, 2002 from http://cwr.utoronto.ca/cultural/.

Kemp, C. (2002). *Infectious Diseases*. Retrieved April 12, 2003 from http://www3.baylor.edu/~Charles_Kemp/Infectious_Disease.htm.

Lang, H. J. (1995). Women as refugees: perspectives from Burma. *Cultural Survival Quarterly*, **19**. Retrieved October 7, 2002 from http://www.culturalsurvival.org/newpage/publications/csq/back_issue_ toc.cfm.cfm?id=19.1.

Okada, S., Taketa, K., Ishikawa, T. *et al.* (2000). High prevalence of hepatitis C in patients with thalassemia and patients with liver diseases in Myanmar (Burma). *Acta Med Okayama*, **54**, 137–8.

Petersen, H., Lykke, J., Hougen, H. P., & Mannstaedt, M. (1998). Results of medical examination of refugees from Burma. *Danish Medical Bulletin*, **45**, 313–16.

Population Reference Bureau (2002). *2002 World Population Data Sheet*. Retrieved May 12, 2003 from http://www.prb.org/pdf/WorldPopulationDS02_Eng.pdf.

Skidmore, M. (2002). Menstrual madness: women's health and well-being in urban Burma. *Women and Health*, **35**, 81–99.

Way, R. T. (1985). Burmese culture, personality and mental health. *Australian and New Zealand Journal of Psychiatry*, **19**, 275–82.

Win, T. T., Lin, K., Mizuno, S. *et al.* (2002). Wide distribution of *Plasmodium ovale* in Myanmar. *Tropical Medicine and International Health*, **7**, 231–9.

Wongsrichanalai, C., Sirichaisinthop, J., Karwacki, J. J. *et al.* (2001). Drug resistant malaria on the Thai–Myanmar and Thai–Cambodian borders. *Southeast Asian Journal of Tropical Medicine and Public Health*, **32**, 41–9.

World Health Organization (2002a). *World Health Report*. Retrieved June 5, 2003 from http://www.who.int/whr/2002/en/.

   (2002b). *Myanmar*. Retrieved December 15, 2002 from http://www.who.int/country/mmr/en/.

10

Cambodia

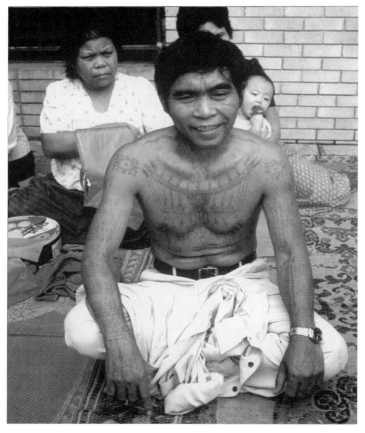

Tattoos such as these are thought to confer protection, power, or have other magical attributes. (Photograph by courtesy of Lance A. Rasbridge.)

Refugee and Immigrant Health: A Handbook for Health Professionals, Charles Kemp and Lance A. Rasbridge. Published by Cambridge University Press. © C. Kemp and L. A. Rasbridge 2004.

Introduction

Once the dominant military and economic force of Southeast Asia, Cambodia was, by the late 1800s, a French colony. From the beginning of colonial rule, there was resistance to the French. With the Geneva Convention of 1954, Cambodia became independent, with a government ruled by Prince Norodom Sihanouk. Communist and other dissident activities were repressed from that point until the late 1960s when the Khmer Rouge, led by Maoist extremists, in particular Pol Pot, became active. A brutal and complex armed struggle ensued, and in 1970, a *coup d'état* replaced Prince Sihanouk with right wing military rulers. Fighting escalated and in 1975, a deeply divided Cambodia fell to the Khmer Rouge.

Within days of victory, the Khmer Rouge initiated a radical restructuring of Cambodian society. Liquidation of all non-communist leaders began immediately and eventually encompassed not only military and political leaders, but also monks, teachers, people who wore glasses, and anyone else judged to be a "new person" or corrupted by capitalism. The cities were emptied of all residents, who then were put to work on agricultural communes. Families were separated according to the needs of work units and a deliberate effort was made to replace traditional relationships and structures such as family, village, and Buddhism with absolute obedience to the communist party or *Angka*.

By 1979, when the Khmer Rouge were overthrown by the Vietnamese army, approximately two million people out of a population of eight million had been murdered or allowed to die from starvation or disease (Glover, 1999).

That night Robona, Ton Ny's six-year-old sister, had a dream in which she saw someone very much like an angel who carried an armful of five lotus blossoms and spoke to her, "Don't be afraid my little girl, I'm keeping your Mama with me. But you shall go on living." In fact, one would have said that all the children were hurrying to join their mother. The first to die were the two five-year-old twins, three days apart, lying silently on a bamboo pallet; then two other brothers, Youthevy and Vouthinouk, nine and seven years old, the first at the hospital, the second when he came home from the hospital. Kosol, the four-year-old, and Robona died three months later, on the same day. All of them starved to death. After they died, Mitia Mir dreamed that he saw four columns still standing from a house in ruins. I thought that they were my uncle and his three surviving children, but now I know that the fourth column was myself . . . No one had the strength to work, so we were given no more food (Szymusiak, 1986, p. 113).

Like Jews who survived Nazi terror, many Khmer experience significant and long-term effects from the years under Khmer Rouge terror. Many feel that, "For us its too late" (as a man said to us at a recent New Year ceremony) to deal with the long-term effects of these traumas.

History of immigration

Beginning in late 1978, Cambodian refugees began fleeing to the relative safety of Thailand. From 1981–1985, approximately 200 000 Khmer were resettled in the United States, France, Australia and Canada.

Once in the West, the Khmer have tended to follow one of several paths. Some have enjoyed financial success (through salaried jobs as often as entrepreneurship) and have become homeowners in mixed middle-class neighborhoods. Others have scattered to suburban apartments. Still others have stayed in the neighborhoods in which they were originally resettled and have become a generally hidden part of inner-city urban life. In many cases, there has been little assimilation. In most cases, regardless of external appearances, there is great pain related to past trauma and current difficulties, and hence risk of mental health problems is higher than virtually all other immigrant groups (Boehnlein, 1987). On the whole, the resettlement experience for Cambodian refugees has been less successful than most other refugee groups, with nearly one-half of all Cambodians in the United States living below the poverty line (Taylor *et al.*, 2002).

Culture and social relationships

Extended families living together or in close proximity are the cultural ideal, but nuclear families are common. Men are the heads of the household, but increasing numbers of households are headed by widowed, divorced, or separated women. In reality, the power in some families is with the wife rather than the husband. Extended families usually are headed by an older parent or grandparent. Because of the inevitable adjustments and changes resulting from living in a foreign land, decision-making may fall to younger family members.

Khmer youth are a matter of concern to many community leaders and workers. Self-destructive behavior such as involvement in gangs is increasingly common. This is due, at least in part, to the destruction of much of the Cambodian culture by the Khmer Rouge and the long-term effects of the war and holocaust on individuals and families. Living in poor inner-city neighborhoods is part of the problem, but gangs and related behavior are a problem for many Khmer living in suburbs as well.

In many respects Khmer society in Cambodia and overseas is deeply divided and has been so for more than a quarter of a century. The pressures on individuals and families are profound and have a marked effect on individual and community health. While few Khmer will say to a Westerner, "I am overwhelmed and lost," there is little doubt that many are exactly that.

Communications

Khmer is the name of the language (as well as the people) of Cambodia, which is mutually unintelligible from neighboring Laotian, Thai, and Vietnamese. Khmer, written and spoken, is related to Sanskrit. Many older Cambodians are illiterate, and increasing numbers of youth, born in the West, have limited spoken Khmer skills.

Traditional Cambodian naming places the family name before the given name. Women retain their father's family name after marriage. The spelling of names sometimes changes due either to reclaiming an original spelling changed during the refugee registration process or taking on a new name when becoming a citizen. Cambodians often speak to one another by honorary relationship, e.g., uncle or by full name rather than informally by first name.

As with most other cultures, respect is essential. Older people should be greeted first and last. Communication is often indirect and requests or questions may be couched in seemingly vague terms. It is unusual for older people to make a direct "no" response to a question or request. Responses that may mean "no" include no response, a change in subject, or statements such as "it's okay" or "no problem," or even an unconvincing "yes." When an answer is not forthcoming, it is of little value to continue to press for a response.

Greeting is typically through the *sompeah* gesture, of hands brought together in a bowing motion, but the more acculturated will be comfortable with hand-shaking. The soul is believed to reside in the head, so incidental touching of the head is discouraged. Similarly, the sole of the foot is considered profane. Many Cambodians will demonstrate respect by maintaining a physical position with their head lower than the one being honored.

While Khmer appreciate children as least as much as others, they do not gush over babies or children. In fact, complimenting and praising babies and children may bring bad luck to the child. Effusive, loud, or overly familiar behavior toward others is seldom in good form, nor is showing anger or involvement in confrontation.

Religion

Most adult Khmer in the West are Buddhist. Worship is at a temple or *wat*, and at altars in individual homes. Worship at temples is usually led by one or more monks, often with assistance by a lay elder or *achar*. Worship includes monks and the congregation chanting in *Pali* (the liturgical language of Theravada Buddhism), burning incense, and prayer. Worship may be concluded by the monks eating food (always before midday) brought by the congregation. The congregation then eats and gradually disburses. The Cambodian Buddhist temple in the West plays an important role in cultural preservation and is typically the site of cultural celebrations, such as the Khmer New Year. See Chapter 5 for a discussion of Buddhism.

Evangelical Christian churches and The Church of Jesus Christ of Latter Day Saints (Mormon) are very active in most Khmer communities. The success of such churches is due in part to the presence of missionaries in refugee camps and the effectiveness and compassion of those missionaries in caring for refugees. Another factor that helps Christian churches is their willingness to go into the community and take an active and ongoing part in the lives and difficulties of refugees. This active outreach and caring is in contrast to the more detached Buddhist groups. Many Khmer are comfortable with attending both Christian and Buddhist worship.

Health beliefs and practices

In general, the Khmer are comfortable with cosmopolitan or Western medicine and with traditional or indigenous healing practices, both spiritual and medicinal (and often both). Illness may be attributed to imbalance in natural forces, i.e., a humoural theory of causation. However, few Khmer will directly express this concept. A common expression of the concept(s) is for people to note the influence of "wind" or *kchall* on blood circulation and thus on illness. There may also be discussion of body conditions called "cold" or "hot." These are not necessarily temperatures, but rather are body states leading to or caused by illness or other changes such as childbirth.

Traditional healing or indigenous practices are carried out by family members and some by traditional healers or *kruu Khmer*. Some *kruu Khmer* specialize in medicinal practice with a spiritual component, while others specialize in magic with a medicinal component. Regardless of who carries out the procedure below or other procedures, they are often accompanied by prayer and other spiritual activities (Buchwald *et al.*, 1992; Kemp & Rasbridge, 1999; Frye, 1991).

- *Kol* (rub) *kchall* (wind) is used to treat a variety of ailments, including fever, upper respiratory infection, nausea, weak heart, and malaise. A coin is dipped in a mentholated medicine. The coin is rubbed in one direction (away from the center of the body) on the patient's chest, back, and/or extremities. This practice is believed to "release the wind" built up in the body by opening skin pores and enhancing blood circulation. *Kol kchall* is usually referred to in Western literature as "coining" or "dermabrasion."
- *Jup* (pinch) *kchall* is used to treat headache and malaise. The first and second fingers are used to pinch and thus bruise the bridge of the nose, neck, or chest. *Jup* also refers to the practice of "cupping," where a candle or a wad of cotton

soaked in alcohol is briefly burned in a small glass, which is then immediately placed on the skin, usually on the back or the forehead. The flame consumes the oxygen and creates a vacuum, thus causing a circular contusion.

- *Oyt pleung* (known as "moxibustion" in the literature) is used to treat gastrointestinal and other disorders. *Oyt pleung* is seldom done in the West, but many adults will have four to six 1–2 cm scars on the abdomen resulting from the procedure.
- Massage or manipulation is practiced by *kruu Khmer* and others.
- Traditional or natural medicines are available in stores and from individuals. Such medicines include a wide variety of plant (leaves, bark, extracts) and other substances. These are often taken or applied topically in some combination of medicines and/or mixed with "wine" (usually vodka).

Spiritual healing practices are often incorporated in other practices, but some illnesses or conditions are viewed as primarily or even only due to spirit problems or possession. These practices (Kemp & Rasbridge, 1999) include the following.

- Magico-religious articles such as amulets, strings, and Buddha images are common. *Katha* (amulets or what appears to be a piece of string) are commonly worn around the neck by children or around the waist by adults. Types of amulets include a small piece of metal inscribed with sacred words written in *Pali* and rolled around string, Buddha images attached to a gold chain, and braided knotted string (with the knots incorporating magical substances).
- *Yuan* are magical pictures/words placed over doors, worn on clothing, or sometimes folded in pockets. They usually are written in *Pali*.
- Buddha images may be seen as charms mentioned above or as statues or pictures in homes. They are found on altars placed high on a wall. Incense, flowers, food, cigarettes, or fetishes such as hair may also be placed on the altar.
- Tattoos are a means of protection against harm or illness. Magical designs and/or words written in *Pali* are found on the chest, back, neck, and arms of some men.
- Other spiritual or magical means of treating illness include blowing on the sick person's body in a prescribed manner and showering or rubbing with lustral or blessed water.

Many Khmer take a syncretic approach to health care as well as other issues in life. Often traditional measures will be tried in the home before seeking health care outside the home and/or be used simultaneously with Western medicine.

Communication is a major issue in assessment and all other phases of care. Communication barriers may be due to language or to cultural issues. The latter include attempting to use a translator who, for gender, age, social status, or past relationship incompatibilities, may be rejected or not listened to.

Most Khmer are oriented more to illness treatment than prevention of illness. Medicines are sought to relieve symptoms and discontinued when symptoms resolve. Childhood immunizations are accepted, but adult immunizations (influenza, pneumonia) are of little interest until illness strikes.

As discussed earlier, resettled Cambodians, due to their collective experience with severe trauma, are at very high risk for mental health disorders. However, most Cambodians are reluctant to acknowledge mental illness *per se*. Primarily, psychological distress is believed to result from spirit possession or from past misdeeds and accrued "bad" karma, and hence is usually associated with "shame" (Ethnomed, 1995). Usually, help for emotional problems is sought from within the Buddhist community or through *kruu Khmer* and traditional medicine. As a last resort, Cambodians experiencing emotional problems may access Western care, but typically they present with physical symptomatology, i.e., somatization (Muecke, 1983).

There are several illnesses within the Cambodian community, with some emotional etiology, that can be considered culture-bound syndromes. Examples include:
- "thinking too much illness," characterized by headaches, chest pain, excessive sleeping, and withdrawal (Frye & D'Avanzo, 1994),
- "sore-neck syndrome," similar to panic attacks, manifesting in shortness of breath, trembling, and diaphoresis (Hinton *et al.*, 2001).

Western care providers must address both the underlying stress-related indices, together with the physical manifestations for successful treatment outcomes.

Pregnancy and childbirth

Early on in the resettlement process, Cambodian refugee births were often assisted by a traditional midwife, *chmop*, in the home (Sargent *et al.*, 1983), but presently virtually all births are hospital based. Modesty issues lead to a marked preference for female providers in obstetric care (Sargent & Marcucci, 1988). Birth control, particularly Depo-Provera injections and oral contraceptives, is gaining acceptance in the West (Ethnomed, 1995), although many women express concern of potential side effects, particularly since most Western medications are understood as humorally "hot."

Pregnancy and the postpartum are periods of heightened awareness of humoral balance. The pregnant state is considered a "hot" condition, primarily because of fetal development and subsequent blood "build-up," evidenced by the cessation of menses. Humorally hot foods and medicines are avoided during pregnancy, particularly ginger and black pepper.

Parturition with consequent blood loss leaves a postpartum woman extremely and immediately susceptible to cold. If humoral balance were not restored, long-term deleterious health consequences such as arthritis, poor blood circulation and skin disorders, collectively known as *toa*, are believed to result. The traditional practice of laying on a bamboo-slatted bed over buckets of hot coals (*ang pleung*) to restore humoral balance is no longer performed in the West, but several other substitute practices are commonly employed.

- A warming medicine (*tnam sraa*) of special herbs steeped in vodka or some other alcohol is consumed.
- Patent medicines, in particular, a powder believed to contain tiger bone is considered the most warming of all is taken.
- Medicinal steam baths are taken by the woman draping herself over a pot of boiled herbs.
- A heated brick or stone wrapped in a towel, may be placed on the abdomen.

Dietary prescriptions in the postpartum include ginger, red pepper, black pepper, sugar, and various meats, all considered to restore "heat." Commonly, sexual relations (and physical exertion in general) are proscribed from the third trimester of pregnancy through at least the first month postpartum, and sometimes longer (Kulig, 1998).

Some pregnant women are reluctant to undergo prenatal screening, due to fear or embarrassment over pelvic exams (Ethnomed, 1995), or lest they are confronted with "bad news" about their unborn baby (Liamputtong & Watson, 2002). Similarly, prenatal screening would seem superfluous for some, as abortion of a damaged fetus would not be considered anyway because of the overriding Buddhist concept of *bap*, the negative karma that would result in such an act of killing (Liamputtong & Watson, 2002).

Breastfeeding was the norm in Cambodia, but most infants born in the West are bottle-fed from birth. It is not uncommon for bottle-feeding to be lengthy and excessive, such as the use of a bottle as a pacifier, with consequent nutritional deficiencies (Rasbridge & Kulig, 1995). The fontanel is sometimes covered with an herbal poultice to prevent the infant's soul from escaping.

End of life

For Cambodians in the West (and to some extent, those elsewhere), dying is often accompanied by more "baggage" than most other people. Besides the usual physical, personal, interpersonal, and spiritual issues, there also may be issues alluded to above, such as survivor guilt, guilt over decisions made during the Holocaust, unresolved grief, lack of cultural support, lack of family support, and others. As with other persons going through the process, Cambodians may experience a wide range of emotions, but acceptance or resignation are the most commonly displayed.

Most families prefer that discussion of end-of-life issues be with the family rather than with the patient. There are often family attempts to "protect" the patient from knowledge of a poor prognosis. In some families there is an almost mystical faith in Western medicine and thus a reluctance to forgo even the most futile treatment. Withdrawal of treatment usually requires extended discussion with all family members and in many cases, repeated explanations.

Pain and other symptoms are often endured with stoicism. This is a critical issue in caring for Cambodians with advanced disease. One must ask very directly and specifically about each symptom that a Cambodian patient (especially older ones) may be experiencing. General or passing questions are meaningless. Equanimity in the face of death is highly valued.

Family expressions of grief after death may be open and unrestrained, or may be inhibited. We have noticed that persons in acute mourning often are extensively and even severely coined – as if to say, without words, "See this terrible pain." White is traditionally the color of mourning clothes.

Ideally, the body should be washed and prepared by the family. The hands are placed in a prayerful position and candles and incense placed in the hands. Some families place a coin in the mouth of the deceased. After the death, neighbors and friends visit in large numbers and are expected to make monetary contributions to the family for the funeral and related ceremonies. Donations are also given at the ceremony.

Cremation is preferred, though some Cambodians in America are buried. Ceremonies are usually held the weekend after the death and again at 100 days after the death. Offerings commemorating the deceased are also made at the New Year in April and at other times as well (Kemp *et al.*, 2000).

Health problems and screening

The healthy life expectancy or HALE in Cambodia is 46.4 years and the full life expectancy is 56 years (Population Reference Bureau, 2002; World Health Organization (WHO), 2002). Infectious diseases are the leading causes of death and disability in Cambodia. Cambodia is one of 22 countries worldwide with a "high burden" of tuberculosis (WHO, 2003). Health risks for new Cambodian immigrants or refugees (Hawn & Jung, 2003; Kemp, 2002; Pickwell *et al.*, 1994; WHO, 2002) include:

- amebiasis
- angiostrongyliasis
- anthrax
- capillariasis
- chikungunya
- cholera
- cryptococcosis
- cryptosporidiosis
- cysticercosis (tapeworm)

- dengue fever
- encephalitis (Japanese)
- filariasis (Bancroftian filariasis and Malayan filariasis)
- gnathostomiasis
- helminthiasis (ascariasis, echinococcosis/hydatid disease, schistosomiasis)
- hepatitis B (15% carriage rate)
- hookworm
- leishmaniasis
- leprosy
- leptospirosis
- malaria, including multidrug resistant (MDR) from *Plasmodium falciparum*-resistant parasites and especially from malaria re-infection
- melioidosis
- mycetoma
- sexually transmitted infections, including HIV/AIDS, chancroid, chlamydia, gonorrhea, granuloma inguinale, lymphogranuloma venereum, syphilis)
- strongylodiasis
- thalassemias
- trematodes (liver-dwelling: clonorchiasis and opisthorchiasis; blood-dwelling: schistosomiasis or bilharzias; intestine-dwelling; and lung-dwelling: paragonimiasis)
- tropical sprue
- tuberculosis (Cambodia is one of 22 countries worldwide designated by WHO as "high burden" for tuberculosis)
- typhus
- yaws (frambesia)
- post-traumatic stress disorder, chronic
- betel nut chewing is associated with oral cancer
- nutritional deficits

REFERENCES

Boehnlein, J. (1987). Clinical relevance of grief and mourning among Cambodian refugees. *Social Science and Medicine*, **25**, 765–72.

Buchwald, D., Panwala, S., & Hooton, T. (1992). Use of traditional health practices by Southeast Asian refugees in a primary care clinic. *Western Journal of Medicine*, **156**, 507–11.

Ethnomed (1995). *Cambodia Cultural Profile*. Retrieved August 8, 2003 from http://ethnomed. org/ethnomed/cultures/cambodian/camb_cp. html.

Frye, B. (1991). Cultural themes in health-care decision making among Cambodian refugee women. *Journal of Community Health Nursing*, **8**, 33–44.

Frye, B. & C. D'Avanzo (1994). Themes in managing culturally defined illness in the Cambodian refugee family. *Journal of Community Health Nursing*, **11**, 89–98.

Glover, J. (1999). *Humanity: A Moral History of the Twentieth Century*. New Haven: Yale University Press.

Hawn, T. R. & Jung, E. C. (2003). Health screening in immigrants, refugees, and internationally adopted orphans. In *The Travel and Tropical Medicine Manual*, 3rd edn., ed. E. C. Jong & R. McMullen, pp. 255–65. Philadelphia, PA: W. B. Saunders.

Hinton, D., Um, K., & Ba, P. (2001). A unique panic disorder presentation among Khmer refugees: The sore neck syndrome. *Culture, Medicine and Psychiatry*, **25**, 297–316.

Kemp, C. (2002). Infectious diseases. Retrieved April 12, 2003 from http://www3.baylor.edu/~Charles_Kemp/Infectious_Disease.htm.

Kemp, C. & Rasbridge, L. (1999). *Refugee Health – Immigrant Health*. Retrieved October 20, 2002 from http://www.baylor.edu/~Charles_Kemp/refugee_health.htm.

Kemp, C., Keovilay, L., & Rasbridge, L. (2000). Culture and the end of life: Cambodians and Laotians – health beliefs and practices related to the end of life. *Journal of Hospice and Palliative Nursing*, **2**, 143–51.

Kulig, J. (1998). Cambodians (Khmer). In *Cultural Assessment*, 2nd edn., ed. E. Geissler, pp. 125–9. St. Louis: Mosby.

Liamputtong, P. & Watson, L. (2002). The voices and concerns about prenatal testing of Cambodian, Lao, and Vietnamese women in Australia. *Midwifery*, **18**, 304–13.

Muecke, M. (1983). In search of healers: Southeast Asian refugees in the American health care system. *Western Journal of Medicine*, **39**, 31–6.

Pickwell, S., Schimelpfening, S., & Palinkas, L. (1994). 'Betelmania': Betel quid chewing by Cambodian women in the United States and its potential health effects. *Western Journal of Medicine*, **160**, 326–31.

Population Reference Bureau (2002). *2002 World Population Data Sheet*. Retrieved May 12, 2003 from http://www.prb.org/pdf/WorldPopulationDS02_Eng.pdf.

Rasbridge, L. & Kulig, J. (1995). Infant feeding among Cambodian refugees. *Maternal Child Nursing*, **20**, 213–18.

Sargent, C. & Marcucci, J. (1988). Khmer prenatal health practices and the American clinical experience. In *Childbirth in America: Anthropological Perspectives*, ed. K. Michaelson, pp. 79–89. South Hadley, MA: Bergin and Garvey Publishers.

Sargent, C., Marcucci, J., & Elliston, E. (1983). Tiger bones, fire and wine: Maternity care in a Kampuchean refugee community. *Medical Anthropology*, **7**, 67–79.

Szymusiak, M. (1986). *The Stones Cry Out*. New York: Hill and Wang.

Taylor, V., Jackson, C., Chan, N., Kuniyuki, A., & Yasui, Y. (2002). Hepatitis B knowledge and practices among Cambodian American women in Seattle, Washington. *Journal of Community Health*, **27**, 151–63.

World Health Organization (WHO) (2002). World health report. Retrieved June 5, 2003 from http://www.who.int/whr/2002/en/.

(2003). Global TB control report 2003. Retrieved June 1, 2003 from http://www.who.int/gtb/publications/globrep/index.html.

11

Caribbean Islands

Introduction

The Caribbean Islands are a group of 21 island nations located in the Gulf of Mexico south of the United States and north of South America. These islands/nations include Anguilla, Antigua and Barbuda, Bahamas, Barbados, Bermuda, Cayman Islands, Cuba, Dominica, Dominican Republic, Grenada, Guadeloupe, Haiti, Jamaica, Martinique, Montserrat, Netherlands Antilles, Puerto Rico, St. Kitts-Nevis, St. Lucia, St. Vincent and the Grenadines, Trinidad and Tobago, Turks and Caicos, and the Virgin Islands. Approximately 37 000 000 people live in the Caribbean Islands, with the largest numbers in Cuba (11.3 million), the Dominican Republic (8.8 million), and Haiti (7.1 million) (Population Reference Bureau (PRB), 2002). Cuba and Haiti are each discussed in separate chapters.

History of immigration

The Caribbean Islands are, on the whole, densely populated and poor, hence outmigration and migration within the islands is common. In most cases, migration is to the United States or to present or former colonizing countries, e.g., Jamaicans migrating to the United Kingdom. In some cases (Cuba and Haiti) there have also been significant numbers of political refugees.

Culture and social relations

The Caribbean Islands are diverse ethnically and racially, with many people descended from African slaves, and also significant numbers of people of Spanish, British, East Indian, and Chinese heritage. Tourism, with its exposure to other cultures and values is a major influence on many in the Caribbean.

Refugee and Immigrant Health: A Handbook for Health Professionals, Charles Kemp and Lance A. Rasbridge. Published by Cambridge University Press. © C. Kemp and L. A. Rasbridge 2004.

Families tend to be nuclear, but with close ties to the extended family. Males are usually the head and breadwinner of the family, but there are also many matrifocal families with women the primary decision-makers, including in health matters. Additionally, there are many unstable sexual unions with significant numbers of children born out of marriage and a lack of paternal involvement in parenting. Traditional age-related roles are held by many, e.g., respect for elders, but tourism, migration, and other factors are breaking down some traditional roles. Because the cultures of the Caribbean Islands are so diverse, some summary data are presented in Table 11.1 (Johnstone & Mandryk, 2001; PRB, 2002; St. Hill, 1996).

Communications

The largest percentage of people in the Caribbean Islands speak Spanish (e.g., Cubans, Dominicans, Puerto Ricans), with others speaking one of several languages.
- French and Creole are spoken in Haiti.
- English and English Patwah (a type of slang) are spoken in Jamaica.
- English with some Creole is spoken in Jamaica, Trinidad, and Barbados.
- Patwah is spoken in St. Lucia, Dominica, and Martinique.

"Creole" as it applies to the language spoken in Haiti and as a linguistic concept, denotes a type of Pidgin language. Creole and Patwah are unique languages and are not mutually intelligible (Rose Jones, personal communication, June 9, 2003).

In general, communications are characterized by respect and formality. New immigrants, in particular, tend to be reserved, shy, and formal in their interactions with health providers. The majority of people in the Caribbean Islands, especially the young, are literate.

Religion

As in other multi-ethnic societies, there are many religions practiced in the Caribbean, and in some cases, religions are blended. Catholicism has the largest number of adherents. There are large numbers of Anglicans living in British-influenced cultures; and in all Caribbean societies, there are increasing numbers of Protestant evangelicals. Though difficult to quantify, there are also spiritualist religions such as Santeria and Obeah practiced throughout the Caribbean Islands and in most cases alongside or combined with other religions such as Catholicism. Rastafarianism, the practice of which includes natural foods and *ganja* (marijuana) use, is growing among black Caribbean Islanders (Koffman & Higginson, 2002).

Health beliefs and practices

Traditional beliefs in the Caribbean Islands about health and illness are related to traditional African beliefs as well as to biomedical or allopathic beliefs and practices.

Table 11.1 Caribbean Islands*

Country	Population (approximate in millions)	Ethnic group(s)	Religion(s)	Government	Language and Language and
Anguilla	.08	African-Caribbean	Protestant, Anglican	British dependency	English, Creole.
Antigua and Barbuda	0.1	African-Caribbean	Protestant, Anglican, spiritist	Independent	English, Creole. One of the four most prosperous CIs
Bahamas	0.3	African-Caribbean, Euro-American	Protestant, Catholic	Independent	English. One of the four most prosperous CIs
Barbados	0.3	African-Caribbean	Protestant, Anglican	Independent	English. One of the four most prosperous CIs
Bermuda	.06	African-Caribbean, Euro-American	Protestant, Anglican, Catholic	Dependent territory of UK	English
Cayman Islands	.05	African-Caribbean, Euro-American	Protestant, spiritist, non-religious	Dependent territory of UK	English. Wealthiest CI. Economy based on banking and tourism
Cuba	11.3	Hispanic, African-Caribbean	Catholic, spiritist, non-religious	Independent communist	Spanish. Impoverished, but advanced in terms of health and health-care
Dominica	.07	African-Caribbean, indigenous	Catholic, Protestant, spiritist	Independent	English
Dominican Republic	8.8	Hispanic, African-Caribbean, Haitian	Catholic, Protestant, spiritist	Independent	Spanish. Impoverished
Grenada	0.1	African-Caribbean	Catholic, Protestant, Anglican	Independent	English
Guadeloupe	0.5	African-Caribbean, Asian-Caribbean	Catholic, Protestant	Overseas department of France	French, Creole
Haiti	7.1	African-Caribbean,	Catholic, Protestant, spiritist	Independent	Haitian Creole. Impoverished. High HIV rate

(*cont.*)

Table 11.1 (cont.)

Country	Population (approximate in millions)	Ethnic group(s)	Religion(s)	Government	Language and Language and
Jamaica	2.6	African-Caribbean, Asian-Caribbean	Protestant, spiritist, unaffiliated	Independent	Jamaican Creole. Declining economy, high crime rate
Martinique	0.4	African-Caribbean, Asian-Caribbean	Catholic, Protestant, unaffiliated	Overseas department of France	French Creole
Montserrat	0.003	African-Caribbean	Protestant, Anglican, unaffiliated	Dependent territory of UK	English
Netherlands Antilles	0.2	African-Caribbean, Euro-American, Hispanic	Catholic, Protestant	Part of the Kingdom of Netherlands	Papiamento, Dutch, English
Puerto Rico	3.9	Hispanic (Euro-American, African-Caribbean)	Catholic, Protestant. Rapidly growing evangelical movement	Related to the US	Spanish, English. Controversy about relation with US
St. Kitts-Nevis	0.04	African-Caribbean, Asian-Caribbean	Protestant, Catholic, Anglican	Independent	English
St. Lucia	0.2	African-Caribbean, Asian-Caribbean	Catholic, Protestant, Anglican	Independent	French Creole, English
St. Vincent and the Grenadines	0.1	African-Caribbean, Asian-Caribbean, indigenous	Protestant, Anglican, independent	Member of British Common-wealth	English and Creole
Trinidad and Tobago	1.3	African-Caribbean, Asian-Caribbean (East Indian)	Catholic, Protestant, Anglican, Hindu, Muslim	Independent	English, Hindi. Racial and religious conflict present, but lessening
Turks and Caicos	0.12	African-Caribbean, Haitian, Euro-American	Protestant, Catholic, Anglican	Dependent territory of UK	English, Creole
Virgin Islands	0.1	African-Caribbean, Euro-American, Hispanic	Protestant, Catholic, Anglican	Self-governing territory of US	English, Spanish

* Geissler, 1994; Johnstone, & Mandryk, 2001, Pan American Health Organization, 2002; Population Reference Bureau, 2002.

Among most people, there is little awareness of health as a concept – other than a lack of illness. Moderate obesity and clear skin are generally seen as signs of good health in adults, children, and infants. Among educated people, there is understanding of biomedical causation and treatment of illness (Juarbe, 1996; St. Hill, 1996).

The concept of balance or "hot and cold dichotomy" is prevalent throughout the region and tends to cut across ethnic and cultural boundaries. There also is widespread use of indigenous or "bush medicine" (Rose Jones, personal communication, June 9, 2003).

Supernatural forces are thought by many to play a central role in illness. Such beliefs are strongest in Haiti, where supernatural forces are believed by many people to be the cause of most illness. Though not as strong nor as openly acknowledged in other islands, a belief in supernatural causation (and treatment) is common throughout the region. Among immigrants in developed countries, there is enormous faith in biomedical treatments (though noncompliance is common) (Juarbe, 1996; Scott, 1974; St. Hill, 1996). Culture-bound illnesses found in the Caribbean (American Psychiatric Association (APA), 2000; Guarnaccia, 1993) include the following.

- *Ataques de nervios* is a dramatic outburst of negative emotion (shouting, crying, intense anxiety, breaking things, losing consciousness) – usually in response to a current stressor such as bereavement. After the *ataque*, the person does not remember the episode.
- *Mal de pelea* is a dissociative episode occurring among Puerto Ricans and similar to *amok*, in which a period of brooding and often paranoia or persecutory thinking precedes a violent and sometimes homicidal outburst.
- *Rootwork* is the explanation for illness attributed to witchcraft or hexing. The hex is the "root." The illness commonly includes anxiety, fatigue, and a variety of gastrointestinal symptoms. Treatment is through a "root doctor."
- *Falling out* is a sudden physical collapse in which the person's eyes are open but he or she does not see, but the ability to hear remains.

Also see the chapter on Haiti. In addition, some of the culture-bound syndromes found among Mexicans and other Latinos may also be found in some Caribbean cultures.

As is common in other tropical climates, the largest meal of the day is usually the noon meal. Foods tend to be spicy on many islands, with Jamaica the source of the incendiary Scotch bonnet pepper. Meat is highly valued and, finances allowing, is eaten in large amounts. Fish is less expensive and for many people, is the primary source of protein. Rice is a staple and fried foods are common. Immigrants to developed nations tend to eat large quantities of meat and fast foods, and thus develop attendant problems such as obesity and hypertension (Pan American Health Organization (PAHO), 2003; Sharma *et al.*, 2002).

Sick people tend to stay in bed and take on a passive and dependent role. Herbal remedies and "tonics" or patent medicines are common and widely available in the home islands and urban areas of developed nations with large numbers of Caribbean immigrants (Scott, 1974; St. Hill, 1996).

Personal hygiene is important to most Caribbean Islanders and its importance continues in the host country. Modesty is important to both genders and same sex health providers are appreciated (Juarbe, 1996; St. Hill, 1996).

Health problems and screening

Cuba has the highest healthy life expectancy or HALE (66.6 years) in Latin America and Haiti, the lowest (42.9 years). The HALE of Haitians has *decreased* by more than 2 years from 2001 to 2002, due at least in part, to the high rate of HIV/AIDS in Haiti (Lamptey *et al.*, 2002; World Health Organization (WHO), 2002). HIV/AIDS is the leading cause of death in some parts of the region, with about 2.4% of adults infected and the highest infection rate in the world after Africa. Haiti has the highest prevalence, with about 6% of adults infected, and is followed by Bermuda, where nearly 4% are infected. Multiple sex partners, lack of condoms and other protective devices, reluctance to use protection, and migration and frequent travel among Caribbean islands and the United States help spread HIV (Lamptey *et al.*, 2002; WHO, 2002)

Though not problems in every Caribbean island, a variety of infectious diseases are found in the Caribbean, and these diseases appear and disappear in various islands through the years (Centers for Disease Control, 2003). In the Caribbean and among immigrants from the Caribbean to other countries, chronic non-infectious diseases such as hypertension, heart disease, stroke, diabetes, and early disability are increasingly common (Lane *et al.*, 2002; PAHO, 2003). Health risks in refugees and immigrants from the Caribbean Islands (Centers for Disease Control, 2003; Hawn & Jung, 2003; Kemp, 2002; Lane *et al.*, 2002; PAHO, 2002) include:

- amebiasis
- angiostrongyliasis
- anisakiasis
- arbovirus encephalitis (Eastern equine encephalomyelitis (EEE))
- Chagas' disease
- cholera
- chromomycosis
- cryptococcosis
- cryptosporidiosis
- dengue fever
- dracunculiasis (Guinea worm disease)

- filariasis (Bancroftian filariasis, Malayan filariasis, and to a lesser extent, onchocerciasis
- granuloma inguinale or Donovanosis
- hepatitis B
- leishmaniasis
- leprosy
- leptospirosis
- malaria
- mucocutaneous leishmaniasis (*Espundia*)
- mycetoma
- paracoccidioidomycosis (South American blastomycosis)
- STDs, including HIV/AIDS, cervical cancer, chancroid, chlamydia, gonorrhea, granuloma inguinale, lymphogranuloma venereum, syphilis)
- strongylodiasis
- toxoplasmosis
- trematodes (liver-dwelling, including clonorchiasis and opisthorchiasis; blood-dwelling, including schistosomiasis or bilharzias; intestine-dwelling; and lung-dwelling, including paragonimiasis)
- trichuriasis (trichocephaliasis or whipworm)
- tuberculosis
- tungiasis
- typhoid fever
- yaws (frambesia)
- yellow fever
- cardiovascular and related diseases, e.g., obesity, hypertension, diabetes, and COPD

Acknowledgement

Rose Jones, Ph.D.

REFERENCES

American Psychiatric Association (APA) (2000). *Diagnostic and Statistical Manual of Mental Disorders*, 4th edn., text revision. Washington, DC: Author.

Centers for Disease Control (2003) *Health Information for Travelers to the Caribbean*. Retrieved May 12, 2003 from http://www.cdc.gov/travel/caribean.htm.

Geissler, E. M. (1998). *Cultural Assessment*. St. Louis: Mosby.

Guarnaccia, P. J. (1993). *Ataques de nervios* in Puerto Rico: culture-bound syndrome or popular illness? *Medical Anthropology*, **15**, 157–70.

Hawn, T. R. & Jung, E. C. (2003). Health screening in immigrants, refugees, and internationally adopted orphans. In *The Travel and Tropical Medicine Manual*, 3rd edn., ed. E. C. Jong and R. McMullen, pp. 255–65. Philadelphia, PA: W. B. Saunders.

Johnstone, P. & Mandryk, J. (2001). *Operation World*. 21st century edn. Waynesboro, GA: Paternoster USA.

Juarbe, T. (1996). Puerto Ricans. In *Culture and Nursing Care*, ed. J. G. Lipson, S. L. Dibble and P. A. Minarik, pp. 222–38. San Francisco: UCSF Nursing Press.

Kemp, C. (2002). *Infections Diseases*. Retrieved April 12, 2003 from http://www.3.baylor.edu/~Charles_Kemp/Infections_Disease.htm.

Koffman, J. & Higginson, I. J. (2002). Religious faith and support at the end of life: a comparison of first generation black Caribbean and white populations. *Palliative Medicine*, **16**, 540–1.

Lamptey, P., Merywen, W. Carr, D., & Collymore, Y. (2002). *HIV hits marginal populations hardest in Latin America, leading cause of death for some Caribbean nations*. Population Reference Bureau. Retrieved March 18, 2003 from http://www.prb.org/.

Lane, D. Beevers. D. G., & Lip, G. Y. H. (2002). Ethnic differences in blood pressure and the prevalence of hypertension in England. *Journal of Human Hypertension*, **16**, 267–73.

Pan American Health Organization (PAHO). (2002). *Country Health Profiles*. Retrieved April 24, 2003 from http://www.paho.org/.

(2003). New study shows enormous burden of diabetes. Retrieved May 30, 2003 from http://www.paho.org/English/DD/PIN/pr030328.htm.

Population Reference Bureau (PRB) (2002). *2002 World Population Data Sheet*. Retrieved May 12, 2003 from http://www.prb.org/pdf/WorldPopulationDS02_Eng.pdf.

Scott, C. S. (1974). Health and healing practices among five ethnic groups in Miami, Florida. *Public Health Reports*, **89**, 824–32.

Sharma, S., Cade, J., Landman, J., & Cruickshank, J. K. (2002). Assessing the diet of the British African–Caribbean population: frequency of consumption of foods and food portion sizes. *International Journal of Food Sciences and Nutrition*, **53**, 439–44.

St. Hill, P. (1996). West Indians. In *Culture and Nursing Care*, ed. J. G. Lipson, S. L. Dibble & P. A. Minarik, pp. 291–303. San Francisco: UCSF Nursing Press.

World Health Organization (2002). *World Health Report*. Retrieved June 5, 2003 from http://www.who.int/whr/2002/en/.

12

Central America

Introduction

Central America lies between South America and North America, and includes Mexico, Guatemala, Belize, Honduras, El Salvador, Nicaragua, Costa Rica, and Panama (Table 12.1). Approximately 140 million people live in Central America, with the great majority (102 million) in Mexico (Population Reference Bureau (PRB), 2002). Mexico and Guatemala are discussed in separate chapters.

History of immigration

Central America has a long history of dictatorships, revolutions (leading usually to another dictatorship), human rights violations, and poverty. These factors have led to great outmigration of both refugees and immigrants to Latin America, the United States, and to a lesser extent, Europe. The route up through Mexico and across the US border is very dangerous, with extortion, robbery, and murder common before arriving in the USA; death from exposure and dehydration is common when crossing desert areas of the USA Even so, the economy in most of Central America is moribund, and the risks of immigration are a small deterrent.

Culture and social relations

People from Central America prefer to be perceived as coming from their particular country as opposed to the region of Central America. Some indigenous people, e.g., Mayans, Aztecs, and Miskitus, may appreciate being perceived as being of their particular group. While some cultural differences exist among Central Americans (especially between Hispanic and indigenous groups), there are significant similarities among the various peoples and cultures.

Refugee and Immigrant Health: A Handbook for Health Professionals, Charles Kemp and Lance A. Rasbridge. Published by Cambridge University Press. © C. Kemp and L. A. Rasbridge 2004.

Table 12.1 Central America*

Country	Population (approximate in millions)	Ethnic group(s)	Religion(s)	Government	Language and comments
Belize	0.3	Hispanic, African-Caribbean, Indigenous	Catholic, Protestant	Independent	Spanish, English, Mayan (several languages)
Costa Rica	3.9	Hispanic, Indigenous, numerous Nicaraguans	Catholic, Protestant	Independent	Spanish
El Salvador	6.6	Hispanic, indigenous	Catholic, Protestant	Independent	Spanish. Most densely populated Central American country. History of brutal conflicts
Guatemala	12.1	Indigenous (Mayan), Hispanic	Catholic, Protestant	Independent	Spanish, numerous Mayan languages. History of brutal conflicts and human rights violations – especially against Mayans
Honduras	6.7	Hispanic	Catholic, Protestant	Independent	Spanish. 1998 hurricane destroyed infrastructure. Great outmigration to USA and Latin America
Mexico	101.7	Hispanic, Indigenous (Aztec, Mayan, other), but culturally Mestizo	Catholic, Protestant	Independent. Transition from single-party system in 2000.	Spanish. Please see separate chapter on Mexico.
Nicaragua	5.4	Hispanic, Caribbean, indigenous	Catholic, Protestant	Independent	Spanish, English. Poorest Central American country
Panama	2.9	Hispanic, Asian, indigenous	Catholic, Protestant, Muslim	Independent	Spanish

* Geissler, 1994; Johnstone & Mandryk, 2001, Pan American Health Organization, 2002; PRB, 2002.

In the home countries, especially rural areas, extended families are the norm. However, there is a strong migratory trend toward urban areas (67% of the regional population), so the percentage of nuclear families is increasing – as is the number of single-parent families (PRB, 2002; Rundle *et al.*, 1999). Single-parent families are often the result of men migrating to other locales seeking employment.

Men are the heads of most two-parent households and are usually the breadwinners. Women's roles are family and home-focused. Changes in work and migration patterns, as well as other social phenomena are changing these centuries-old social roles. Physical and sexual abuse of women is common in at least some countries – and is likely a region-wide problem (Pan American Health Organization, 2001).

Traditionally, elders are highly respected and cared for within the family, and children are protected by the family. These age-related roles and expectations are also changing, with increasing numbers of elders and children abandoned by their families. Street children, in particular, are a rapidly growing population with attendant problems of drug abuse, prostitution, and crime.

Communications

With the exception of some rural indigenous people, Spanish is the language of Central America. Communications are characterized by respect (*respeto*) and what might be described as warm reserve where strangers are concerned. As relationships deepen, the reserve diminishes, but there remains a core of dignity within most Central Americans. Most much prefer to be called by Mr. or Mrs. (*senor or senora*), especially by younger people.

Central Americans are generally loathe to complain of illness or pain unless the problem is great or concerns the family – especially children. Personal/emotional problems are seldom discussed outside the family or church.

Naming is an important aspect of Central American cultures and a source of confusion where medical records are concerned. Most people have two first names, e.g., Ana María + the father's family name (*primer apellido*), e.g., Camacho + the mother's family name (*segundo apellido*), e.g., Pérez. Her full or legal name is thus Ana María Camacho Pérez, but she may also be known as Ana María Camacho. If she marries (Juan Carlos Guerrero Martinez, for example), she will take her husband's *primer apellido* as follows: Ana María Pérez de Guerrero (Guerrero being the husband's father's family name). In the USA, she will likely be known as Ana María Guerrero or perhaps Ana Guerrero or María Guerrero.

Religion

Roman Catholicism is the primary religion of Central America. Protestant evangelical (*Cristiana*) missionaries are very active throughout Central and South America, with 10–25% of the population now being classified as Protestant, e.g., Baptist,

Pentecostal, or independent "Bible believer." Some indigenous people may also be classified as "Christo-pagan," with Mayan or Aztec gods combined with Catholic saints (Boyle, 1996; Johnstone & Mandryk, 2001)

Health beliefs and practices

Health is generally seen as the absence of illness. A person who is thought to appear healthy is likely to be moderately obese (seldom slender), have smooth skin and glossy hair, and feel good.

Influences on health include emotional, spiritual, and social state, as well as physical factors such as humoral imbalance expressed as too much "hot" or "cold" (or "weak") (Boyle, 1996). Such belief is usually held concurrently with a belief in biomedical treatments. "Hot" and "cold" are intrinsic properties of various foods, medicines (herbal or allopathic), or conditions, and there are sometimes differences of opinion about what is hot and what is cold. Folk or ethnomedical illnesses or conditions one might encounter in a Central American patient (American Psychiatric Association, 2000; Boyle, 1996; Levine & Gaw, 1995; Lieberman *et al.*, 1997; Neff, 1998; Schechter *et al.*, 2000; Spector, 1996) are as follows.

- *Antojos* are cravings in a pregant woman. It is thought by many that failure to satisfy the cravings may lead to injury to the baby, including genetic defects.
- *Ataque de nervios* are episodic, dramatic outbursts of negative emotion – usually in response to a current stressor (but often related to a significant childhood stressor).
- *Barrevillos* are obsessions.
- *Bilis* and *colera* is thought to be bile flowing into the blood stream after a traumatic event, with the end result of nervousness and/or rage.
- *Caida de la mollera* is the presence of a sunken fontanelle in an infant.
- *Colera* (see *bilis* above).
- *Decaiminientos* is fatigue and listlessness from a spiritual cause.
- *Dercernsos* are fainting spells.
- *Empacho* is intestinal obstruction and is characterized by abdominal pain, vomiting, constipation, anorexia, or gas and bloating. Postpartum women and infants and children are most susceptible.
- *Frio de la matriz* is coldness of the womb. Symptoms include pelvic congestion, menstrual irregularities and loss of libido; all of which may last for several years postpartum if treatment is not successful. The cause is inadequate rest after delivery.
- *Grisi siknis* occurs among the *Miskitu* people living on the Atlantic coast of southern Central America. *Grisi siknis* is a dissociative disorder that affects primarily

young women, and is manifested by the belief that she is being attacked by "devils" and must run and hide. Aggression is also a feature.

- *Mal de Ojo* is the "Evil Eye" that may affect infants or women. It is caused by a person with a "strong eye" (especially green or blue) looking with admiration or jealousy at another person. *Mal de Ojo* is avoided by touching an infant when admiring or complimenting him or her.
- *Mareos* is associated with *nerviosimo* and includes dizziness and/or vertigo.
- *Muina* (see *Bilis* and *colera* above).
- *Nerviosimo* (or *nervios*) is "sickness of the nerves" and is common and may be treated spiritually and/or medicinally.
- *Pasmo* is paralysis or paresis of extremities or face and is treated with massage.
- *Susto* is fright resulting in "soul loss." *Susto* may be acute or chronic and includes a variety of vague complaints. Women are affected more than men.

Cold conditions are treated with hot medications and hot with cold medications, thus bringing the individual back into balance. Problems that are primarily spiritual in nature are treated with prayer and ritual. However, few Central Americans who use folk means of treating illness are troubled by simultaneously using cosmopolitan treatments such as antibiotics, antidepressants, and so on.

The array of lay and other healers used by Central Americas are similar to those used by Mexicans, and include *yerberos* (herbalists), *sobador* (massage therapists), *parteras* (midwives who may also treat young children), *cuaranderos total* (lay healers who intervene in multiple dimensions, e.g., physical and spiritual) (Neff, 1998; Zapata & Shippee-Rice, 1999; Scott, 1974). A *doctor naturalista* (naturalist doctor) may also be utilized as may the services of a *botánica* (store selling medicinal herbs and religious amulets, candles, statues, and the like). Regardless of the source of care, the patient (and family) are likely to include faith in God as a vital component of understanding of the problem and the cure (Zapata & Shippee-Rice, 1999). Common folk remedies from Mexico and Central America are shown in Table 12.2.

The diet of Central Americans is variable according to the country of origin, but commonly includes rice and beans (black or pinto), usually prepared with lard. Tamales and soups are common throughout Central America and are prepared differently according to regional tradition. Fast foods, both American-style such as hamburgers and Mexican such as *tacos de fajita* are enjoyed by many.

Pregnancy and childbirth

Prenatal care is valued where available and despite Catholic proscriptions against birth control, family planning/spacing is widely accepted – again, where available (PAHO, 2002). "Hot" foods, cool air, strong moonlight, and especially eclipses are avoided by many Central American women during pregnancy (Boyle, 1996).

Table 12.2 Common folk remedies from Mexico and Central America*

Remedy	Uses
Garlic (*ajo*)	Hypertension, antibiotic, cough syrup, *tripaida*
Lead/mercury oxides (*Azarcón/Greta*)	*Empacho*, teething (note that these are heavy metal poisons)
Damiana (*Damiana*)	Aphrodisiac, *frio en la matriz*, chickenpox
Wormwood (*Estafiate*)	Aphrodisiac, *frio en la matriz*, chickenpox (intoxicant and poisonous in sufficient quantity)
Eucalyptus, e.g., Vicks Vapor Rub (*Eucalipto*)	Rhinitis, asthma, bronchitis, tuberculosis
Chaparral (*Gobernadora*)	Arthritis (poultice); tea for cancer, sexually transmitted disease, tuberculosis, cramps, *pasmo*, analgesic (poisonous if taken internally in sufficient quantity)
Mullein (*Gordolobo*)	Cough suppressant, asthma, coryza, tuberculosis
Chamomile (*Manzanilla*)	Nausea, flatus, colic, anxiety; eyewash
Oregano (*Orégano*)	Rhinitis, expectorant, menstrual difficulties, worms
Passion flower (*Pasionara*)	Anxiety, hypertension
Bricklebush (*Rodigiosa*)	Adult onset diabetes, gallbladder disease
Rue (*Ruda*)	Antispasmodic, abortifacient, *empacho*, insect repellent (poisonous in sufficient quantity)
Sage (*Salvia*)	Prevent hair loss, coryza, diabetes (poisonous with chronic use)
Linden flower (*Tilia*)	Sedative, hypertension, diaphoretic (poisonous with chronic use)
Trumpet flower (*Tronadora*)	Adult onset diabetes, gastric symptoms, chickenpox
Peppermint (*Yerba buena*)	Dyspepsia, flatus, colic, *susto*
Aloe vera (*Zábila*)	External – cuts, burns; internal – purgative, immune stimulant (poisonous if taken internally in sufficient quantity)
Sapodilla (*Zapote blanco*)	Insomnia, hypertension, malaria

* Neff, 1998.

Hospitals are much preferred for delivery. As is common throughout Latin America, labor often includes vocalization of discomfort with moaning and crying out. The laboring woman is likely to appreciate her mother's presence. The husband's presence is of less importance.

After delivery, some mothers will practice *la cuarenta* (specified rest and dietary practices). Postnatal mothers are viewed as being in a "cold" and weak state, hence should be given "hot" foods and drinks, and avoid "cold" substances as well as exposure to cold – especially cold winds (Boyle, 1996).

Health problems and screening

Healthy life expectancies (HALE) in Central America ranges from 64.8 years in Costa Rica to 54.3 years in Guatemala (World Health Organization (WHO), 2001). Infant mortality rates ranged from a low of 13/1000 live births in Costa Rica to 45.2/1000 live births in Nicaragua and 48/1000 in Guatemala (Pan American Health Organization (PAHO), 2002). Acute respiratory infections and acute diarrhea with dehydration are the leading causes of death in children under five years.

Chronic non-communicable diseases are emerging as health problems of growing significance in Central America. These include cardiovascular disease, malignant neoplasms (for women, cervical), cerebrovascular disease, chronic obstructive pulmonary disease and asthma, and diabetes (PAHO, 2002). Health risks in refugees and immigrants from Central America (Hawn & Jung, 2003; Kemp, 2002; Lane *et al.*, 2002; PAHO, 2002; Centers for Disease Control, 2003; PAHO, 2003) include:

- amebiasis
- angiostrongyliasis
- anisakiasis
- arbovirus encephalitis (Eastern equine encephalomyelitis (EEE))
- Chagas' disease
- chromomycosis
- cryptococcosis
- cryptosporidiosis
- dengue fever (including dengue hemorrhagic fever)
- dracunculiasis (Guinea worm disease)
- filariasis (Bancroftian filariasis, Malayan filariasis, and to a lesser extent, onchocerciasis)
- granuloma inguinale or donovanosis
- hepatitis B
- leishmaniasis
- leprosy
- leptospirosis
- malaria
- mucocutaneous leishmaniasis (*Espundia*)
- mycetoma
- paracoccidioidomycosis (South American blastomycosis)
- STDs, including HIV/AIDS, cervical cancer, chancroid, gonorrhea, granuloma inguinale, lymphogranuloma venereum, syphilis

- strongylodiasis
- trichuriasis (trichocephaliasis or whipworm)
- tuberculosis
- tungiasis
- typhoid fever
- yaws (frambesia)
- yellow fever
- cardiovascular and related diseases, e.g., obesity, hypertension, diabetes

REFERENCES

American Psychiatric Association (2000). *Diagnostic and Statistical Manual of Mental Disorders*, 4th edn, text revision. Washington, DC: Author.

Boyle, J. S. (1996). Central Americans. In *Culture and Nursing Care*, ed. J. G. Lipson, S. L. Dibble and P. A. Minarik, pp. 64–73. San Francisco: UCSF Nursing Press.

Centers for Disease Control (2003). *Health Information for Travelers to the Caribbean*. Retrieved May 12, 2003 from http://www.cdc.gov/travel/caribean.htm.

Geissler, E. M. (1998). *Cultural Assessment*. St. Louis: Mosby.

Hawn, T. R. & Jung, E. C. (2003). Health screening in immigrants, refugees, and internationally adopted orphans. In *The Travel and Tropical Medicine Manual*, 3rd edn., ed. E. C. Jung and R. McMullen, pp. 255–65. Philadelphia, PA: W. B. Saunders.

Johnstone, P. & Mandryk, J. (2001). *Operation World, 21st Century edn*. Waynesboro, GA: Paternoster USA.

Kemp, C. E. (2002). *Infectious Diseases*. Retrieved April 29, 2003 from http://www3.baylor.edu/~Charles_Kemp/Infectious_Disease.htm.

Lane, D. Beevers, D. G., & Lip, G. Y. H. (2002). Ethnic differences in blood pressure and the prevalence of hypertension in England. *Journal of Human Hypertension*, **16**, 267–73.

Levine, R. E. & Gaw, A. C. (1995). Culture-bound syndromes. *Cultural Psychiatry*, **18**, 523–36.

Lieberman, L. S., Stoller, E. P., & Burg, M. A. (1997). Women's health care: Cross-cultural encounters within the medical system. *Journal of the Florida Medical Association*, **84**, 364–73.

Neff, N. (1998). *Folk Medicine in Mexicans in the Southwestern United States*. Accessed 9/24/2000 from http://192.147.157.49/galaxy/Community/Health/Family-Health/Mexican-Health.html (no longer available on the internet).

Pan American Health Organization (2001). *Women's Network against Violence, Nicaragua*. Retrieved April 29, 2003 from http://www.paho.org/english/hdp/hdw/nicaragua.pdf.

(2002). *Country Health Profiles*. Retrieved April 24, 2003 from http://www.paho.org/.

(2003). New study shows enormous burden of diabetes. Retrieved May 30, 2003 from http://www.paho.org/English/DD/PIN/pr030328.htm.

Population Reference Bureau (2002). *2002 World Population Data Sheet*. Retrieved May 12, 2003 from http://www.prb.org/pdf/WorldPopulationDS02_Eng.pdf.

Rundle, A., Carvalho, M., & Robinson, M. (1999). *Cultural Competence in Health Care*. San Francisco: Jossey-Bass.

Schechter, D. S., Marshall, R., Salman, E., Goetz, D., Davies, S., & Liebowitz, M. R. (2000). Ataque de nervios and history of childhood trauma. *Journal of Trauma and Stress*, **13**, 529–34.

Scott, C. S. (1974). Health and healing practices among five ethnic groups in Miami, Florida. *Public Health Reports*, **89**, 824–32.

Spector, R. E. (1996). *Cultural Diversity in Health and Illness*, 4th edn. Stamford, CT: Appleton & Lange.

World Health Organization (2001). *Healthy Life Expectancies*. Retrieved March 25, 2003 from http://www3.who.int/whosis/hale/hale.cfm?path=whosis,burden_statistics, hale& language=english.

Zapata, J. & Shippee-Rice, R. (1999). The use of folk healing and healers by six Latinos living in New England. *Journal of Transcultural Nursing*, **10**, 136–42.

13

China

Bi-Jue Chang and Charles Kemp

This chapter is dedicated with love and respect to the memory of Eric Wang (1984–2002), and to his loving family.

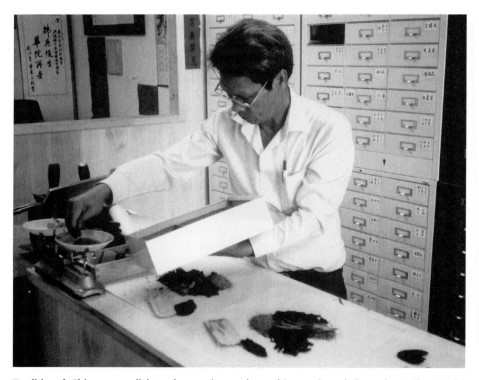

Traditional Chinese medicine pharmacies such as this are found throughout the World. (Photograph by courtesy of Lance A. Rasbridge.)

Refugee and Immigrant Health: A Handbook for Health Professionals, Charles Kemp and Lance A. Rasbridge. Published by Cambridge University Press. © C. Kemp and L. A. Rasbridge 2004.

Introduction

In this chapter the term Chinese refers to people of Chinese ancestry, regardless of whether they are from the Republic of China (Taiwan), the People's Republic of China (mainland China), or are "overseas" Chinese from any of the world's other countries. Chinese culture and social structures are very old – dating to as long ago as around 2500 BC or about the same time as the beginning of the Pharonic Dynasties of Egypt (Char *et al.*, 1996; Grun, 1982). For millennia the Chinese have followed precepts laid out by the earliest teachers and written out by the Sages, especially Lao Tsu and Confucius around 500 BC (Hummel, 1962).

History of immigration

The Chinese have a long history of outmigration from China, and as a result, there are few places in the world where there are not Chinese people living. It is not widely recognized (except by Chinese) that there is a long history of discrimination against the Chinese, such as the United States Chinese Exclusion Act of 1882, exclusion of Chinese serving in the military in several Southeast Asian countries today, and institutionalized violence against Chinese in, for example, Indonesia (Braun & Nichols, 1997; Landler, 1998). Chinese immigration (especially from Taiwan) to the west increased in the 1940s and further increased after 1965 and again increased from 1980–1990. Prior to 1965, most Chinese immigrants were working class; after 1965, most have been professionals (Chang, 1999). Currently there are significant numbers of Chinese entering western countries legally and illegally (Braun & Nichols, 1997; US Department of State, 2000 & 1991). In the year 2000 there were 2.3 million people in the USA who claimed Chinese ancestry exclusively and another 0.4 million who claimed Chinese and other ancestry (US Census Bureau, 2002).

Culture and social relations

The continuous primary theme or value in social structure among Chinese throughout history is the centrality of the family (Chin, 1996; Kim *et al.*, 2001; Tong & Spicer, 1994). From the centrality of the family (Kim *et al.*, 2001) arise the following.
- Filial piety (or duty) – manifested by respect and even reverence for parents.
- Conformance to norms – evidenced by adherence to family and societal norms, and especially by not bringing shame to the family.
- Family recognition through achievement – shown by individuals striving to succeed and not accepting praise for their achievement.

- Emotional self-control – manifested by reserved and formal public verbal and nonverbal communications. Arguments, disagreements, or demands are kept to a minimum.
- Collectivism – evidenced by people keeping the focus on family and community over self.
- Humility – manifested by a lack of striving for individual achievement except as achievement relates to the family.

Although extended families are the ideal and are relatively common in China, nuclear families are also common – especially in the West.

Family structure is traditionally hierarchal and patriarchal, with the oldest adult male the primary decision-maker in health and other matters. Older children have precedence over younger children and male children over female (Chang, 1999). In family matters there also is significant influence from elders – including women. Families tend to be very private, and few are willing to discuss family issues or conflict with non-family members.

The family is often the first and sometimes only source of health care. Health decisions may be made by the family based as much or more on what is best for the family as on what is best for the patient (Tong & Spicer, 1994). In most Chinese immigrant homes, both Chinese and English are spoken. Many youth go to "Chinese school" where they learn etiquette, calligraphy, and other cultural matters important in maintaining the culture in a foreign land.

Communications

China is an enormous country with at least 58 indigenous ethnic groups, a number of which speak different languages or dialects (Yusuf & Byrnes, 1994). There are seven major Chinese language groups, with numerous dialects within each. The seven groups are Mandarin (spoken by the largest number of people), Cantonese, Hakka, Xiang, Min, Gan, and Wu. Mandarin, Wu, and Gan are mutually intelligible, while the others are not – except that written characters are the same throughout. Mandarin (also called *Guoyu*) is the official language of the People's Republic of China and Taiwan (Chinalanguage, n.d.).

Communications are complex and based on context, social status, intuition, and other matters not readily discernible to Westerners (Chang, 1999; Chin, 1996; Kagawa-Singer & Blackhall, 2001). For example, if a young patient is asked by an older health provider if she or he would like a glass of cold water, the answer would likely be yes, even though cold drinks traditionally are undesirable to ill persons. In general, yes–no questions should be avoided when possible, as the polite response is nearly always, "yes."

Religion

Religion, as commonly practiced among many Chinese, blends religious beliefs and practices with philosophical systems. Religion (Buddhism) and philosophical systems (Taoism and Confucianism) are integrated with cultural identity to the extent that it is difficult to understand or examine one without the other (Kagawa-Singer & Blackhall, 2001).

The primary religion is Buddhism. Virtually all Chinese Buddhists practice one of many branches of Mahayana Buddhism. In Mahayana Buddhism, there is belief in a vast array of saints and Buddhas stretching over time incomprehensible or ages (*kalpas*) of the universe. Buddhism is discussed more fully in the chapter on religions.

The primary philosophical influences on Chinese culture are Confucianism and Taoism (the latter pronounced, and sometimes spelled Daoism). Confucianism teaches the proper relationship of people to one another, i.e., child to parent, student to teacher, and so on. Confucianism, then, is the basis for veneration of ancestors and respect for elders. Taoism teaches the proper relationship of people to nature, yet also addresses in a deep way, the relationship of people to one another.

Knowing others is wisdom;
Knowing the self is enlightenment.
Mastering others requires force;
Mastering the self needs strength.

He who knows he has enough is rich.
Perseverance is a sign of will power.
He who stays where he is endures.
To die but not perish is to be eternally present.

Chapter 33 of the *Tao Te Ching*
(Lao Tsu with translation by Gia-Fu & English, 1972)

Buddhism, Confucianism, and Taoism all affect the health/illness experience and health decision-making.

Health beliefs and practices

A first concept to understand in Chinese approaches to health and illness is that of balance, as expressed by the *yin–yang* symbol (☯). The Chinese *yin–yang* symbol is well known and mightily misunderstood in the West. Misunderstood, *yin* and *yang* are presented as opposites, with yin representing female, cold, or negative force; and *yang* representing male, hot, or positive force. A more complete understanding is that these are dynamic and complementary forces. One cannot exist without the other. Within *yin* there is *yang* and within *yang* there is *yin*; and when either reaches its extreme, it becomes the other. There is no completeness without *yin* and *yang* in harmony (Ji *et al.*, 2001). In terms of health and illness, a lack of harmony or balance leads to trouble and illness.

Medicines and foods are often considered as either "hot" or "cold." Western medicines are more often hot than cold, while traditional Chinese medicines may be either. Food properties are sometimes subject to debate with respect to which are hot and which are cold. Hot foods are generally high in protein, fat, and calories. Examples of hot foods include chicken, pork, organ meats, eggs, brown sugar, ginger, and alcohol beverages. Cold foods include cold drinks, fruits, most vegetables, and soy products (Chan *et al.*, 2000; Cheung, 1997; Liu & Moore, 2000).

A second important (and related) concept is that of traditional Chinese medicine (TCM). The origins of TCM reach back more than 3000 years and the best-known (old) text was first published in 300 BC. TCM is based philosophically on Taoism (Kagawa-Singer & Blackhall, 2001) and operationally on a channel (meridian) system, in which various body channels carry vital or life energy called *qi* or *ch'i*, blood, and other body fluids (Nestler, 2002). There are numerous channels, with internal organs connected to these channels, and acupuncture points determined by the channels. Imbalance or disruption in the channels leads to illness, and the treatment goal of TCM is to restore balance. The two primary means of TCM treatment are acupuncture and the use of compounds (Nestler, 2002). While some of the latter are herbal in nature, heavy metals are also used, and may, in some cases lead to toxicity – most commonly lead and mercury poisoning (Ernst & Coon, 2001). In the West, the practice of medicinal TCM is not as open as in Asia, but there are TCM practitioners and medications available in most large metropolitan areas.

A third concept important in understanding Chinese approaches to health and illness is a belief in western allopathic medicine. In China, TCM and Western medicine may be practiced side by side, with patients utilizing one or the other – or both – according to illness or patient inclination (Nestler, 2002). Indeed, in much of Southeast Asia, a typical pharmacy has one (physical) side of the business devoted to Western medicine and the other side devoted to compounding and dispensing TCMs.

Culture-bound syndromes that may affect Chinese (American Psychiatric Association, 2000; Jilek & Jilek-Aall, 1985; Kua *et al.*, 1986; Levine & Gaw, 1995) include the following.

- *Suo yang* (or *Koro*) is the perception that the penis (or sometimes, female genitalia) is retracting into the body, which is thought to then result in death. This syndrome has occurred in localized epidemics in Asia. *Koro* is more often thought of as a Chinese culture-bound illness, but has occurred among Indians, Thai, and others. *Suo yang* has sometimes occurred in epidemics, especially in rural areas.

- Possession-trance is a trance-like state in which the person is believed to be possessed by a spirit or goddess (usually recognizable to witnesses).
- *Shenjing shuairuo* matches the outdated (in Western psychiatry) psychiatric diagnosis of neurasthenia and includes a wide variety of somatic complaints: physical and mental fatigue, difficulty concentrating, insomnia, headache, dizziness, memory loss, irritability, sexual dysfunction, gastrointestinal distress, and other non-specific complaints. *Shenjing shuairuo* is thought by many researchers to mirror major depression.
- *Shenkui* is a state of anxiety or panic with complaints including physical and mental fatigue, weakness, dizziness, backache, insomnia, frequent dreams, and sexual dysfunction. These are attributed to semen loss from any of several reasons, including the perception of semen in the urine, frequent sex, frequent masturbation, or nocturnal emission. *Shenkui* may be considered by the patient to be life-threatening.
- *Qi-gong* is a brief psychotic episode that may include dissociation, paranoia, or other features. *Qi-gong* also refers to a Chinese health-enhancing exercise, the participation in which sometimes leads to the disorder by the same name – especially among frequent practitioners of the exercise.
- *Hsieh-ping* is the brief possession by an ancestral ghost and is accompanied by hallucinations, tremor, and delirium.

Pregnancy and childbirth

Prenatal care is highly valued among Chinese women, as evidenced by the third highest rate among women in 17 ethnic groups in the United States in seeking prenatal care in the first trimester of pregnancy (Leigh & Lindquist, n.d.,). TCM remedies may be used for nausea, fatigue, edema, and other conditions of pregnancy.

Postpartum, many women practice *Zuo yuezi* (sitting in for the first month) for 30 days. *Zuo yuezi* includes staying in the house; avoiding cold foods, drinks, wind, water, and any other cold substance or contact; diet based on balance (of *yin-yang*) as discussed earlier; abstinence for physical work; and abstinence from excessive pleasurable activities (e.g., sex, parties, etc.). Bathing (and especially washing the hair) is limited and may include a warm bath with ginger wine or other "hot" alcoholic beverage (Cheung, 1997).

End of life

End-of-life care for Chinese patients and families centers around family and communications (Tang, 2001). Symptom management may be complicated by patient and family reluctance to complain and respect for others – especially those in positions of authority. Barriers to pain and other symptom management by family caregivers may also be related to other issues, including a lack of knowledge about pain and pain management, fatalism, fear of addiction, desire to be a good patient, and fear of distracting the physician from treating the disease (Lin, 2000; Lin *et al.*, 2000; Tang, 2001).

Communications related to end of life issues are often complicated by reluctance to discuss prognosis and in some instances, diagnosis (Kagawa-Singer & Blackhall, 2001; Tong & Spicer, 1994). To a greater extent than in other cultures, it remains a norm among Chinese patients and families for (a) the family to withhold information or even lie to the patient and (b) for the patient to pretend that she or he does not know what is really happening (Kleinman, 1988; Lapine *et al.*, 2001). The family is expected to help prepare the body for burial. Traditionally, there is always an older relative or person from the temple to instruct the oldest son or daughter on what to do regarding washing and dressing the body.

Burial is preferred by most, but not all Buddhists. In the homeland, the body may be disinterred at 5 years or longer after burial, and the remains placed in a large urn, which is kept at home, in a temple, or is reburied.

"My disciples, my end is approaching, our parting is near, but do not lament. Life is ever changing; none can escape the dissolution of the body. This I am now to manifest by my own death, my body falling apart like a decaying cart." (From The last teaching of Buddha, in *The Teaching of Buddha* Bukkyo Dendo Kyokai, p. 24, [translation] 1981)

Health problems and screening

China is a vast country and conditions and health problems vary widely. Overall, the healthy life expectancy (HALE) is 63.2 years; and the life expectancy at birth is 71 years (Population Reference Bureau, 2002; World Health Organization (WHO), 2002a). Infectious diseases have been greatly reduced over the past several decades, e.g., reported cases of measles dropped from 1.2 million in 1980 to less than 90 000 in 2000. However, China is one of 22 countries worldwide designated by WHO as "high burden" for tuberculosis. The number of TB cases in China is the highest in Asia, but the rate (per 100 000) of new cases in China is 18th among 41 Asian countries (WHO, 2002). With declining rates of infectious diseases, the rates of chronic non-infectious diseases (e.g., cancer and cardiovascular disease) are increasing. Infectious disease risks for new immigrants from China (Hawn & Jung, 2003; Kemp, 2002; WHO, 2002b) include:

- amebiasis
- dengue fever
- filariasis

- gnathostomiasis
- hemorrhagic fever with renal syndrome
- hepatitis
- histoplasmosis
- HIV/AIDS
- hookworm
- leprosy:
- malaria
- schistosomiasis
- strongylodiasis
- trachoma
- trematodes (several varieties, e.g., blood, intestine, liver)
- tuberculosis

REFERENCES

American Psychiatric Association (2000). *Diagnostic and Statistical Manual of Mental Disorders*, 4th edn, text revision. Washington, DC: Author.

Braun, K. L. & Nichols, R. (1997) Death and dying in four Asian–American cultures: a descriptive study. *Death Studies*, **21**, 327–59.

Bukkyo Dendo Kyokai (Buddhist Promoting Foundation) (1981). The last teaching of Buddha. In *The Teaching of Buddha*, pp. 18–26. Tokyo: Author.

Chan, S. M., Nelson, E. A. S., Leung, S. S. F., Cheung, P. C. K., & Li, C. Y. (2000). Special postpartum dietary practices of Hong Kong Chinese women. *European Journal of Clinical Nutrition*, **54**, 797–802.

Chang, K. (1999). Chinese Americans. In *Transcultural Nursing: Assessment and Intervention*, ed. J. N. Giger and R. E. Davidhizer, pp. 385–401. St. Louis: Mosby.

Char, D. F. B., Tom, K. S., Young, G. C. K. Murakami, T., & Ames, R. (1996). A view of death and dying among the Chinese and Japanese. *Hawaii Medical Journal*, **55**, 286–95.

Cheung, N. F. (1997). Chinese zuo yeuzi (sitting in for the first month of the postnatal period) in Scotland. *Midwifery*, **13**, 55–65.

Chin, P. (1996). Chinese Americans. In *Culture and Nursing Care*, ed. J. G. Lipson, S. L. Dibble and P. A. Minarik, pp. 74–81. San Francisco: UCSF Nursing Press.

Chinalanguage. (n.d.). *Languages*. Retrieved March 3, 2003 from http://www.chinalanguage.com/Language/index.html.

Ernst, E. & Coon, J. T. (2001). Heavy metals in traditional Chinese medicines: a systematic review. *Clinical Pharmacology and Therapeutics*, **70**, 497–504.

Grun, B. (1982). *The Timetables of History*. New York: Simon and Schuster.

Hawn, T. R. & Jung, E. C. (2003). Health Screening in immigrants, refugees, and internationally adopted orphans. In *The Travel and Tropical Medicine Manual*, ed. E. C. Jong and R. McMullen, 3rd edn., pp. 255–65. Philadelphia, PA: W. B. Saunders.

Hummel, A. W. (1962). Foreward: *Tao Teh Ching* (Translated by J. C. H. Wu, 1962). Boston: Shambala.

Ji, L.-J., Nisbett, R. E., & Su, Y. (2001). Culture, change, and prediction. *Psychological Science*, **12**, 450–6.

Jilek, W. G. & Jilek-Aall, L. (1985). The metamorphosis of 'culture-bound' syndromes, *Social Science and Medicine*, **21**, 205–10.

Kagawa-Singer, M. & Blackhall, L. J. (2001). Negotiating cross-cultural issues at the end of life. Journal of the American Medical Association, **286**, 2993–3002.

Kemp, C. (2002). *Infectious Diseases*. Retrieved July 25, 2003 from http://www3.baylor.edu/~Charles_Kemp/Infectious_Disease.htm.

Kemp, C. & Rasbridge, L. (2000). *Refugee Health – Immigrant Health*. Retrieved July 22, 2003 from http://www.baylor.edu/~Charles_Kemp/refugee_health.htm.

Kim, B. S., Yang, P. H., Atkinson, D. R., Wolfe, M. M., & Hong, S. (2001). Cultural value similarities and differences among Asian–American ethnic groups. *Cultural Diversity and Ethnic Minority Psychology*, **7**, 343–61.

Kleinman, A. (19880. *The Illness Narratives*. New York: Basic Books.

Kua, E. H., Sim, L. P. & Chee, K. T. (1986). A cross-cultural study of the possession-trance in Singapore. *Australian and New Zealand Journal of Psychiatry*, **20**, 361–4.

Landler, M. (1998, May 16). Indonesia's ethnic Chinese feel their neighbors' wrath. *New York Times*. Retrieved June 30, 2003 from http://www.mtholyoke.edu/acad/intrel/indochin.htm.

Lao Tsu (translation, 1972). *Tao Te Ching* (Translated by Gia-Fu F. & English J.). New York: Vintage Books.

Lapine, A., Wang-Cheng, R., Goldstein, M., Nooney, A., Lamb, G., & Derse, A. R. (2001). When cultures clash: physician, patient, and family wishes in truth disclosure for dying patients. *Journal of Palliative Medicine*, **4**, 475–80.

Leigh, W. A. & Lindquist, M. A. (n.d.). *Women of Color Health Data Book*. US Department of Health & Human services: Hyattsville, MD. Retrieved June 15, 2003 from http://www.4woman.gov/owh/pub/woc/toc.htm.

Levine, R. E. & Gaw, A. C. (1995). Culture-bound syndromes. *Cultural Psychiatry*, **18**, 523–36.

Lin, C.-C. (2000). Barriers to the analgesic management of cancer pain: a comparison of attitudes of Taiwanese patients and family caregivers. *Pain*, **88**, 7–14.

Lin, C.-C., Wang, P., Lai, Y.-L., Lin, C.-L., Tsai, S.-L., & Chen, T. T. (2000). Identifying attitudinal barriers to family management of cancer pain in palliative care in Taiwan. *Palliative Medicine*, **14**, 463–70.

Liu, H. G. & Moore, J. F. (2000). Perinatal care: cultural and technical differences between China and the United States. *Journal of Transcultural Nursing*, **11**, 47–54.

Nestler, G. (2002). Traditional Chinese medicine. *Medical Clinics of North America*, **86**, 63–73.

Population Reference Bureau (2002). *2002 World Population Data Sheet*. Retrieved May 12, 2003 from http://www.prb.org/pdf/WorldPopulationDS02_Eng.pdf.

Tang, S. T. (2001). Taiwan. In *Textbook of Palliative Nursing*, pp. 747–56. New York: Oxford.

Tong, K. L. & Spicer, B. J. (1994). The Chinese palliative patient and family in North America: a cultural perspective. *Journal of Palliative Care*, **10**, 26–8.

US Census Bureau (2002). *The Asian Population 2000.* Retrieved July 23, 2003 from http://www.census.gov/prod/2002pubs/c2kbr01-16.pdf.

US Department of State (1991). *Three Charged in Smuggling of Aliens from China.* Retrieved July 2, 2003 from http://usinfo.state.gov/regional/ea/chinaaliens/reprint4.htm.

  (2000). *More Nations Cooperate to Fight Alien Smuggling, Trafficking.* Retrieved July 4, 2003 from http://www.usemb.gov.do/IRC/immigr/smuggle.htm.

World Health Organization (2002a). *World Health Report.* Retrieved June 5, 2003 from http://www.who.int/whr/2002/en/.

  (2002b). *China.* Retrieved March 5, 2003 from http://www.who.int/country/chn/en/.

Yeung, A., Howarth, S., Chan, R., Sonawalla, S., Nierenberg, A. A., & Fava, M. (2002). Use of the Chinese version of the Beck Inventory for screening depression in primary care. *Journal of Nervous and Mental Disease,* **190**, 94–9.

Yusuf, F. & Byrnes, M. (1994). Ethnic mosaic of modern China: an analysis of fertility and mortality data for the twelve largest ethnic minorities. *Asia–Pacific Population Journal,* **9**, 25–46.

14

Cuba

Introduction

From 1511 to 1898 Cuba was a Spanish colony populated largely by Spanish and black African slaves (slavery was abolished in 1886). Once free of Spanish rule, as a result of the Spanish–American War, the Cuban republic came quickly under the rule of dictators such as Gerardo Machado and Fulgencio Batista y Saldivar. Despite significant corruption and repression under these regimes, the United States remained significantly involved in Cuban affairs, and a relatively large middle and professional class developed.

After years of guerilla war, communist revolutionaries led by Fidel Castro overthrew the Batista regime in 1959. Castro and the communist government have remained in power since 1959. Communist changes in government and society led to positive developments for the common people, such as increased access to basic health care and increased literacy rates, but to the middle and upper classes came increased repression and loss of land and material wealth (Robson, 2000). The country remains impoverished, even more so since the collapse of the Soviet Bloc in the early 1990s.

History of immigration

One outcome of communist victory in Cuba has been a dramatic increase in immigration to the USA, with large Cuban communities in Miami, Tampa, and New York City. The population of Cubans in the United States exceeds one million, or about one-tenth of the population of Cuba itself (Robson, 2000). Since the Revolution, there have been three distinct waves of immigration, each having in general terms different socioeconomic profiles and different acculturation experiences.

Refugee and Immigrant Health: A Handbook for Health Professionals, Charles Kemp and Lance A. Rasbridge. Published by Cambridge University Press. © C. Kemp and L. A. Rasbridge 2004.

The first group, which fled immediately after the 1959 revolution, often referred to as Cuban exiles, was made up largely of capitalists, professionals, and the wealthy, many of whom already had business and family ties in the USA. Most originally viewed their stay as temporary, but have by now gone on to integrate into American society (Robson, 2000).

The second distinct wave of Cuban immigrants overall can be characterized as refugees, those in theory escaping political repression, but in reality fleeing from economic deprivation as well. This group tends to be less educated and less wealthy than the earlier Cuban immigrants, with many risking their lives on the perilous journey on the open seas in makeshift boats or rafts. The largest single influx arrived in 1980, when the Cuban government allowed 125 266 Cubans, including a number of criminals as well as persons with mental illness, to leave Cuba in the "Mariel boat lift." While most "*Marielitos*" were healthy and guilty only of wanting to leave a repressive system, this extraordinary event is often seen only as a means of Cuba ridding itself of the mentally ill and criminals. In the 20 years since the Mariel boat lift, 1425 of the *Marielitos* have been sent back to Cuba and 1750 remain in the custody of the U.S. Immigration and Naturalization Service (INS) (Ojito, 2000). Most *Marielitos* have enjoyed success in the USA, while others have had greater difficulty than earlier Cubans in establishing themselves.

The most recent large influx of Cubans was in 1994, when about 30 000 "rafters" reached the USA. Since then, the INS has sent all Cubans stopped in the water back to Cuba, detaining many in the US base at Guantanamo Bay, while allowing those who reach land to stay.

In the mid-1990s, US policy reversed, due in part to political and humanitarian pressures, initiating more orderly paths to US immigration. This process demarcates the third distinct wave of Cuban immigrants. For one, the USA allowed the 31 000 Cubans detained at Guantanamo to be "paroled" into the USA. Furthermore, additional immigration visas were allotted, allowing for a more systematic mode of entry through diplomatic channels in Havana.

From the beginning of modern Cuban immigration in 1959 and continuing until today, there have been large numbers of family reunification cases. Most early Cuban immigrants to the USA were of Spanish origin, while later refugees and immigrant groups have included more people of mixed or African origin.

Culture and social relations

As with other cultures, differences among Cubans exist according to social class, background, ethnicity, immigration generation, and other factors. These differences can manifest in health-seeking behaviors and many other acculturation indices. Although many Cuban refugees are from urban backgrounds, significant numbers will have lived in the city for less than one generation, and hence may have more rural than urban outlook on life. Almost 40 years of communist rule has resulted in a culture that is definitely Latino in nature, yet to some extent has moved away from such traditional influences as the Catholic Church. For example, in a startling testimony to the power that necessity and Marxism can exert over religion, large numbers of Cuban women (in Cuba) have had multiple abortions as a means of birth control.

The extended family is idealized and relatively common among Cubans of all social classes (Blank & Torrechila, 1998). However, in many cases, the nuclear family is the basic unit of social structure. Men usually have the dominant role, but many Cuban women are outspoken and assertive in public and private. Age, social status, and education are respected. Both within and without families, deference may be given to the elderly, persons of higher social status (especially male), and to those with higher education.

Communications

The language of Cuba is Spanish, though there are many idiosyncratic differences between Spanish spoken by Cubans and the Spanish of Mexicans, for example. Many new refugees and immigrants speak only Spanish. Conversation tends to be animated, fast, and may seem loud, and communications within families and among friends often seem warm and affectionate. Direct eye contact is the norm in almost all interactions. Men greet one another with hand shakes and women are often physically affectionate with one another.

Both women and men tend to be passionate and express themselves in a way that may seem demanding to more reserved people. This may result in negative perceptions by health care providers who sometimes expect docility in refugees or immigrants. Bear in mind that all Cuban immigrants since the Revolution come from a Communist state where their needs were routinely, if perhaps inadequately, met by the system (Robson, 2000).

Religion

Cubans traditionally are Catholic, but many younger recent refugees and immigrants have had little exposure to religion of any sort. Protestant missionaries (often of "Bible church" or Pentecostal orientation) are very active in Cuban communities in the USA.

Although Catholicism is the primary religion of Cubans, *Santeria* is practiced by some Cubans (and others from the Caribbean) in Cuba and the USA. There is evidence that *Santeria* is practiced by persons from middle and upper-class backgrounds as well as those with less education. *Santeria* is based on the *Lacumi* beliefs of the Yoruba people who came to Latin America as slaves. *Santeria* incorporates Yoruba gods (the "Seven African Deities") or *orishas*, Catholic saints, and variations on Catholic ritual. *Santeria* rituals, a few including animal sacrifice, are conducted by *Santeros* (priests) or less commonly, by *Babalawos* (high priests). Herbal formulations and prayer are most commonly used. Healing by blessing rituals (*santiquo*) include supplications to one of the following *orishas* and corresponding saint (Pasquali, 1994).

- *Chango*/Saint Barbara (Although S. Barbara is female, *Chango* is male)
- *Oggun*/Saint Peter
- *Orunla*/Saint Francis
- *Yemaya*/Our lady of Regla
- *Oshun*/Our Lady of Charity of Cobre
- *Obatala*/Our Lady of Mercy
- *Eleggua*/Saint Anthony

Santeros intervene in both physical and mental illnesses and seldom operate in conflict with biomedical treatments. When treating mental illness, *Santeros* may ascribe the problem as a special attribute or strength (*facultade*) of the person being treated.

Health beliefs and practices

Traditional Cuban culture holds that mind, body, and spirit are inextricably intertwined. Health is viewed as a sense of well-being, freedom from discomfort, and a robust appearance. Traditionally, many Cubans believe that moderate obesity indicates good health and thinness indicates poor health (Varela, 1996). Traditional diet (fried foods, beans, sweets) contributes to obesity and the wide availability of colas, sweets, and fast foods in the USA promotes obesity and attendant health problems. Meat is a valued part of the Cuban diet. Meat was less available in Cuba, but of course is affordable in the USA, hence large quantities may be consumed, with attendant health problems. Infants and children are often comforted with food and plump infants are viewed as healthy.

While biomedical or allopathic medical practices are widespread in Cuba and germ theory is accepted and understood by most Cubans, traditional and other theories of illness causality are also frequently incorporated in health beliefs and practices. Stress is thought to cause a variety of physical and mental health problems. Supernatural forces (e.g., *mal de ojo* or evil eye) or a lack of balance are thought by some, especially the less educated, to cause or contribute to physical and mental health problems. Among people who understand germ theory, imbalance may still be seen as the reason why some people become ill from microorganisms and some do not.

Amulets may be worn as protection against supernatural harm. *Santeros* are utilized in some cases to treat or prevent illness, especially those related to supernatural forces (see discussion under religion above). Regardless of a person's faith (Catholic, Protestant, *Santeria*, or a blend of these), spiritual care/belief is often incorporated in treatment or explanation of illness. Children, pregnant women, and postnatal women are thought to be especially vulnerable to supernaturally influenced health problems (Pasquali, 1994; Varela, 1996).

Persons who are sick tend to take on a passive and dependent role. Self-care is poorly understood and little accepted. The physician is highly respected and expected to be in a more directive than partnership role. Decision-making usually includes older or more respected family members. Some expect bad news such as a poor prognosis to be shared with the family (oldest immediate family member) before the patient is told. HIV/AIDS and other STD diagnoses should be shared only with the patient and only with staff (vs. family or community) translators. Women are expected to provide and be in charge of sick care within the family, including when the patient is hospitalized (Varela, 1996).

The desire for family to be informed about a terminal illness or poor prognosis before the patient has at least the potential to lead to conflict. To avoid conflict, it is best to clarify with the patient and family in early contacts that such information is given to the patient unless she or he expressly requests otherwise. It is difficult for patients and families to agree to do not resuscitate (DNR) orders as such orders and acceptance of terminal status may represent giving up and abandonment of the patient.

Hospitalized patients are likely to be attended by family around the clock. Hygiene is important and is best given by the patient her or himself, or by family members. Some will resist shampooing during an illness. Patients will struggle to use the toilet rather than a bedpan. Although Cubans are not excessively modest, modesty for persons who are ill may be an important issue. Both men and women express pain openly, though both may tolerate painful procedures without complaint (Varela, 1996).

Pregnancy and childbirth

Pregnant women are expected to stay inside if possible and avoid over-exertion. Contact with persons who have deformities or health problems, as well as discussion of these should be avoided during pregnancy. In general, it is best to avoid any potentially stressful or negative discussion with a pregnant woman. Cubans in America are well aware of the value of prenatal care and tend to be early seekers of care. Men may be surprised at the prospect of participating or being present at delivery and the pregnant woman's mother may be surprised at not being allowed to direct the proceedings. The traditional postnatal practice is for the new mother and infant to remain inside the home for about 40 days after delivery. Women from the family or neighbor women are responsible for caring for both (and providing food for the father as well) during this time. Potentially stressful or negative discussions should be avoided or treated delicately. Breastfeeding is common (Varela, 1996).

Many Cubans prefer circumcision, which is available in public hospitals in Cuba, but is not in some public hospitals in the USA. Families in which a woman is pregnant should be made aware of this potential problem.

Health problems and screening

Most health indicators in Cuba have shown a general improvement over the past several decades. In fact, Cuba has the highest healthy life expectancy or HALE (66.4 years) in Latin America. The full life expectancy at birth for Cubans is 76 years (Population Reference Bureau, 2002; World Health Organization (WHO), 2002). The infant mortality rate is the same in Cuba as in the United States (7.2 per 1000) (Pan American Health Organization (PAHO), 2002). Childhood immunizations (a key reason for improved child mortality rates) are a bright spot in Cuba, with the percentage of children less than 1 year of age and up to date with immunizations exceeding the same population in the USA. (PAHO, 2002). General mortality in Cuba since the 1950s and 1960s is characterized by a shift from communicable diseases to marked predominance of causes associated with chronic noncommunicable diseases. Mortality from diabetes, for example, has more than doubled from 9.9 per 100 000 in the 1970s to 23.4 per 100 000 in 1996 (PAHO, 2002).

Tuberculosis and dengue fever are the infectious diseases of greatest concern among recent refugees and immigrants from Cuba (Guzman et al., 2002; Marrero et al., 2000; Centers for Disease Control and Prevention (CDC), 2002). Among Cubans there also has been found an unusual "epidemic neuropathy," which manifests as optic neuropathy with loss of central vision, peripheral neuropathy and mixed optic and peripheral neuropathy, due probably to nutritional deficiencies (Carelli et al., 2002; Rodriguez-Hernandez et al., 2001). Health risks in refugees and immigrants from the Caribbean Islands, including Cuba are found below. However, note that risks for infectious diseases are lower in Cuba than in any other Caribbean Island (Centers for Disease Control, 2002; Guzmán & Kourí, 2002; Hawn & Jung, 2003; Kemp, 2002; Lane et al., 2002; Marrero et al., 2000; PAHO, 2002):

- chronic noncommunicable illnesses including (in decreasing order of importance as cause of death) cardiovascular disease, malignant neoplasms, cerebrovascular disease, chronic obstructive pulmonary disease and asthma, and diabetes. The prevalence of hypertension in Cuba is 30.6%.

- amebiasis
- angiostrongyliasis
- anisakiasis
- arbovirus encephalitis (Eastern equine encephalomyelitis (EEE))
- Chagas' disease
- cholera
- chromomycosis
- cryptococcosis
- cryptosporidiosis
- dengue fever
- dracunculiasis (Guinea worm disease)
- filariasis (Bancroftian filariasis, Malayan filariasis, and to a lesser extent, onchocerciasis)
- hepatitis B
- leishmaniasis
- leprosy
- leptospirosis
- malaria
- mucocutaneous Leishmaniasis (*Espundia*)
- mycetoma
- paracoccidioidomycosis (South American blastomycosis)
- STDs, including HIV/AIDS, cervical cancer, chancroid, chlamydia, gonorrhea, granuloma inguinale, lymphogranuloma venereum, syphilis
- strongylodiasis
- toxoplasmosis
- trematodes (liver-dwelling: clonorchiasis and opisthorchiasis; blood-dwelling: schistosomiasis or bilharzias; intestine-dwelling; and lung-dwelling: paragonimiasis)
- trichuriasis (trichocephaliasis or whipworm)
- tuberculosis (low risk)
- tungiasis
- typhoid fever
- yaws (frambesia)
- yellow fever (very low risk)

Acknowledgement

Manuel Balbona, Ph.D.

REFERENCES

Blank, S. & Torrechila, R. S. (1998). Understanding the living arrangements of Latino immigrants: a life course approach. *International Migration Review*, **32**, 3–19.

Carelli, V., Ross-Cisneros, F. N., & Sadun, A. A. (2002). Optic nerve degeneration and mitochondrial dysfunction: genetic and acquired optic neuropathies. *Neurochemistry International*, **40**, 573–584.

Centers for Disease Control and Prevention (CDC) (2002). *Medical Examinations of Aliens (Refugees and Immigrants)*. Retrieved November 11, 2002 from http://www.cdc.gov/ncidod/dq/health.htm.

Guzmán, M. G. & Kourí, G. (2002). Dengue: an update. *The lancet Infectious Diseases*, **2**, 33–42.

Guzmán, M. G., Kouri, G., Valdes, L., Bravo, J., Vazquez, S., & Halstead, S. B. (2002). Enhanced severity of secondary dengue-2 infections: death rates in 1981 and 1997 Cuban outbreaks. *Pan American Journal of Public Health*, **11**, 223–7.

Kemp, C. (2002). *Infectious Diseases*. Retrieved April 12, 2003 from http://www3baylor.edu/~Charles_Kemp/Infectious_Disease.htm.

Lane, D., Beevers, D. G., & Lip, E. Y. H. (2002). Ethnic differences in blood pressure and the prevalence of hypertension in England. *Journal of Human Hypertension*, **16**, 267–73.

Marrero. A., Caminero, J. A., Rodriguez, R. & Billo, N. E. (2000). Towards elimination of tuberculosis in a low income country: the experience of Cuba, 1962–97. *Thorax*, **55**, 39–45.

Ojito, M. (April 23, 2000). You are going to El Norte. *The New York Times Magazine*, 68–73, 78.

Pan American Health Organization (2002). *Cuban (Country Health Profile)*. Accessed November 25, 2002 from http://www.paho.org/English/SHA/prflCUB.htm.

Pasquali, E. A. (1994). Santeria. *Journal of Holistic Nursing*, **12**, 380–90.

Population Reference Bureau (2002). *2002 World Population Data Sheet*. Retrieved May 12, 2003 from http://www.prb.org/pdf/WorldPopulationDS02_Eng.pdf.

Robson, B. (2000). Cubans – their history and culture. *The Cultural Orientation Project*. Retrieved August 22, 2003 from http://www.culturalorientation.net.

Rodriguez-Hernandez, M., Hirano, M., Naini, A., & Santiesteban, R. (2001). Biochemical studies of patients with Cuban epidemic neuropathy. *Ophthalmic Research*, **33**, 310–13.

Varela, L. (1996). Cubans. In *Culture and Nursing Care*, ed. J. G. Lipson, S. L. Dibble and P. A. Minarik. San Francisco: UCSF Nursing Press.

World Health Organization (2002). *World Health Report*. Retrieved June 5, 2003 from http://www.who.int/whr/2002/en/.

15

Egypt

Zbys Fedorowicz and Wael Wagih Hamed

Introduction

Egypt, officially the Arab Republic of Egypt, is located in north-eastern Africa and includes the Sinai Peninsula which is located in the Middle East. It is bordered to the North by the Mediterranean Sea, to the east by Israel and the Red Sea, to the south by Sudan, and to the west by Libya. In 2002 Egypt's population was more than 70 million people and growing at the rapid rate of about 1.66% (Central Intelligence Agency (CIA), 2002).

Egypt is bisected north to south by the River Nile. Its waters and rich sediments provided the foundation for the development of one of the world's first great civilizations, that of ancient Egypt with a history dating back to about 3200 BC. Ancient Egypt's history is divided into three distinct historical periods or Kingdoms, pre-eminently the Pharaonic. The word pharaoh in Egyptian means "great house" and was the name originally used by the ancient Egyptians for the palace of their king. This honorific term, used as a way of referring to the king, dates to as far back as 1400 BC. The pharaoh was considered to be the son of Osiris, the god of the underworld; as the religious, civil, and military leader on Earth he acted as a mediator between gods and men. During this Pharaonic period some of the most renowned pharaohs, Thutmose I, Thutmose II, and Ramses II, were responsible for a sizeable increase in Egypt's power and territory.

The word Egypt is derived from the Greek *Aigyptos* or in arabic, *qubt*, the stem for the word Copt. The Copts, although in the minority, consider themselves to be the indigenous peoples of this land. It was their liberation from the oppressive rule of the Romans by Arab Muslims in the 7th century that would presage the subsequent demographic changes from a Christian to a Muslim majority.

Modern Egypt has both sedentary urban and nomadic traditions that are relics of its long history of intermingling between Arab invaders and native inhabitants of

Refugee and Immigrant Health: A Handbook for Health Professionals, Charles Kemp and Lance A. Rasbridge. Published by Cambridge University Press. © C. Kemp and L. A. Rasbridge 2004.

the Nile Valley region. The majority of Egyptians are descended from the indigenous pre-Muslim population (the ancient Egyptians) and the Arabs, who conquered the area in the 7th century AD. Elements of other conquering peoples (Greeks, Romans, Turks) are also present, especially in Lower Egypt. About 45% of the Egyptian population lives in urban areas, although some nomadic and semi-nomadic herders, mostly Bedouins, continue to live in the desert regions. The Bedouins typify the Arab share of the population who entered the region after the conquest of Egypt by the caliphate of Islam.

History of immigration

Egyptians have a long history of immigration to the West and their educated classes are to be found well distributed throughout the legal, medical and engineering professions. Egypt's universities, Ain Shams, Cairo University and Al Azhar, have created a remarkable succession of notable thinkers, artists, writers, authors, and poets. Since the oil-boom of the 1960s, the adaptability and dedicated work ethic of Egyptians has made them much sought after "gastarbeiters" (guestworkers) throughout the Arabian Gulf.

A nationalist movement in 1952 ousted the Egyptian monarchy from power and transformed Egypt into a republic. This unique style of nationalism, initiated by the Free Officers led by Gamal Abdel Nasser remains to the present day as an important force in Egyptian politics. Nasser's policies, which also included a dalliance with communism, heralded the start of an era of repression and human rights violations that precipitated a hemorrhagic loss of skilled professionals. In addition, the exodus of a large percentage of the medical profession during the 1970s was a direct result of "over supply" of medical graduates. This departure of intellectuals was accompanied by the flight of religious groups such as the Muslim Brotherhood and many Coptic Christians.

The Muslim Brotherhood, founded in Egypt in 1928 by Hassan al-Banna, expanded, achieving a following estimated at 2 million. They developed political ambitions, and posed a threat to the survival of the Egyptian political system. In 1954 the Brotherhood was suppressed by the new Free Officer regime, and many of their adherents found shelter in Kuwait, the United Arab Emirates and later the United Kingdom, from whence they would continue their political activities in the years to come. There was a simultaneous emigration of Copts, who had become increasingly insecure as a result of Nasser's avowed links to communist Russia.

Militant Islamists have remained active in Egypt since the late 1970s and succeeded in assassinating President Anwar Sadat in 1981. They continue their attacks on government, the Coptic community, and foreign tourists to the present day.

A rapidly expanding divide between the upper and lower socioeconomic groups has left an almost nonexistent middle class, prompting a new wave of mainly economic migrants. Two categories of immigrants predominate: the professional and the laboring classes. The professionals are increasingly marginalized by the oversupply in the skilled disciplines and the laborers are shackled to a life of hardship and deprivation.

Culture and social relations

The extended family occupies a position of great importance in Egyptian society; and older male members (grandfather, father, eldest son, eldest uncle, etc.) play significant roles in the process of decision-making in the health care of individual family members. Even though their knowledge may be rudimentary and supported by no more than personal experiences, their opinions are sought and often inordinate weight is attached to their perceived medical wisdom. The oldest or clearly most dominant person present in a healthcare encounter should thus be directly included in discussions and decisions.

While traditional thinking and roles predominate, Egypt has been at the forefront of the Arab world in allowing access to higher education for women. As a result, women have entered the professions, including medicine. Professional-class immigrants to other countries in the West often have a cosmopolitan world outlook.

Peasant farming on a subsistence level is widespread, but with increased urbanization the failing rural economies are driving poverty-stricken, landless peasants to the cities. This rural migration has produced an exponential growth of cities leading to serious problems in these urban areas, with increasing unemployment, housing shortages, and the proliferation of vast slums. The capital city of Cairo exemplifies the best and the worst in this perspective. With a population of around 16 million people (Johnstone & Mandryk, 2001), Cairo is struggling to cope with the problems generated by massive population growth, urban sprawl, and a deteriorating infrastructure. Though rich in culture and history, the city reveals Egypt's growing poverty.

Egypt has an agrarian-based economy, which exports its products worldwide. There is a developing heavy industry and burgeoning technology sector. Industrial activities include the manufacture of iron and steel (at Hulwan), and the refining of oil at several locations, with new fields in the El Alamein and Gulf of Suez areas, and a major exploration effort to the West. In recent years the clothing manufacture industry has suffered from incessant competition from the Asian subcontinent and has seen dwindling demand for Egyptian cotton, long considered to be the finest.

Communications

Arabic is the official language of Egypt. Communication between different genders may be constrained by religious tradition, and touch between genders outside marriage is rare, except for less religious upper-class persons. Many Egyptians look directly into the eyes of others, and some place great importance on whether the other person's eyes dilate (indicates interest) or contract (indicates uninterest).

Religion

Islam is the official religion, and almost 90% of all Egyptians are Sunni Muslims. About 7% of the population belongs to the Coptic Church, a Christian denomination which is the largest religious minority. Around 3% of the population belongs to the Greek Orthodox, Roman Catholic, Armenian, and various Protestant Churches. Additionally, the country has a very small Jewish community (Johnstone & Mandryk, 2001). See Chapter 5 for a discussion of Islam.

Health beliefs and practices

Egyptian health beliefs are an admixture of distinctive and unique components: modern biomedical, Islamic *shariaa* (values and beliefs), Bedouin (Arabic), and some residual Pharaonic traditions. Concepts of health and illness are strongly shaped by the strong religious beliefs of the community. Egyptians, as indeed most Muslims, are fatalistic about health and disease and look upon these as preordained by God and therefore beyond individual control. It is this submission to the will and orders of God, the provider of health, that guides the conduct of life in this world, while the role of disease is to test patience and faith and will erase sins in preparation for the next world. Accordingly, most Egyptians are remarkably stoic and enduring towards disease, even those diseases that are relentless or incurable.

Islamic rules, traditions, and lifestyle practiced by the more devoutly religious sector of the community have helped to limit the spread of many infectious diseases which, considering the levels of poverty and illiteracy, are notably lower than would normally be expected.

- Performing *Wadoo* or ritual ablution (washing hands, face and feet) five times a day helps to reduce eye and skin infections.
- The use of *miswak* or twigs of Persica trees for oral hygiene, although not universally used, before each prayer assists in reducing oral disease.
- Strict moral and social barriers in extramarital relations and prohibition of homosexuality limit the prevalence of sexually transmitted infections.

Bedouin beliefs incorporate *djinn* (or *jinn*) and aspects of animism that are not accepted by mainstream Islam. They are often characterized by harsh treatment modalities: branding, cutting and use of purgatives, emetics and other powerful potions. With increased urbanization and easier access to modern healthcare facilities the demand for this type of service is dwindling, but demand still exists especially when other measures fail.

As in other orthodox religions, Egyptian Copts have strong beliefs in the healing powers of saints and religious figures. In Cairo there is a church dedicated to Mary, the mother of Jesus, where Copts (and many Muslims) pray and light candles seeking remedies for their ailments. Infertile couples also visit this church, believing that Mary can cure their infertility. There have been numerous claims of sightings of the Virgin Mary in the sky above the church.

Female genital cutting (FGC) is a common practice among both Muslim and Coptic populations especially in rural areas and may have origins as far back as the Pharaonic times. Types of FGC practiced in Egypt include type I (17%), type II (72%), and type III (9%) (Toubia, 1999) (see Chapter 6). The Egyptian government indicated its commitment to the eradication of this practice and in 1959 issued a ministerial decree making it a punishable offence. However, it is still performed by barbers and traditional healers. See Chapter 6 for details and definitions of FGC.

Egypt is a land of diversity where it is possible to find state of the art healthcare facilities with highly skilled clinicians providing world standard medicine alongside general practitioners practicing rudimentary primary medical care reminiscent of the 1950s and 1960s, and a large number of traditional healers and herbal medicine experts (*Attar, Hawaj*) using alternative or complementary medicine. The only recognized culture-bound syndrome identified by the authors as occurring in Egypt (American Psychiatric Association, 2000) is *Zar* possession, a spirit possession characterized by dissociative episodes in which the person may shout, sing, cry, speak incomprehensibly, hit the head against a wall, or become mute. As noted above, *Zar* possession may be episodic, in which case it can be viewed as a culture-bound syndrome. However, it may be long term, in which case it can be viewed as chronic mental illness – though local perception is often that the condition is nonpathological.

Pregnancy and childbirth

Family planning is actively encouraged by the government to combat the rapidly increasing population and the burden it places on the healthcare services. However, the multiple successive intensified campaigns called for by either governmental mass media or the many nongovernmental organizations (NGOs) working in that field find a receptive audience only among a relatively small sector of the population.

Most Egyptians, especially the very religious and/or the enormous under-class, see pregnancy as the will of Allah.

Most Egyptian immigrants in the West readily seek prenatal care, but are uncomfortable with male providers at any level of obstetric care. Abortion, unless medically justified, is regarded as 'sinful' and is expressly forbidden by the authorities.

Health problems and screening

Despite progress in the 20th century, particularly in the health of urban populations, health services still lag behind the Egyptian population's needs, especially in rural areas. Substantial progress has been made in eradicating cholera, smallpox, and malaria, but diseases such as schistosomiasis or bilharzia (a parasitical disease) remain widespread. Fresh water is scarce away from the Nile, which remains the country's only year-round water source. Rapid population growth is straining natural resources and depleting agricultural land. Pollution from the country's oil sector threatens coral reefs, beaches, and marine habitats. In addition, raw sewage and industrial and agricultural by-products pollute the country's water supplies.

Without concerted efforts to control environmental pollution and population growth, the health and social services in Egypt will come under increasing pressure with the potential for civil unrest fomented by fundamentalist groups and resulting in further waves of emigration.

The average life expectancy at birth in Egypt is 62 years for men and 66.2 years for women. The healthy life expectancy (HALE) at birth for males is 56.4 years and 57.0 years for females. The infant mortality rate is 37/1000 and the child mortality per 1000 is 46 for males and 44 for females (CIA, 2002; World Health Organization (WHO) (2002a). Infectious diseases are the leading causes of death and disability in Egypt. Egypt is one of nine countries in the world with indigenous transmission of polio (low transmission rate) (WHO, 2002b). As with many other immigrants (vs. refugees), Egyptians are likely to present in the West with chronic lifestyle diseases such as hypertension and cancer. Health risks for new Egyptian immigrants (Hawn & Jung, 2003; Kemp, 2002; WHO, 2002a) include:

- amebiasis
- anthrax
- boutonneuse fever
- brucellosis or undulant fever
- cholera
- Crimean–Congo hemorrhagic fever
- cysticercosis (tapeworm)

- dracunculiasis (Guinea worm disease)
- familial Mediterranean fever (Mediterranean area, primarily among persons of Sephardic Jewish, Armenian, and Arab ancestry)
- giardia
- helminthiasis (ascariasis, echinococcosis/hydatid disease, schistosomiasis – see trematodes below)
- hepatitis
- hookworm
- leishmaniasis
- malaria
- plague
- Rift Valley (hemorrhagic) fever
- sickle cell disease or sickle cell hemoglobulinopathies (occurs primarily in people of African lineage, but also to a lesser extent among people from the Mediterranean area, Arabs, and Indians)
- thalassemias
- toxocariasis
- trachoma
- trematodes (liver-dwelling: clonorchiasis and opisthorchiasis; blood-dwelling: schistosomiasis or bilharzia; intestine-dwelling; and lung-dwelling: paragonimiasis). Schistosomiasis is a problem of great significance in Egypt.
- trichinosis (trichinella)
- tuberculosis
- typhus
- chronic noninfectious diseases such as cardiac disease and related, cancer, diabetes, COPD

REFERENCES

American Psychiatric Association (2000). *Diagnostic and Statistical Manual of Mental Disorders*, 4th edn, text revision. Washington, DC: Author.

Central Intelligence Agency (2002). *World Factbook*. Author. Retrieved June 16, 2003 from http://www.cia.gov/cia/publications/factbook/geos/eg.html.

Hawn, T. R. & Jung, E. C. (2003). Health screening in immigrants, refugees, and internationally adopted orphans. In *The Travel and Tropical Medicine Manual*, 3rd edn., ed. E. C. Jong and R. McMullen, pp. 255–65. Philadelphia, PA: W. B. Saunders.

Johnstone, P. & Mandryk, J. (2001). *Operation World: 21st Century edn*. Waynesboro, GA: Paternoster USA.

Kemp, C. E. (2002). *Infectious Diseases*. Retrieved April 12, 2003 from http://www3.baylor.edu/~Charles_Kemp/Infectious_Disease.htm.

Toubia, N. (1999). *Caring for Women with Circumcision.* New York: Rainbo Publications. www.rainbo.org.

World Health Organization (2002a). *World Health Report: Egypt.* Retrieved June 5, 2003 from http://www.who.int/whr/2002/en/.

——— (2002b). *Global Polio Status 2002.* Retrieved May 9, 2003 from http://www.polioeradication.org/all/global/.

16

Ethiopia and Eritrea

Introduction

Ethiopia is an arid country located on the Horn of (East) Africa at the Red Sea. Ethiopia was never colonized, but in 1935 suffered terribly at the hands of Italy's army as a prelude to World War II. The country was ruled from 1930 until 1973 by the Emperor Haile Selassie. In 1973, the Emperor was overthrown by a group of army officers, who established a repressive marxist military regime. Along with the repression came drought, famine, a secessionist movement in Eritrea, and other conflicts.

Ethiopia and Eritrea are now separate countries whose relationship is characterized by conflict. Major cultural groups living in Ethiopia include the Oromo (the largest group in Ethiopia) and the Amhara. In Eritrea, Tigreans are the largest group. Other groups living in Ethiopia/Eritrea include the Afad-Isas, Somalis, Wolaitas, Sidamas, Kimbatas, and Hadiyas. Despite the diversity, the ethnic groups living in the region are culturally similar (Beyene, 1996; Ethnomed, n.d. a, b).

History of immigration

Prior to the 1973 coup, there were very few Ethiopians living in the West. Outmigration began immediately after the coup. Migration to the West began in 1980, with the greatest number of Ethiopians coming to the West from 1983–1993. A common experience was for a small group of 5–20 people to travel across the desert by night and hide by day. The journey to the country of first asylum was dangerous and many died on the way. There were major airlifts of more than 55 000 Ethiopian Jews to Israel in 1985 and 1991 (Operations Moses and Solomon). Most of these were illiterate farmers.

Refugee and Immigrant Health: A Handbook for Health Professionals, Charles Kemp and Lance A. Rasbridge. Published by Cambridge University Press. © C. Kemp and L. A. Rasbridge 2004.

Ethiopians living in the West are most often from urban backgrounds and many came with, or obtained, college degrees in their host countries. Many Eritreans are from rural backgrounds and thus came with little education – but in many cases, are now in school. Most live in large urban areas in the USA or Western Europe (Ethnomed, n.d. b).

Culture and social relations

Ethiopians wish to be called Ethiopians, and Eritreans much prefer to be known as Eritreans. Influences operational to varying degrees in the lives of Ethiopians/ Eritreans include traditional thinking (especially among the Oromo and those from rural backgrounds), the Coptic Church, Islam, and now, Western culture.

The ideal family structure and living arrangement is the extended family. However, there are few truly extended Ethiopian/Eritrean families living in the West. In most families, men are dominant, although the roles of some Ethiopian/Eritrean women are changing rapidly in the West. At least in the early days of outmigration, there were many more men than women coming to the USA and other countries of refuge. The imbalance of men and women is changing, with more women than men now leaving Ethiopia (Ethnomed, n.d. b).

Ethiopian/Eritrean women are perceived as needing protection by their husband or male family members. Men make most of the decisions, especially those in relation to the outside world. The emancipation of Ethiopian/Eritrean women in the West is changing family and interpersonal dynamics – including decision-making and other male/female roles. Factors promoting women's emancipation include (a) the power of Western culture and the women's movement and (b) the early lack of Ethiopian/Eritrean women living in the West, i.e., with an abundance of men, women do not have to tolerate being dominated.

Traditionally, disputes are settled by community (male) elders. Originally in the West there were few such men, but leaders and elders have emerged in the Ethiopian/Eritrean communities in host countries (Beyene, 1996; Ethnomed, n.d. a, b).

Communications

Amharic is the official language of Ethiopia, and Tigrinya the language of Eritrea. A third language, Oromigna is used by the Oromo people. Most Ethiopians/Eritreans prefer translations and other assistance be provided by persons from their own ethnic or linguistic group – thus translation by an Ethiopian for a Tigrean will not be as effective as a Tigrean translating for a Tigrean.

Communication tends to be direct, with most people usually speaking softly. Among those who live in the West, eye contact is usually direct. Little emotion or affect is shown to strangers, but physical affection is common between friends (Ethnomed n.d. a & b).

Religion

Most Ethiopians (65%) are Coptic Christians (or Ethiopian Orthodox). Approximately 30% are Muslims and there are a few Jews – with many of the later migrating to Israel in 1985 or 1991. Eritreans are about evenly divided among Christians and Muslims (Johnstone & Mandryk 2001). As discussed in the chapter on religions, the Coptic Church is a part of Eastern Orthodoxy, but is considered by some Christians to be heretical. The Ethiopian Orthodox faith views the spiritual and physical worlds as similarly sacred and makes wide use of icons. Intercessory prayer is used to obtain God's healing in physical and mental illness.

Both Coptic Christians and Muslims practice restriction of some foods. Coptic Christians, for example, do not consume meat or dairy products for more than half of each year. The latter is probably more closely followed in the homeland than in the West. Muslims are forbidden pork and other flesh not properly killed. Muslims also do not eat from vessels in which pork may have been served or cooked.

Health beliefs and practices

Traditional Ethiopian/Eritrean belief is that health results from equilibrium between the body and the outside world, and illness from disequilibrium. The external world may be either the physical (sun, temperature, foods, etc.) or the spiritual world. The relationship between the person and the supernatural world is very important in maintaining health and happiness. Emotional state is thought to influence health, with interpersonal conflict adversely affecting health. Those who live in the Western world are more likely to understand biomedical principles of causation (Beyene, 1996; Hodes, 1997; Ethnomed, n.d. b).

Traditional herbal medicine is highly developed and widely used in Ethiopia/Eritrea. Analyses of extracts/fractions taken from traditional herbal medicines show that many such substances have significant activity against disorders for which they are used, e.g., parasites, infections, and other medical problems. There are at least 21 types of specialized traditional healers operating in Ethiopia/Eritrea. These include tooth extractors, cuppers (i.e., suctioning or cupping – sometimes involving large amounts of blood), amulet writers, seers, herbalists, and uvula cutters (Beyene, 1996; Hodes, 1997).

As with many others from the developing world, Ethiopians/Eritreans put great stock in medications, with injections more valued than oral medications. Many patients are dissatisfied if medications are not given while diagnostic tests are pending or if the illness does not necessarily call for medication.

In some cases, Ethiopians/Eritreans tend to take less fluids than is healthy. Fluids are preferred at room temperature. Fluids are particularly a problem when a patient is in the hospital where hydration is most important and drinks are often offered with ice (Ethnomed, n.d. a, b).

Ritual female genital cutting (FGC) is practiced by Ethiopians/Eritreans from all three major religions (Coptic, Muslim, Jewish). Cutting usually is done in infancy or childhood and 90–95% of women from Eritrea and Ethiopia have had FGC performed, usually Types I (the removal of the prepuce and/or part or all of the clitoris) or II (the removal of prepuce and clitoris together with the partial or complete excision of the labia minora); and in some cases, slight ritual scarring (Grisaru, Lezer, & Belmaker, 1997b; Sark, 1995; Toubia, 1999). See Chapter 6 for further discussion of FGC.

Magico-religious practices are common in Ethiopia/Eritrea, and some continue among refugees in the West. Amulets (*kitab*) are worn by some, usually under clothing. A person's mental condition is thought to play an important role in her or his physical health, hence shocking or potentially traumatic news should be given with care and with family or other social support at hand. Many will prefer that a poor prognosis or other such news be given first to a (male) family member. Open discussion of terminal illness is not desired by most, and acceptance of a poor prognosis is unusual (Beyene, 1996; Ethnomed, n.d. a, b).

Mental illness is attributed to evil spirits by both Muslims and Christians. Mental illness is sometimes attributed to *long-term* possession by the *Zar* spirit, especially among newer refugees or immigrants (see below on culture-bound syndromes). *Zar* possession is more common among women in Ethiopia/Eritrea and among men in refugees and immigrants living in the Western world. Spirit possession is treated with prayer and herbal preparations or holy water, depending on whether the patient is Muslim or Christian. Some people may utilize different sources of religious and medical help for mental disorders, with the reputation of the healer of greater importance than his religious orientation (Beyene, 1996; Hodes, 1997).

Culture-bound syndromes found among Ethiopians (American Psychiatric Association, 2000; Grisaru *et al.*, 1997a; R. Hodes, personal communication 1/2000) include the following.

- *Zar* possession is spirit possession characterized by dissociative episodes in which the person may shout, sing, cry, speak incomprehensibly, hit the head against a wall, or become mute. As noted above, *Zar* possession may be episodic, in which case it can be viewed as a culture-bound syndrome; or may be long term, in which case it can be viewed as chronic mental illness – though local perception is often that the condition is nonpathological.

- *Buda* is the power of the evil eye and may be used to inflict harm on others, especially infants.
- *Moygnbaggen* or "get a fool" presents with symptoms of syncope, fever, headache, abdominal cramps, or stiff neck. The syndrome is treated by bloodletting (brachial vein).

Somatic complaints as a manifestation of emotional distress are common. These complaints are often vague and/or difficult to treat. Therapy in mental illness or distress should be more active and include the family. Hodes (1997) suggests low doses of antidepressants as especially helpful.

Hospitalized or sick patients take on a passive and dependent role. Physicians are expected to know and convey to the patient what is best for the patient. As with many others from third-world countries (especially those with less education), large amounts of information and frequent decision-making by the patient or family may induce anxiety. Healthcare providers are expected to be warm and friendly (but to not act as partners in the health relationship). In Ethiopia/Eritrea the extended family plays a significant role in the care of hospitalized patients, but in the West, few Ethiopian/Eritrean families are of sufficient size to take on such a role and the healthcare system does not accommodate extensive involvement in care. As among other refugees and immigrants, being in a sick role intensifies whatever difficulties an Ethiopian patient may have in adjustment to a different culture (Ethnomed, n.d. a, b).

Most Ethiopians/Eritreans are stoic with respect to physical (and emotional) pain. Pain medications may be refused and pain control in advanced disease such as cancer is difficult to achieve (Ethnomed, n.d. a). Specific Ethiopian/Eritrean beliefs about health and illness (Hodes, 1997; R. Hodes, personal communication 1/2000) include the following.

- Excess sun causes *mitch*, which is translated as sunstroke, but causes rash, itching, or herpes (especially if sun strikes a part of the body that is sweating or unclean).
- The heart is thought to regulate other organs by producing heat and is not involved with blood. Complaints of a "heart problem" (vs. complaints of cardiac symptoms) may be related to dyspepsia or other genitourinary problem.
- The uvula is believed to put infants at risk for suffocation, hence is excised in many Ethiopians/Eritreans.
- Eye problems may be treated with incisions of the eyelids or eyebrows.
- Amulets to treat or prevent disease are called *kitab*.
- Diarrhea in infants may be treated by extracting the milk teeth.
- Menopause that leads to increase in abdominal girth may be attributed to pregnancy which "stays bone."
- Wind (cold) may cause pleuritic chest pain or *wugat*. Treatment is with cupping.

- The stomach is believed to be an inert organ in which ascaris worms live and process food.
- Sexually transmitted diseases may be attributed to urinating under a full moon, urinating on a hot stone, contact with an infected dog, or other means. HIV infection is increasing in Ethiopia.
- Having sex weakens tuberculosis medicines. Responses to this belief may include divorce, ceasing sex, or discontinuing the medications.

Among rural people, pregnancy is thought to be a time of increased vulnerability for the mother. The fetus is also at risk for harm from evil spirits and sorcery. In Ethiopia/Eritrea, most deliveries are performed by a midwife or female family members. In the West, Ethiopians/Eritrean women prefer female physicians. Some feel that Western physicians are too quick to perform Cesarean sections and may attempt to prevent such intervention by waiting as long as possible to go to the hospital for delivery.

Some women practice a brief symbolic rejection of the infant for the discomfort and pain caused by pregnancy and delivery. After delivery, the mother may stay in the home for 2–6 weeks. Breast-feeding (for up to 3 years) is the norm in Ethiopia and also is practiced in the West, but for a shorter time. Many mothers introduce other foods at about 4 months. Family planning was not widely available in Ethiopia/Eritrea, but is well accepted by many Ethiopians/Eritreans in the West (Beyene, 1996; Ethnomed, n.d. b; Hodes, 1997).

Health problems and screening

Healthy life expectancies (HALE) in Ethiopia are 38 years and in Eritrea 44 years, while full life expectancies are 44.2 years in Ethiopia and 56.5 years in Eritrea. The infant mortality rate in Ethiopia is 98.6/1000 live births and in Eritrea is 73.6/1000 live births (Central Intelligence Agency (CIA), 2003; World Health Organization (WHO), 2003a, b).

Few Ethiopians/Eritreans arrive in the West with the dramatic health problems and malnutrition seen in the early days of displacement. Nevertheless, health problems are common, and may include the long-term effects of malnutrition, war trauma (physical and psychological), and a variety of infectious diseases, most notably hepatitis, tuberculosis, intestinal parasites, and HIV/AIDS. In Ethiopia, 10% of the population is HIV positive and in Eritrea the rate is 2.9% (CIA, 2003). Ethiopia/Eritrea is also one of 11 countries accounting for more than 66% of world deaths from measles (Stein *et al.*, 2003). Health risks in refugees and immigrants from Ethiopia/Eritrea (Ackerman, 1997; Gavagan & Brodyaga, 1998; Hawn & Jung, 2003; Kemp, 2002; WHO, 2003a, b) include

- amebiasis
- anthrax

- boutonneuse fever (African tick fever, Marseilles fever, tick typhus)
- cholera
- Crimean–Congo hemorrhagic fever
- dengue fever
- dracunculiasis (Guinea worm disease)
- echinococcosis (hydatid disease)
- filariasis (Bancroftian filariasis, Malayan filariasis, loiasis or loa loa, onchocerciasis hemorrhagic fevers (HFs): Lassa HF, Crimean–Congo HF, Chikungunya fever, dengue fever and HF, and Rift Valley fever)
- hepatitis B (9% carriage rate)
- hookworm
- leishmaniasis
- leprosy
- malaria
- malnutrition
- measles
- plague
- relapsing fevers (louse-borne relapsing fever (LBRF) is a public health problem primarily in the highlands of Ethiopia; while tick-borne relapsing fever (TBRF) has a much wider distribution)
- Rift Valley fever
- schistosomiasis or bilharzia
- sickle cell disease or sickle cell hemoglobinopathies
- STDs, including HIV/AIDS, cervical cancer, chancroid, gonorrhea, granuloma inguinale, lymphogranuloma venereum, syphilis
- strongylodiasis
- trachoma
- trematodes (liver-dwelling: clonorchiasis and opisthorchiasis; blood-dwelling: schistosomiasis or bilharzias; intestine-dwelling; and lung-dwelling)
- tuberculosis
- typhoid and paratyphoid fever
- typhus
- yaws (frambesia)
- malnutrition
- post-traumatic stress disorder

REFERENCES

Ackerman, L. K. (1997). Health problems of refugees. *Journal of the American Board of Family Practice*, **10**, 337–48.

American Psychiatric Association (2000). *Diagnostic and Statistical Manual of Mental Disorders*, 4th edn, text revision. Washington, DC: Author.

Beyene, Y. (1996). Ethiopians and Eritreans. In *Culture and Nursing Care*, ed. J. G. Lipson, S. L. Dibble and P. A. Minarik, pp. 101–14. San Francisco: UCSF Nursing Press.

Central Intelligence Agency (2003). *World Factbook*. Retrieved June 3, 2003 from http://www.cia.gov/cia/publications/factbook/geos/et.html.

Ethnomed (n.d. a). *Eritrean Cultural Profile*. Retrieved May 1, 2003 from http://ethnomed.org/ethnomed/cultures/eritrean/eritrean_cp.html.

   (n.d. b). *Ethiopian Cultural Profile*. Retrieved May 1, 2003 from http://ethnomed.org/ethnomed/cultures/eritrean/eritrean_cp.html.

Gavagan, T. & Brodyaga, L. (1998). Medical care for immigrants and refugees. *American Family Physician*, **57**, 1061–8.

Grisaru, N., Budowski, D., & Witzum, E. (1997a). Possession by the "Zar" among Ethiopian immigrants to Israel: psychopathology or culture-bound syndrome? *Psychopathology*, **30**, 223–33.

Grisaru, N., Lezer, S., & Belmaker, R. H. (1997b). Ritual female genital surgery among Ethiopian Jews. *Archives of Sexual Behavior*, **26**, 211–15.

Hawn, T. R. & Jung, E. C. (2003). Health screening in immigrants, refugees, and internationally adopted orphans. In *The Travel and Tropical Medicine Manual*, 3rd edn., ed. E. C. Jong and R. McMullen, pp. 255–65. Philadelphia, PA: W. B. Saunders.

Hodes, R. (1997). Cross-cultural medicine and diverse health beliefs: Ethiopians abroad. *Western Journal of Medicine*, **166**, 29–36.

Johnstone, P. & Mandryk, J. (2001). *Operation World: 21st Century edn*. Waynesboro, GA: Paternoster USA.

Kemp, C. (2002). *Infectious Diseases*. Retrieved April 12, 2003 from http://www3.baylor.edu/~Charles_Kemp/Infectious_Disease.htm.

Sark, M. (1995). Female genital mutilation: an introduction. *FGM Research On-line*. Retrieved September 30, 1999 from http://www.fgmnetwork.org/intro/fgmintro.html.

Stein, C. E., Birmingham, M., Kurian, M., Duclos, P., & Strebel, P. (2003). The global burden of measles in the year 2000 – a model that uses country-specific indicators. *Journal of Infectious Diseases*, **187** *(Suppl. 1)*, S8–S14.

Toubia, N. (1999). *Caring for Women with Circumcision*. New York: Rainbo Publications.

World Health Organization (2003a). *Ethiopia*. Retrieved May 30, 2003 from http://www.who.int/country/eth/en/.

   (2003b). *Eritrea*. Retrieved May 30, 2003 from http://www.who.int/country/eri/en/.

17

Guatemala

Rachel H. Adler

Introduction

For a country that is only about the size of the state of Kentucky, Guatemala is remarkably diverse with a rich and interesting history. The story of the Guatemalan immigration movement of sizeable numbers can be traced back to 1954, when the government of Jacobo Arbenz Guzmán was overthrown by a violent coup (Barry, 1991; Carmack, 1992). The new government, aligned with the USA, actively sought to purge communist elements in Guatemalan society by identifying and eliminating leftist groups. As a result, civilians came under attack and human rights abuses became commonplace.

Although violations of human rights have occurred regularly since 1954, they intensified in the 1980s. Counterinsurgency offensives were carried out against rural populations, especially indigenous communities, church workers, health-care providers, teachers, and development workers. Unspeakable horrors, such as public massacres, were routine during the 1980s. The public display of mangled bodies was a tactic used by the army and the police to instill fear into civilian populations.

During the 1980s an estimated 150 000 indigenous Maya were killed (Loucky & Moors, 2000) and between 500 000 and 1 000 000 Guatemalans were forced from their homes due to political violence (Barry, 1991). Many of these refugees fled north to United Nations-sponsored refugee camps in southern Mexico. Others escaped to the USA, Canada or other Central American countries. Peace accords ending the civil war were finally signed in the late 1990s, allowing some refugees to return.

History of immigration

The history of Guatemalan immigration to the USA is replete with legal complexity. Guatemalans leaving their homeland because of fear of persecution during the civil war were clearly refugees under the 1951 United Nations Convention. However, the vast majority of Guatemalans seeking political asylum in the USA have been denied because of US support of the Guatemala regime, leaving most Guatemalan refugees with undocumented legal status (Adler, 2001). This is important because these Guatemalans do not have the access to medical care, employment, or social service benefits granted to official refugee populations in the USA. Moreover, even before the end of the civil war, many Guatemalans left the country not out of fear of persecution but rather because relatives and friends were already established in the USA, a trend continuing to the present. And many Guatemalans who were not able to adjust their status under the amnesty provisions of the Immigration Reform and Control Act of 1986 are still likely to be undocumented. While the issue of who is a genuine refugee is complex and politicized, it should be assumed by healthcare practitioners that most Guatemalans in the USA were at least somewhat adversely affected by the events of the horrific civil war.

The major receiving areas for Mayan Guatemalans in the 1980s were California, Texas and Florida. Secondary migration from those areas to Kansas, Alabama, North Carolina and Colorado ensued and today there are Guatemalans in most regions of the USA (Loucky & Moors, 2000). Most rural Guatemalans worked in agriculture in Guatemala, both as peasant farmers and as wage laborers on agro export plantations. Thus, upon arrival in the USA, particularly in rural areas, they often end up doing farm work. Guatemalans in urban areas of the USA are concentrated in the service sector as gardeners, maids and restaurant employees. Those Guatemalans without legal residency are seriously limited in the employment options available to them, helping to explain the concentration of Guatemalans in poorly paid, insecure and undesirable sectors of the economy.

Culture and social relations

The major ethnic distinction in Guatemala is between Mayan and Ladino. Mayan refers to indigenous groups in Guatemala, of which there are many, represented by the linguistic diversity of the country. Ladino is the term used for Guatemalans who do not identify themselves as Mayan. The distinction between Ladino and Mayan is ethnic rather than racial. That is, whether a person is Ladino or Mayan is not based on phenotypical characteristics, but on self-identification and the display of ethnic boundary markers such as language, dress and food preference. The difference between Mayan and Ladino in Guatemala is hierarchical. Ladinos have more access to wealth, power and prestige in Guatemalan society and there is a social stigma attached to being Mayan. Yet culturally, there are many similarities among rural Guatemalan peasants, whether they are Ladino or Mayan.

There are both Ladino and Mayan populations in the USA. The well-studied population in Indiantown, Florida, for example, was at first populated completely by Q'anjob'al Maya. Although they are still the majority, today there are Ladinos, other Mayans and other Central American immigrants in Indiantown as well (Burns, 2000). Other areas of the country, such as Trenton, New Jersey, have always had predominantly Ladino populations.

When Guatemalans arrive in the USA they become part of a larger Latino ethnic group, at least from the perspective of the dominant society. Yet besides a common language, they do not always share much in common culturally with other Latino groups. There is variation in this regard depending on the region of the country in which they settle. In California, for example, Guatemalans are surrounded by a large Mexican population with whom they do share cultural similarities because of the parallel history and geography between Mexico and Guatemala. In places like New Jersey, however, Guatemalans are surrounded by Puerto Rican and Dominican populations with which they have much less in common. Their refugee experience also distinguishes Guatemalans from many other Latino ethnic groups.

Communications

There is great linguistic variety in Guatemala but the *lingua franca* is Spanish. In the USA there are Guatemalans who are monolingual speakers of indigenous languages such as Q'anjob'al, Mam or K'iche', but the majority of Guatemalans in the USA can speak at least some Spanish.

Whether encountering Mayan- or Spanish-speaking Guatemalans, monolingual English health practitioners should use translators. However, even with a translator there can be miscommunication when clinicians use technical language. Miralles (1989) suggests that doctors and nurses should not assume that patients or translators understand the questions being asked. Rather, patients should be asked for their own self-diagnosis (Miralles, 1989). Also, gestures should be used to indicate which areas of the body are experiencing problems (Miralles, 1989).

Religion

Historically, Guatemala is a Catholic country. There is some variation between how Catholicism is practiced by Ladinos and Mayans, with the Mayan version of Catholicism containing elements of indigenous religion tied in for good measure. The belief in *nahuales,* animal spirits which protect people throughout their lives, is an exclusively Mayan idea (Shea, 2001). Protestant evangelists, however, have converted a large segment of the Catholic population of Guatemala since the 1970s. Under the leadership of born-again Christian General Efraín Ríos Montt during the height of the counterinsurgency of the 1980s, there was pressure for people to convert to Protestantism because Catholics were suspected of being opposed to the military regime (Zur, 1998). There is tension between adherents of Catholicism and Protestantism for political reasons and also because the latter eschew some traditional and revered religious practices such as veneration of the saints. Since saints' day festivals are community-defining events, refusal to participate in such rituals is often interpreted by traditional Catholics as a slight against the community. Refugees in the USA are Catholic or one of several Protestant denominations. Protestant refugees who converted during the counterinsurgency of the 1980s, however, were often coerced into their new religion (Zur, 1998). Therefore, they may retain traditional views of spirituality, as well as health and illness.

Health beliefs and practices

There are two systems of medicine in Guatemala: the Western biomedical model and traditional ethnomedicine. There is often a disparaging attitude towards traditional ethnomedicine on the part of biomedical practitioners. Yet Guatemalans are likely to use traditional remedies first and only consult biomedical practitioners if the traditional cures are not working. A similar approach exists among Guatemalan refugees. Moreover, the undocumented status of many Guatemalan refugees may lead Guatemalans to wait until it is absolutely necessary to consult a physician, since it is potentially dangerous and expensive for them to do so.

In traditional Guatemalan medicine, illness represents disequilibrium between the processes of the body and the physical, social and cosmological orders (Lipp 2001). Unlike the biomedical model, illness etiology is often social and so treatment involves social factors as well (Lipp, 2001). For example, when illness occurs, the patient may attribute the cause of illness to witchcraft or sorcery (Adams & Rubel, 1967). When someone in the family is sick, he or she is treated first at home with medicinal plants, massage and/or sweat baths. If these treatments do not work, a *curandero* (traditional healer) may be consulted (Lipp, 2001). *Curanderos* can determine whether the illness was caused by witchcraft and, if so, perform rituals to heal the patient. Some of the traditional medical practitioners in Guatemala include the following.

Curanderos

Curanderos diagnose illness by taking the pulse of the patient and by using techniques to divine the cause of sickness (Lipp, 2001). *Curanderos* treat their patients with medicinal plants in the form of teas, baths and poultices, and also with prayer, spraying patients' bodies with liquid, rubbing an egg over patients' bodies, prescribing dietary restrictions, and practicing elaborate curing rites (Lipp, 2001). The animal companion soul (*nahual*) is believed to be vulnerable to harm, especially when a person is dreaming, and can become dislodged, stolen, injured or even eaten (Lipp, 2001). This can happen as a result of sorcery, which is viewed as a punishment for behavior that violates the social norms of the community. Thus, the *curandero's* treatment of illness often emphasizes the future social conduct of the patient.

Parteras

Parteras (midwives) deliver the majority of babies throughout rural Guatemala, especially in Mayan communities. However, midwives also deliver a substantial number of births in urban areas and among Ladinos (Cosminsky, 2001). In order for midwives to practice legally in Guatemala, they are required to be licensed (Cosminsky, 2001). To become licensed, *parteras* must enroll in a training course in which they learn biomedical procedures. This training does not preclude traditional midwifery since some women use unlicensed midwifes and because even those with training do not necessarily dismiss traditional birthing practices in favor of medicalized ones (Cosminsky, 2001).

Pharmacists

Unlike in the USA, pharmacists in Guatemala often diagnose and treat illness. In fact, people will often go to the pharmacist first, before seeking the help of a physician. Patients describe their symptoms and pharmacists distribute medication accordingly and without a prescription from a doctor. It should be assumed that Guatemalans in the USA have access to medicines that in the USA require a physician's prescription, and that they may self-medicate before seeking medical assistance.

An important aspect of health and illness found in Guatemala and throughout Latin America is humoral medicine theory. According to this system all foods and medicines are believed to fall along a metaphoric hot–cold distinction (Foster, 1994). Actual temperature does come in to play in this scheme, but many foods, remedies, and physical states are also said to be either "hot" or "cold" regardless of actual temperature.

A healthy body is perceived to maintain a state of equilibrium in regard to body temperature. When illness occurs, the body's temperature is lowered or raised and a healthy state cannot be achieved without restoring its equilibrium. In the case of illness, remedies that are purported to have the opposite humoral value as the illness are used to get the body back into balance. For example, a toothache is considered to be a hot state so one remedy is the application of a poultice made with grape leaves, which have a metaphoric cold value (Foster, 1994). A body that is too thermally or metaphorically hot or cold is also susceptible to illness, so it is important to avoid anything that upsets the natural body temperature. Thermally cold foods, such as iced drinks, taken immediately after a thermally hot food, such as soup, is said to cause illness. Likewise, it is common for medical personnel in the USA to observe Latino parents covering up a sick baby with blankets, especially if the child is running a fever. Health workers remove the blankets only to have the child's parents replace them the instant that they are alone. This behavior can be explained by the humoral theory to which the parents subscribe. An overheated child will become more ill if exposed to cold air. Even though illness is most often treated with a principle of opposites (cold remedy for hot illness) the transition to a healthy body temperature must be done gradually. Exposing a baby to cold air when she is already too hot is therefore antithetical to the restoration of health. The avoidance of a sudden shift from thermal heat to cold is common and can also help explain why Guatemalan patients may be wary to follow certain recommendations, such as drinking cold fluids when they have a fever.

The specifics of the humoral system, that is which foods and remedies are classified as hot or cold, varies somewhat within Latin America. Regardless of the disparities of this system, health practitioners should be aware of the importance given to humoral states by Guatemalan patients.

A final aspect of Guatemalan health beliefs and practices are the traditional syndromes. Traditional syndromes are often caused by emotional states or problematical social relations. For example, *mal de ojo* (the evil eye) is directly caused by envy. If someone looks at a baby with too much admiration, the child is vulnerable to *mal de ojo*. Babies falling victim to this illness will cry constantly, exhibit a sad expression, have one eye larger than the other and experience vomiting and diarrhea (Foster, 1994). A way to prevent *mal de ojo* is for the admirer to slap the child lightly to symbolically disavow the compliment (Foster, 1994). Other culture-bound illnesses are *susto* (caused by fright), *bilis* (caused by anger and fright) and *chipil* (caused by jealousy). These traditional syndromes are treated based on the humoral principles discussed above. People seek the help of a *curandero* if they are unable to cure these illnesses on their own.

Pregnancy and childbirth

Pregnancy is considered to be a "hot" time and women must avoid becoming overheated when they are pregnant (Cosminsky, 1994). Pregnant women are warned against lifting anything heavy and are encouraged to eat a healthy diet. In Mayan communities, a kneeling position is favored for delivery (Cosminsky, 1982). There is a special relationship between the placenta and the baby and the placenta should be burned and the ashes buried. The umbilical cord is often saved and used as a remedy for women who cannot have children (Cosminsky, 1982). After birth a woman is in a cold state and should eat and drink hot foods to restore balance (Cosminsky, 1982; 1994).

Guatemalans generally view pregnancy and birth as normal life events rather than as medical problems to be cured in a hospital (Miralles, 1989). Among refugees in Indiantown, Florida, there are ambivalent attitudes towards hospital delivery because it is expensive and also because women fear that tubal ligations would be performed on them without their consent (Miralles, 1989). There are midwives among the Guatemalans in Indiantown and some women opt to employ their services and deliver their babies at home.

Among Indiantown refugees, many women who did not use birth control in Guatemala do begin using it in the USA (Miralles, 1989). Abortion is also practiced among the refugees; the older the woman, the more likely she is to use birth control or have an abortion (Miralles, 1989). In Guatemala, injections are used to induce abortion and the refugee population in Indiantown does have access to this medical intervention (Miralles, 1989).

Medical practitioners should be aware that economic constraints and legal status may prevent Guatemalan women from seeking prenatal care. Furthermore, some women plan to give birth at home with the assistance of a midwife and will only show up at the hospital if problems occur.

End of life

According to *K'iche'* Mayan belief, a good death is one that is expected and planned for whereas a bad death is one that happens suddenly with no advance warning and without the traditional funerary ceremonies performed (Zur, 1998). Thus, health practitioners should provide patients and family members with sufficient information so that a terminal patient can get their affairs in order before they die. Relatives may want to prepare for the impending death of loved ones by having diviners perform rituals over them before they die (Zur, 1998). It is important to perform the appropriate rituals for a deceased person because the good or bad fate of the spirit is determined not by his or her actions in life but rather by how people venerate his or her death (Zur, 1998). Dying away from home is considered negative, and burial in the home village is traditionally preferred (Zur, 1998); unfortunately, refugees may not be able to afford to send the body back to Guatemala or even be able to attend a funeral there for reasons of personal security.

During the civil war in Guatemala, death was unexpected, sudden, and the proper rituals did not happen. Many refugees had loved ones who disappeared, making it impossible for funerary rituals to take place. Others lost loved ones in massacres after which bodies were burned or buried *en masse*, also prohibiting appropriate funerary rites. The pain and trauma suffered by people who lost loved ones may lead to somatization of grief whereby people experience physical pain as a result of the suppression of emotional pain (Zur, 1998). Death is a potentially sensitive issue for Guatemalan refugees because of the traumas that they have experienced in their homeland. Medical practitioners should be aware of the powerful negative psychological consequences of refugees' experiences with death during the civil war.

Health problems and screening

At 54.3 years, the healthy life expectancy (HALE) in Guatemala is the second lowest (after Honduras) in Central America (World Health Organization (WHO), 2002). Infant mortality rates are high at 48/1000 live births (Pan American Health Organization (PAHO), 2002). Acute respiratory infections and acute diarrhea with dehydration are the leading causes of death in children under 5 years.

Chronic noncommunicable diseases are emerging as health problems of growing significance in Guatemala and elsewhere in Central America. These include cardiovascular disease, malignant neoplasms (for women, cervical), cerebrovascular disease, chronic obstructive pulmonary disease and asthma, and type 2 diabetes (PAHO, 2002). Health risks in refugees and immigrants from Guatemala (Hawn & Jung, 2003; Kemp, 2002; Lane *et al.*, 2002; Molesky, 1986; PAHO, 2002) include:

- amebiasis
- angiostrongyliasis
- anisakiasis
- arbovirus encephalitis (Eastern equine encephalomyelitis (EEE))
- Chagas' disease
- chromomycosis
- cryptococcosis
- cryptosporidiosis
- dengue fever (including dengue hemorrhagic fever)
- dracunculiasis (Guinea worm disease)
- filariasis (Bancroftian filariasis, Malayan filariasis, and to a lesser extent, onchocerciasis)
- granuloma inguinale or donovanosis
- hepatitis B
- leishmaniasis
- leprosy
- leptospirosis
- malaria
- mucocutaneous leishmaniasis (*Espundia*)

- mycetoma
- paracoccidioidomycosis (South American Blastomycosis)
- STDs, including HIV/AIDS, cervical cancer, chancroid, gonorrhea, granuloma inguinale, lymphogranuloma venereum, syphilis
- strongylodiasis
- trichuriasis (trichocephaliasis or whipworm)
- tuberculosis
- tungiasis
- typhoid fever
- yaws (frambesia)
- yellow fever
- exposure to chemicals used in agriculture
- post-traumatic stress disorder and/or depression
- cardiovascular and related diseases, e.g., obesity, hypertension, diabetes.

REFERENCES

Adams, R. N. & Rubel, A. J. (1967). Sickness and social relations. In *Handbook of Middle American Indians*, ed. M. Nash, pp. 333–55. Austin: University of Texas Press.

Adler, R. H. (2001). Are you a real refugee? A critique of official classifications of migrant types from a political economy perspective. In *Negotiating Transnationalism: Selected Papers on Refugees and Immigrants*, ed. M. Hopkins and N. Wellmeir, pp. 142–59. American Anthropological Association: Washington DC.

Barry, T. (1991). *Central America Inside Out: The Essential Guide to Its Societies, Politics, and Economics*. New York: Grove Weidenfeld.

Burns, A. F. (2000). Indiantown, Florida: the Maya diaspora and applied anthropology. In *The Maya Diaspora: Guatemalan Roots, New American Lives*, ed. J. Loucky and M. M. Moors, pp. 152–71. Philadelphia, PA: Temple University Press.

Carmack, R. M. (1992). Editor's preface to the first edition. *In Harvest of Violence: The Maya Indians and the Guatemalan Crisis*, pp. ix–xvii. Norman, Oklahoma: University of Oklahoma Press.

Cosminsky, S. (1982). Knowledge and body concepts of Guatemalan midwives. In *Anthropology of Human Birth*, ed. M. A. Kay, pp. 233–52. Philadelphia: F. A. Davis Company.

(1997). Childbirth and change: a Guatemalan study. In *Ethnography of Fertility and Birth*, 2nd edn., ed. C. P. MacCormack, pp. 195–220. Philadelphia, PA: Academic Press.

(2001). Maya midwives of Southern Mexico and Guatemala. In *Mesoamerican Healers*, ed. B. R. Huber and A. Sandstrom, pp. 179–210. Austin, TX: University of Texas Press.

Foster, G. M. (1994). *Hippocrates' Latin American legacy: Humoral Medicine in the New World*. Langhorne, PA: Gordon and Breach Publishers.

Hawn, T. R. & Jung, E. C. (2003). Health screening in immigrants, refugees, and internationally adopted orphans. In *The Travel and Tropical Medicine Manual*, 3rd edn., ed. E. C. Jong and R. McMullen, pp. 255–65. Philadelphia, PA: W. B. Saunders.

Kemp, C. (2002). *Infectious Diseases*. Retrieved April 12, 2003 from http://www3.baylor.edu/~Charles_Kemp/Infectious_Disease.htm.

Lane, D., Beevers, D. G., & Lip, G. Y. H. (2002). Ethnic differences in blood pressure and the prevalence of hypertension in England. *Journal of Human Hypertension*, **16**, 267–73.

Lipp, F. J. (2001). A comparative analysis of Southern Mexican and Guatemalan shamans. In *Mesoamerican Healers*, ed. B. R. Huber and A. Sandstrom, pp. 95–116. Austin, TX: University of Texas Press.

Loucky, J. & Moors, M. M., eds. (2000). The Maya diaspora: introduction. In *The Maya Diaspora: Guatemalan Roots, New American Lives*, pp. 1–10. Philadelphia, PA: Temple University Press.

Miralles, M. A. (1989). *A Matter of Life and Death: Health-seeking Behavior of Guatemalan Refugees in South Florida*. NY: AMS Press.

Molesky, J. (1986). Pathology of Central American refugees. *Migration World Magazine*, **14**, 19–23.

Pan American Health Organization (PAHO) (2002). *Guatemala*. Retrieved from http://www.paho.org/English/DD/AIS/cp_320.htm.

Shea, M. E. (2001). *Culture and Customs of Guatemala*. Westport, CT: Greenwood Press.

Zur, J. N. (1998). *Violent Memories: Mayan War Widows in Guatemala*. Boulder, CO: Westview Press.

FURTHER READING

Benyshek, D. C., Martin, J. F. & Johnston, C. S. (2001). A reconsideration of the origins of the type 2 diabetes epidemic among Native Americans and the implications for intervention policy. *Medical Anthropology*, **20**, 25–64.

Burns, A. F. (1993). *Maya in Exile: Guatemalans in Florida*. Philadelphia, PA: Temple University Press.

Entwistle, B. A. & Swanson, T. M. (1989). Dental needs and perceptions of adult Hispanic migrant farmworkers in Colorado. *Journal of Dental Hygiene*, **63**, 286–92.

Lukes, S. M. & Miller F. Y. (2001). Oral health issues among migrant farmworkers. *Journal of Dental Hygiene*, **76**, 134–40.

McCauley, L. A., Sticker, D., Bryan, C., Lasarev M. R., & Scherer, J. A. (2002). Pesticide knowledge and risk perception among adolescent Latino farmworkers. *Journal of Agricultural Safety and Health*, **8**, 397–409.

McCurdy, S. A., Arretz, D. S., & Bates, R. O. (1997). Tuberculin reactivity among California Hispanic migrant farmworkers. *American Journal of Industrial Medicine*, **32**, 600–5.

Martin, J. F., Johnston, C. S., Han, C. T., & Benyshek, D. C. (2000). Nutritional origins of insulin resistance: a rat model for diabetes-prone human populations. *Journal of Nutrition*, **4**, 741–4.

Mills, P. K. & Kwong, S. (2001). Cancer incidence in the United Farmworkers of America, 1987–1997. *American Journal of Industrial Medicine*, **40**, 596–603.

Population Reference Bureau (2002). *2002 World Population Data Sheet.* Retrieved May 12, 2003 from http://www.prb.org/pdf/WorldPopulationDS02_Eng.pdf.

Ward, M. H., Prince, J. R., Stewart, P. A., & Zahm, S. H. (2001). Determining the probability of pesticide exposures among migrant farmworkers: results from a feasibility study. *American Journal of Industrial Medicine*, **40**, 538–53.

World Health Organization (2002). *World Health Report.* Retrieved June 5, 2003 from http://www.who.int/whr/2002/en/.

(2003). *Global TB Control Report 2003.* Retrieved June 1, 2003 from http://www.who.int/gtb/publications/globrep/index.html.

Wright, A. (1990). *The Death of Ramón González: The Modern Agricultural Dilemma.* Austin, TX: University of Texas Press.

18

Haiti

Background

The Republic of Haiti (hereafter, Haiti) lies on the western third of the Island of Hispaniola in the West Indies. The eastern portion of Hispaniola is the Dominican Republic. Haiti is mountainous, densely populated (>7 000 000 people), and has the lowest per capita income in the Western Hemisphere. Most of the population is black descendents of African slaves brought to the West Indies by French colonists (Pan American Health Organization (PAHO), 1999).

From 1957–1971, "President for Life" Francois "Papa Doc" Duvalier ruled Haiti. Duvalier's secret police, the *tontons macoutes* used terror and repression to control the country. "Papa Doc" Duvalier was succeeded by his son, Jean-Claude "Baby Doc" Duvalier in 1971. In 1990, Jean-Bertrand Aristide was elected president and there was tremendous optimism in Haiti that the Duvalier's reign of terror was finished. In 1991, Aristide was overthrown by elements of the former regime, but in 1994 with assistance from the USA was returned to power. The Aristide administration (later the Preval administration, and then again Aristide) was more democratic and less corrupt than previous administrations, but the country remains impoverished and the military remains powerful. Poverty in Haiti is a result of a matrix of overpopulation, high unemployment rate (60%), high and accelerating inflation rate, high illiteracy rate (55%), destruction of natural resources, no industry or exports, and little viable industrial or government infrastructure.

History of immigration

Haitians come to the USA and to a lesser degree, France and other Western European countries, as legal immigrants, illegal immigrants, and as refugees. Legal immigration tends to be difficult for Haitians, but because of desperate economic conditions

Refugee and Immigrant Health: A Handbook for Health Professionals, Charles Kemp and Lance A. Rasbridge. Published by Cambridge University Press. © C. Kemp and L. A. Rasbridge 2004.

in Haiti, the rate of illegal immigration remains high. Most illegal immigrants to the USA leave Haiti via small boat, despite significant risk of drowning or interdiction in the sea journey. The number of refugees, never very great, has declined since the early 1990s to several thousand/year. Most new Haitian immigrants and refugees are adults or teens (with few infants or old people), and most are poorly educated.

Culture and social relations

Many Haitian refugees and immigrants come from the city of Port-au-Prince, but may actually be from rural backgrounds. Most are poorly educated, speak only Creole, and have marginal or no ability to read or write. Influences on Haitian culture include their West African origins, experiences as slaves, and the crushing poverty of Haiti. The better-educated Haitians tend to be more future oriented, while those with less education tend to be oriented to the present, and, like many refugees, also oriented to a past that may become increasingly romanticized as time passes in the new land. There is a small middle class and a miniscule wealthy class. It should be noted that, despite physical similarities, there is often little interaction or perceived commonality between native-born American Blacks and Haitians.

The extended family is the ideal social unit, but because of previously noted difficulties in immigration, is relatively rare in the USA. In many respects, Haitian society is matriarchal, especially where child-rearing and family life is concerned. Common-law marriage or setting up a household (*plasé*) is the norm – in part, because of the expense of the more desirable legal marraige (Coreil, Barnes-Josiah, & Cayemittes, 1996; Maynard-Tucker, 1996).

Although Haitian culture is considered by many to be matriarchal (e.g., Colin & Paperwalla, 1996), the man in the relationship is likely to hold ultimate control and authority in most matters, especially those related to the world outside the family. Parents are authoritarian and the use of force as a means of discipline is common. Respect for adults, support to the family, and achieving in school are strongly held values that often do not survive in American urban settings (Colin & Paperwalla, 1996).

As noted in the section on communication, relationships and communication may be very affectionate and even unrestrained. Many Haitians live in ethnic enclaves that serve as cultural/emotional support systems to people who have lost their primary support systems.

Communications

Most Haitians speak Creole, a French/pidgin dialect that is seldom written, and the educated also speak French. Communication tends to be relatively direct (except, perhaps, regarding certain religious and personal matters). Some Haitians will indicate agreement with a person of higher socioeconomic status rather than risk conflict in disagreement. In communicating with friends, direct eye contact, expressive or animated tone of voice, and expressive hand gestures are common, as is touching the other person. Personal space is often not as pronounced as among some other cultures, and interaction may be very close. Touch by caregivers is generally appreciated (Colin & Paperwalla, 1996).

Interpreters outside the family may be mistrusted, but use of children to interpret (the most likely English speakers) carries the potential of creating conflict within the family or within the interpreter who may be called on to deal with difficult matters. An interpreter unknown to the patient may be better than a friend. Written materials are often of little use.

Religion

Most Haitians (80%) are Catholic, and many of these also believe to at least some extent in Voodoo (also spelled Voudou, Vodoun, or Vodun) (Brown, 1998). There are increasing numbers of Haitians who have become Protestant because of missionary contact in Haiti or in "Little Haiti" areas in the USA. In either case, religion may play a central role in the life of an individual, especially during illness or other crisis. From a cosmopolitan perspective, even mainstream religion may be seen as akin to magic.

Voodoo beliefs include the presence of a powerful spirit world from which neglected ancestors, malicious spirits, or even the raised or living dead (zombies) may come to the living to bring misfortune or death. Zombification, or more accurately, catalepsy is a result of poisoning with neurotoxins (tetrodotoxins and possibly others) from one or more species of puffer fish or amphibians (Craan, 1988). Spirits are known as *loas, mysteres,* or saints. Some Haitians work to maintain a strong relationship with this spirit world and significant effort is made to ensure that the relationship is protective or at least not damaging. Spirits may be controlled or brought into activity through ritual and/or the efforts of sorcerers or practitioners. Types of Voodoo or related practitioners (Coreil, 1983; Cosgray, 1995) include the following.

- *Houngan* (male), *mambo* (female), or *bokor* (black magician) are terms for a shaman or Voodoo practitioner.
- *Doctè fèy* is an herbalist or leaf doctor, in Haiti, the most commonly used folk healer.
- *Matronn* or *fam saj* is the term for a midwife or traditional birth attendant.
- *Doctè zo* is a bonesetter.
- *Pikirist* is an injectionist.

Catholic saints are incorporated into Voodoo, except that they may have different functions and names in Voodoo. What appear to be Catholic amulets may actually be Voodoo or in some cases (from a Voodoo perspective), both Catholic and Voodoo.

Health beliefs and practices

Educated Haitians or those with experience in modern health care are likely to have a greater understanding from a lay perspective of the scientific basis of illness. Illness may also be attributed to natural causes outside the body, such as cold, heat, winds, or humoral imbalance (Colin & Paperwalla, 1996). Changes in eating, living, or other habits may also influence health and illness. Illness may be seen as punishment (malediction) from God, especially when a person's relationship with God is weakened. A state of depression means generalized weakness, dejection, and worry that make one vulnerable to illness (Martin *et al.*, 1995). As noted earlier, some sickness is thought by some Haitians to be a result of *expedition* or illness sent by another through spirits.

Haitian beliefs about health and illness may also be strongly influenced by life in Haiti where there is limited access to the most basic health care (clean water, immunizations, prenatal/obstetric care, antibiotics, and so on). Thus, a reliance on folk and/or spiritual explanations and treatments for illness may simply be the only option a person has ever had. It is common for Haitians to simultaneously use multiple sources of care for an illness, e.g., a *docte fey*, primary care clinic, and sorcerer.

In seeking health care, the primary focus among most Haitians is on solving a specific problem. In many cases, a Haitian who presents at a primary care or other source of cosmopolitan health care will already have tried home or traditional remedies. Use of modern health resources for prevention of illness and health promotion is uncommon. However, use of traditional or magic-religious measures to prevent illness or harm is almost universal among Haitians (DeSantis & Thomas, 1990). Traditional means of health promotion and disease prevention (Colin & Paperwalla, 1996) are as follows.

- Eating well (being plump), sleeping well, keeping warm, exercising, and keeping clean are important to maintaining strength and avoiding weakness (*febles*).
- Maintaining equilibrium between "hot" and "cold" factors, including "hot" and "cold" or "light" and "heavy" foods helps prevent illness.
- Enemas (*lavman*) are given to children and purgatives to pregnant women and infants. Both are for the purpose of cleansing the inner body of impurities.
- Herbal teas, massage, are used to treat illness in early stages.
- Spiritual practice, especially Catholic ritual, prayer, and Voodoo practices are used to prevent harm or sickness.

The rate of chronic illnesses such as diabetes and hypertension is extraordinarily high among Haitians and treatment is very difficult because of high rates of noncompliance (Preston *et al.*, 1996). Noncompliance may be due to difficulty understanding the nature of chronic illnesses, difficulty accessing and maintaining a relationship with healthcare providers, and reliance on traditional or magical means of treatment. Socioeconomic status plays a well-known role in increased morbidity and mortality in all populations and in all diseases – and such is the case with Haitians. Self-medication, including with black market antibiotics or antibiotics loaned by friends is common.

Specific culture-bound illnesses of Haiti (Colin & Paperwalla, 1996; Coreil *et al.*, 1996; Coreil *et al.*, 1996) include the following.

- *Pedisyon* (perdition) is a common culture-bound illness in which a woman is thought to be pregnant, but the flow of blood to the uterus is diverted to menstrual blood and the pregnancy is thus arrested. The belief is that this state (characterized by menstruation) may last for years until a cure is obtained and the pregnancy then resumes.
- *Maldyok* is the evil eye (but not usually considered serious) and is attributed to an envious glance from another person.
- *Seziman* is fright caused by stress. Problems of *seziman* are thought to include the movement of blood to the head with resulting loss of vision and the potential for stroke.

Pregnancy and childbirth

The first pregnancy is often in the mid-teen years. Prenatal care is uncommon in Haiti, and at least in rural areas, delivery is commonly at home with assistance from a *matronn* or *fam saj*. Among Haitians living in developed countries, prenatal care is more often utilized, though the prenatal care may be perceived as less valuable than care in the postpartum and newborn periods. Spicy foods are avoided during pregnancy and increased dietary intake is common. Purgatives may be used throughout the pregnancy (Barnes-Josiah *et al.*, 1998; Thomas & DeSantis, 1995). Care for the mother during the postpartum period (Harris, 1987) includes the following.

- Warmth is maintained through drinking warm herbal teas, dressing warmly, and taking hot baths and "vapor baths" for 2–4 weeks. After this time, a cold bath may be taken to tighten bones and muscles.
- Dietary guidelines are followed, including eating beans and rice, plantains, and porridge, and avoiding certain foods, especially those that are cold or white in color (though coloring may be added, e.g., adding coffee to milk).
- Abdominal binders are used to help the abdomen return to the nonpregnant shape and help "close" the bones thought to be opened during pregnancy and delivery.

- Gas is a concern in the postpartum period and is avoided by preventing air from entering the vagina or ears, and by using an abdominal binder.

Care for the newborn includes cleaning and dressing the infant to maintain warmth – especially of the head. Some women give a purgative to the infant shortly after birth (or, when delivering in a hospital, after discharge from the hospital). It is common for mothers to keep a band of cloth tied around the infant's abdomen for the first 2–3 months of life to help the infant develop a well-formed body and good sense of balance. Some believe that disposable diapers serve this purpose as well as traditional bands. Breastfeeding is the norm for Haitians, but bottle feeding allows the mother to work outside the home, hence the bottle may be an economic necessity in developed locales. It is common for Haitian mothers to mix starchy additives to formula to promote weight gain and docility in the infant (Harris, 1987; Thomas & DeSantis, 1995).

End of life

Most deaths in Haiti occur in the home, but in developed countries, the hospital is preferred. The family is commonly involved in all nontechnological aspects of care and remains close to the patient. There does not seem to be any strong proscription against informing the patient of terminal status – at least in advanced stages of illness. Spiritual care is provided by family and clergy, and whether Catholic or Protestant, involvement of a hospital chaplain is deeply appreciated. Emotion is expressed without restraint when the patient is imminent and after the patient dies. The family usually prefers to bathe the body after death. Autopsy is accepted if legally required, but is otherwise resisted. However, autopsy may occasionally be requested to be sure that the person has not been zombified.

The funeral may be planned around the travel and work plans of family members living in other cities or countries. The funeral is preceded by a *veye* or wake. Whether Catholic or Protestant, funerals are characterized by the open expression of emotion. Burial is strongly preferred to cremation.

In addition to the funeral service there are 7 days of prayer called *dernie priye*, which serve to facilitate the soul's passage to the next world. These prayers are concluded on the seventh day with a mass called *prise de deuil*. After each of these services there is a reception in memory of the deceased (Colin & Paperwalla, 1996).

Health problems and screening

The healthy life expectancy (HALE) of Haitians is 42.9 years, a *decrease* of more than 2 years from 2001 to 2002, due at least in part, to the high rate of HIV/AIDS in Haiti (Lamptey et al., 2002; World Health Organization (WHO), 2002). With about 6% of adults infected, Haiti has the highest HIV/AIDS prevalence rate in the Western hemisphere. Infant mortality rates (74/1000 live births) are extraordinarily high, as are child death rates (133/1000 < 5 years) (Lamptey *et al.*, 2002; PAHO, 1999; WHO, 2002). More than 50% of all Haitian preschoolers are malnourished; and more than 35% of all Haitian women are anemic and many have experienced complications of pregnancy and/or delivery (PAHO, 1999). Tropical infectious diseases are common, as are obesity and related chronic health problems such as hypertension and diabetes (Molokhia & Oakeshott, 2000; PAHO, 1999). Common health risks or problems of new Haitian immigrants (Ackerman, 1997; Beach *et al.*, 1999; Centers for Disease Control (CDC) 2003; Halstead *et al.*, 2001; Hawn & Jung, 2003; 4A; Holcomb *et al.*, 1996; Kemp, 2002; Molokhia & Oakeshott, 2000; PAHO, 2002; WHO, 2002) include:

- amebiasis
- angiostrongyliasis
- anisakiasis
- arbovirus encephalitis (Eastern equine encephalomyelitis (EEE))
- Chagas' disease
- chromomycosis
- cryptococcosis
- cryptosporidiosis
- dengue fever
- dracunculiasis (Guinea worm disease)
- filariasis (Bancroftian filariasis, Malayan filariasis, and to a lesser extent, onchocerciasis)
- granuloma inguinale or donovanosis
- hepatitis B
- leishmaniasis
- leprosy
- leptospirosis
- malaria
- mucocutaneous leishmaniasis (*Espundia*)
- mycetoma
- paracoccidioidomycosis (South American blastomycosis)
- STDs, including HIV/AIDS, cervical cancer, chancroid, gonorrhea, granuloma inguinale, lymphogranuloma venereum, syphilis
- strongylodiasis
- trichuriasis (trichocephaliasis or whipworm)
- tuberculosis
- tungiasis

- typhoid fever
- yaws (frambesia)
- yellow fever
- cardiovascular and related diseases, e.g., obesity, hypertension, diabetes
- gastrointestinal cancers

REFERENCES

Ackerman, L. J. (1997). Health problems of refugees. *Journal of the American Board of Family Practice*, **10**, 337–48.

Barnes-Josiah, D., Myntti, C., & Augustin, A. (1998). The "three delays" as a framework for examining maternal mortality in Haiti. *Social Science Medicine*, **46**, 981–93.

Beach, M. J., Steit, T. G., Addiss, D. G., Prospere, R., Roberts, J. M., & Lammie, P. J. (1999). Assessment of combined ivermectin and albendazole for treatment of intestinal helminth and *Wucheria bancrofti* infections in Haitian schoolchildren. *American Journal of Tropical Medicine and Hygiene*, **60**, 479–486.

Brown, P. L. (1998). Where the Spirits of voodoo feel at home. *New York Times*. 12/31/98, B1, B18.

Centers for Disease Control (CDC) (2003). *Health Information for Travelers to the Caribbean.* Retrieved from http://www.cdc.gov/travel/caribbean.htm.

Colin, J. M. & Paperwalla, G. (1996). Haitians. In *Culture and nursing Care: A Pocket Guide*, ed. J. G. Lipson, S. L. Dibble, and P. A. Minarik, pp. 139–54. San Francisco: UCSF Nursing Press.

Coreil, J. (1983). Parallel structures in professional and folk health care: a model applied to rural Haiti. *Culture, Medicine and Psychiatry*, **7**, 131–151.

Coreil, J., Barnes-Josiah, D. L., & Cayemittes, A. A. M. (1996). Arrested pregnancy syndrome in Haiti: findings from a national survey. *Medical Anthropology Quarterly*, **10**, 424–36.

Cosgray, R. E. (1995). Haitian Americans. In *Transcultural Nursing: Assessment and Intervention*, ed. J. N. Giger and R. E. Davidhizar, pp. 501–23. St. Louis: Mosby.

Craan, A. G. (1988). Toxicologic aspects of Voodoo in Haiti. *Biomedical and Environmental Sciences*, **1**, 372–81.

DeSantis, L. & Thomas, J. T. (1990). The immigrant Haitian mother: transcultural nursing perspective on preventive health care for children. *Journal of Transcultural Nursing*, **2**, 2–15.

Halstead, S. B., Streit, T. G., LaFontant, J. G. *et al.* (2001). Haiti: absence of dengue hemorrhagic fever despite hyperendemic dengue virus transmission. *American Journal of Tropical Medicine and Hygiene*, **65**, 180–3.

Harris, K. (1987). Beliefs and practices among Haitian American women in relation to childbearing. *Journal of Nurse-Midwifery*, **32**, 149–55.

Hawn, T. R. & Jung, E. C. (2003). Health screening in immigrants, refugees, and internationally adopted orphans. In *The Travel and Tropical Medicine Manual*, 3rd edn., ed. E. C. Jong and R. McMullen, pp. 255–65. Philadelphia, PA: W. B. Saunders.

Holcomb, L. O., Parsons, L. C., Giger, J. N., & Davidhizar, R. (1996). Haitian Americans: implications for nursing care. *Journal of Community Health Nursing*, **13**, 249–60.

Kemp, C. (2002). *Infectious Diseases*. Retrieved April 12, 2003 from http://www3.baylor.edu/~Charles_Kemp/Infectious_Disease.htm.

Lamptey, P., Merywen, W. Carr, D. & Collymore, Y. (2002). *HIV Hits Marginal Populations Hardest in Latin America, Leading Cause of Death For Some Caribbean Nations*. Population Reference Bureau. Retrieved March 18, 2003 from http://www.prb.org/.

Martin, M. A., Rissmiller, P., & Beal, J. A. (1995). Health-illness beliefs and practices of Haitians with HIV disease living in Boston. *JANAC*, **6**, 45–53.

Maynard-Tucker, G. (1996). Haiti: unions, fertility and the quest for survival. *Social Science Medicine*, **43**, 1379–87.

Molokhia, M. & Oakeshott, P. (2000). A pilot study of cardiovascular risk assessment in Afro-Caribbean patients attending an inner city general practice. *Family Practice*, **17**, 60–2.

Pan American Health Organization (1999). *Haiti: Country Health Profile*. Retrieved December 8, 2002 from http://www.paho.org/English/SHA/prflHAI.htm.

Preston, R. A., Materson, B. J., Yoham, M. A., & Anapol, H. (1996). Hypertension in Haitians: results of a pilot survey of a public teaching hospital multispecialty clinic. *Journal of Human Hypertension*, **10**, 743–5.

Thomas, J. T. & DeSantis, L. (1995). Feeding and weaning practices of Cuban and Haitian immigrant mothers. *Journal of Transcultural Nursing*, **6**, 34–42.

World Health Organization (2002). *World Health Report*. Retrieved June 5, 2003 from http://www.who.int/whr/2002/en/.

19

India

Sonal Bhungalia, Stephanie Van De Kieft, and Margaret Young

Introduction

India is the second most populous nation (after China) and is one of the oldest civilizations on Earth. India's history is one of many dynasties, religions, and conquering invaders. The invaders exerted power and imposed their own cultural institutions, resulting in cultural blending. Today there are as many as six different racial strains present in India, making attempts to trace origins of people very difficult.

Among the major influences in India's history are Hinduism/Brahmanism, Hellenism, Buddhism, and Islam. Hinduism began about 1500 BC and has been the unifying thread in India's history. Alexander the Great brought Hellenism to India in 326 BC, and although he died 3 years later, Hellenism continued to influence India for many years. Following the Maura dynasty in 184 BC, Buddhism dominated for over a century. Brahmanism eventually replaced Buddhism, and the Hindu caste system rose. The Islamic Mughal Empire reigned from 1526 to 1707 and exerted considerable influence on Indian culture.

The British entered India in 1608, at first sharing, then dominating a trade organization, the British East India Company. The British replaced the Mughal rule in India in 1858, and remained in control until 1947. Despite some British attempts at reform, hostility grew among Indians, but multiple uprisings against the British government failed. Religious and political conflict also arose between Hindus and Muslims. In 1930, Mahatma K. Gandhi, a Hindu, ordered *Satyagraha* (passive resistance) and led a revolt against the British government. Britain made a truce with Gandhi, but conditions did not improve. The British remained in India until 1947, when the Indian Independence Act gave independence to India and established Pakistan and India as independent nations. The separation of the countries was largely along religious lines, with the majority of Hindus establishing

Refugee and Immigrant Health: A Handbook for Health Professionals, Charles Kemp and Lance A. Rasbridge. Published by Cambridge University Press. © C. Kemp and L. A. Rasbridge 2004.

residency in India and Muslims going to Pakistan. Conflict arose at the partition of India and Pakistan and continues today (Kemp & Bhungalia, 2002; Roberts, 1993).

History of immigration

Because India was a major British colony, there was significant immigration and exchange of culture between the countries. The vast number of Indians and limited opportunities within India also contributed to great numbers of Indians immigrating across the world. A total of around 22 000 000 Indians live outside of India in, for example, Sri Lanka (3.2 million Indians), USA (2.1 million), Malaysia (1.6 million), South Africa 1.1 million), United Kingdom (one million), and in the Middle East (an approximate one million migrant workers) (Johnstone & Mandryk, 2001). In the West, Indians are commonly well-educated, English-speaking individuals. Older, first generation Indian immigrants, though well educated, may not speak the language of their country of immigration, hence need a translator and advocate for healthcare transactions.

Culture and social relations

Within Indian society, extended family members usually live together as a single-family unit that includes grandparents, parents, and children, as well as the families of parental uncles. Among Indians in the West, extended families are still prevalent. Often, the husband's parents move in with the family after retirement or when the family decides to have children or if there is an illness and help is needed. The grandparents' role in raising children is highly valued, as they are the link to Indian culture, religion, and heritage. In families with multiple sons, the parents or grandparents usually choose to live with the youngest son. Also affecting the decision about which son the parents live with are financial capabilities, need for assistance in child-raising, and the relationship with the daughter-in-law (Kemp & Bhungalia, 2002; Rundle et al., 1999).

Relationships between siblings tend to be close. Many times, brothers live together for both financial and familial reasons. After marriage, if families live apart, siblings and their families continue to meet throughout the year for religious holidays and special occasions, as well as for vacations.

Because of the value placed on independence and privacy in Indian culture and the desire to save face, family issues, including healthcare decisions, are usually discussed within the immediate family before outside help is sought. Because of the close-knit family structure, a family can expect many visitors when a family member is in the hospital.

Within Indian society, the roles of men and women are distinct. Women manage the home by keeping all finances, family, and social issues in order. Women are more passive in the Indian culture and men typically are the bread-winners and managers of issues requiring interaction with individuals in the community, e.g., health care. This type of behavior implies that men have a dominant and authoritative role because they are the primary point of contact with society. However, these roles are beginning to change among some educated Indians in the larger cities of India and among some immigrants in progressive or permissive societies such as the United States (Rajwani, 1996).

Respect is highly valued, and children are taught to be respectful of all elders, whether grandparents, siblings, teachers, or family friends. Discipline of children is thought to come naturally, and understanding is used to help the child determine between good and bad. From an early age, children are responsible for helping with household chores on a regular basis. In many cases, when a family has recently come from India, a child is responsible for many adult tasks/issues such as finances, legal forms, and translations. Healthcare providers should take note when scheduling appointments during school time if the child is needed for translation. Healthcare providers can also assess the effects on the child of having adult responsibilities (Bhungalia *et al.*, 2000).

Communications

While there are 407 languages in use in India, Hindi, the national language, is spoken by 66% of the population. There are two main categories of language in India, including the Indo-Aryans in the north and the Dravidians in the south. Indo-Aryans predominantly speak Hindi, but have numerous dialect variations. English is an important second language for many Indians (Bhungalia *et al.*, 2000; Johnstone & Mandryk, 2001).

Emotion is seldom expressed outside of personal relationships; in fact, smiling is usually limited to informal situations and among social equals. Direct eye contact and pointing are considered rude, shaking the head from side to side indicates "yes," and beckoning is done with the palm down (Rundle *et al.*, 1999).

Religion

For millennia, religion, especially Hinduism, has been a pervasive force in India and Indian culture. There is evidence that the worship of Shiva (one of the Hindu trinity) is the oldest surviving religious cult in the world (Roberts, 1993). Approximately 80% of the people in India are Hindu, 12.5% are Muslim, 2.4% are Christian, 2% are Sikh, and 2% are Buddhist, Jain, Zoroastrian, or other (Johnstone & Mandryk, 2001). In the Western world there is probably a slightly greater percentage of

Christians because of a greater outmigration of Christians and the greater influence of missions in the Western world.

Hinduism dates back to around 5000 BC. The major Hindu scriptures are the *Vedas*, the *Upanishads*, and the *Bhagavad-Gita* (often referred to as the *Gita*). The most recent Hindu scripture is the *Bhagavad-Gita*, which was written somewhere around 800–300 BC. Like the Bible, the early Hindu scriptures are a collection of writings by seers or prophets, while the *Bhagavad-Gita* is a dialogue between Lord Krishna and Prince Arjuna.

The goal of Hinduism is freedom (of the soul or *Atman*) from endless reincarnation and the suffering inherent in existence. In popular usage, reincarnation and transmigration (rebirth) of the soul are viewed similarly. The endless reincarnations are the result of *karma*, the actions of the individual in this present life and also the accumulation of actions from past lives. Hinduism is discussed in greater detail in Chapter 5.

Health beliefs and practices

The Indian system of traditional medicine is known as *Ayruveda*, which means "knowledge of life." Indian medicine mixes religion with secular medicine, and involves observation of the patient as well as the patient's natural environment and how these are in (or out of) balance (Kemp & Bhungalia, 2002).

In the *Ayurveda* system, the body is composed of three primary forces, termed *dosha*. The three *dosha* are called *Vata*, *Pitta*, and *Kapha*. Each *dosha* represents characteristics derived from the elements (humors) of wind or air, bile (analogous to fire), and phlegm (analogous to water). The other elements are space and earth. The state of equilibrium between the *dosha* is perceived as a state of health; the state of imbalance is disease. Upon examination, the *Ayurvedic* physician finds out the position of the three *dosha* (*Tridosha*). Once the aggravated or unbalanced *dosha* is known, it is brought into balance by using different kinds of therapies (Kemp & Bhungalia, 2002; Rundle *et al.*, 1999).

Each *dosha* represents certain bodily activities. *Vata* is responsible for breathing, brain activity, circulation, and excretion. It is thought by traditionally minded Indians that people whose constitutions are predominantly *Vata* are thin, quick thinking, with swift action. When in imbalance, they become nervous, anxious, constipated, and insomniac. *Pitta* is responsible for vision, digestion, hunger, thirst, and regulation of body heat and temperature. When in balance, people whose constitutions are predominantly *Pitta* are intelligent, disciplined, sharp, and contented. When in imbalance, they are intolerant to heat, become bald, show short temper, anger and lust, and are prone to heartburn and ulcers. *Kapha* represents solid structure of the body and lubricating mucous. *Kapha* types have strong, well-developed bodies, with the tendency to not gain weight, and are mentally cool. When in imbalance, they are obese, disorganized, and sloppy; and develop allergies with dull activity, speech, and behavior (Kemp & Bhungalia, 2002).

There are approximately 1400 plants used in *Ayurvedic* medicine, none of which is synonymous with instant pain relievers or antibiotics. The herbs used in *Ayurvedic* remedies tend to gradually metabolize and have few side effects on the body.

Common Natural Remedies*

Botanical name	Common name	Use
Andriograohis paniculata	King of Bitters	Hepatoprotective
Boswellia serrata	Olibanum, Farnk incense	Antiarthritic, Antihyperlipid
Cassia angustifilia	Indian senna	Laxative
Coleus forskohlii	Coleus	Antiobesity
Garcinia camogia, Calcium	Garcinia, Kokum	Antiobesity
Garcinia cambogio, Potassium	Garcinia, Kokum	Antidiabetic
Gynema sylvestris	Gymnema	Aphrodisiac, Antioxidant
Shilajit	Asphalt	Aphrodisiac
Tribulus terrestris	Puncture vine	Aphrodisiac
Taxus baccata	Himalayan	Taxol, Ovarian cancer

* Kemp & Bhungalia, 2002.

Most Indians eat two to three meals per day, preferring a large meal at lunch and a small meal at supper. Hindus may prefer to use metal utensils such as copper, brass, and iron for cooking and eating on, as these materials are considered sacred. Most Indians eat with their fingers, but only of the right hand. Hand-washing before meals is important whether eating with hand or utensils. One must avoid any form of distraction while eating, e.g., watching television, reading, or excessive talking. Over-eating is discouraged because it is believed that it decreases one's lifespan (Rajwani, 1996).

Women generally serve the food and may eat separately from men. Food preparation has strict rules. Women are not allowed to cook during their menses. The perception of Hindus is the belief that some foods are "hot" and some are "cold", and therefore, should only be eaten during certain seasons and not in combination. Depending on the region of India and how foods are thought to affect body functions, there are differing perceptions of "hot" and "cold" foods (Kemp & Bhungalia, 2002; Rajwani, 1996).

Culture-bound syndromes that may affect Indians (American Psychiatric Association, 2000: Bhatia, 2000; Chadda & Ahuja, 1990; Jilek & Jilek-Aall, 1985; Krause, 1989; Kua *et al.*, 1986; Morinis, 1985) include the following.

- *Dhat* syndrome is the perceived presence of semen in the urine, accompanied by physical and mental fatigue. Note that urinalysis does not show the presence of semen.
- *Jinjinia bemar* or *Koro* is the perception that the penis (or sometimes, female genitalia) is retracting into the body, which is thought to then result in death. This syndrome has occurred in localized epidemics in Asia. *Koro* is more often thought of as a Chinese culture-bound illness, but has occurred among Indians, Thai, and others.
- God-intoxication is a state of religious ecstasy close to, or indistinguishable from, insanity.
- Possession-trance is a trance-like state in which the person is believed to be possessed by a spirit or goddess (usually recognizable to witnesses).
- Compulsive spitting is a self-descriptive disorder found among a variety of psychiatric patients, but with no unifying diagnosis.
- Ascetic syndrome includes psychosocial withdrawal, religiosity, and lack of concern about personal appearance.
- *Locha* is religion-inspired trichotillomania, in which members of certain sects pluck out their hair.
- *Dil ghirda hai* or sinking heart is the perception that the heart is sinking downward and losing its strength in response to stress, hunger, sunstroke, or stress.

Pregnancy and childbirth

Many Indian women view pregnancy as a "hot" state, or a time of increased body heat. As a result, there is reluctance to becoming "overheated" because it is believed that this may induce miscarriage. Women who have this belief avoid "hot" foods such as meat, eggs, nuts, herbs and spices, and instead, take foods that have a cooling effect, such as milk products, fruits and vegetables. Over-eating is avoided as it is believed to result in a very large baby and a subsequently difficult delivery.

Throughout the pregnancy, it is believed that the developing child is vulnerable to evil spirits. It is therefore the tradition of many Hindu families to perform rituals to protect the mother and the unborn baby. During the fifth month of pregnancy, some of the ceremonies performed may include *Valakappu*, *Puchutal* and *Saddha* and in the eighth month, another ritual, called *Simantam* may also be performed. Indian women may also protect themselves from evil spirits by wearing a type of amulet called a *valai* or *valayal*, which means, "to surround" (with an invisible barrier) to keep the pregnant woman safe from the influence of evil spirits.

The role of the Indian woman in labor is passive. She follows instructions from healthcare providers or family members. A stoic approach by the mother to the labor and delivery process is desirable, and receives praise. Although there is not a cultural standard that prohibits the father from being present during the delivery, men are usually not in the delivery room at the time of birth.

The recuperation time for the mother and baby usually lasts for 40 days after birth. During that time, the mother is encouraged to remain at home, where she is to obtain adequate rest and is offered special ("hot") foods along with regular meals. Cold foods are believed to produce diarrhea, indigestion, and gas and are therefore avoided. External heat as well as internal heat are encouraged for the recuperating mother. The mother should keep herself warm during this time. She will often have back massages with warm oil. She is discouraged from taking more than one bath a week, although she should wash her perineal area with warm water every time she eliminates.

Breastfeeding by Indian women is generally practiced and encouraged (except that colostrum is considered bad for the newborn infant). It is usually continued for anywhere from 6 months to 3 years. It is common for breast milk to be supplemented with cow's milk and diluted with sugar water. The child is given diluted milk because the infant's stomach is believed to be weak initially (Bhungalia *et al.*, 2000; Kemp & Bhungalia, 2002; Rajwani, 1996).

End of life

Many Hindu patients prefer to die at home, and some will go back to India – especially to the sacred city of Varanasi, to die. Consistent with the Western idea of resolving unfinished business, a Hindu person who is elderly or terminally ill may put significant effort into resolving relationships and other such personal matters. Dying full of anger or fear leads to a lower level of rebirth than dying full of love and acceptance. It is important to understand that a devout Hindu believes that she or he has already been born and died many times in the past, and this contributes to increased acceptance of terminal status and suffering (Kemp & Bhungalia, 2002).

The idea that suffering is inevitable and the result of *karma* may result in indifference with reporting symptoms and with symptom control. Many will seek a conscious dying process and death, and hence choose discomfort over clouded sensorium. Difficulties between hospice staff and family or the patient may arise when therapeutic measures are refused, especially when it seems that the patient may want or need the therapy, but the family influences her or him to refuse.

A person near death may be placed with her or his head facing east and a lamp placed near the head. Family members are likely to be present in large numbers as death nears. Chanting and prayer, incense, and various rituals are part of the process. These may include application of sacred ash or paste to the person's forehead, and placing a few drops of milk or water from the sacred Ganges River (or *Ganga Ma*) in the dying person's mouth. Ideally, the person who is dying will chant her or his mantra (a sacred phrase) as death occurs. If this is not possible, a family member may softly chant the mantra in the person's right ear. If there is not a chosen mantra, then *Aum Namo Narayana* or *Aum Nama Sivaya* may be used.

The moment of death is seen by some as similar to falling asleep, with the difference being that, in sleep, the silver cord that connects the body to the soul stays intact, but breaks in death.

After death, the family should be the only ones to touch the body, hence healthcare staff should touch the body as little as possible. Ideally, a family member should clean the body and this person should be of the same sex as the deceased. After being cleaned, a cloth is tied under the chin and over the top of the head, the thumbs and great toes tied together, and the body is wrapped in a red cloth and placed with the head facing south. Embalming and organ donation are prohibited.

When a person dies in a hospital, the family may want the death certificate signed as soon as possible and then transport the body home rather than to a funeral home. At the home, religious pictures are turned to the wall and mirrors may also be covered. The ceremony at the home includes prayer, incense, chanting, and singing sacred songs.

The preference is for cremation and, ideally, the ashes are spread over the holy river, The Ganges (or *Ganga Ma*). The men and boys of the family may shave their hair as a symbol of mourning for the dead. The mourning family may wear all white and wish to have a *Brahman* at the funeral to perform a prayer and blessing (Kemp & Bhungalia, 2002).

Health problems and screening

The healthy life expectancy or HALE in India is 51.4 years and the full life expectancy is 63 years (Population Reference Bureau, 2002; World Health Organization (WHO), 2002a). Infectious diseases are the leading causes of death and disability in India. India is classified by the WHO as a "moderate HIV prevalence country" with 500 000 deaths from HIV/AIDS expected in India in 2005 (WHO, 2001). India is also one of nine countries in the world with indigenous transmission of polio (high transmission rate), and is one of 22 countries with a high burden of tuberculosis (WHO, 2002b, 2003). India is also one of 11 countries accounting for more than 66% of world deaths from measles (Stein *et al.*, 2003). Health risks for new Indian immigrants or refugees (Hawn & Jung, 2003; Kemp, 2002; WHO, 2002a) include:

- amebiasis
- boutonneuse fever
- cholera

- dengue fever
- filariasis (Bancroftian filariasis and Malayan filariasis)
- granuloma inguinale or donovanosis (especially Southern India)
- hepatitis
- hookworm
- hymenolepiasis
- Kyasanur Forest hemorrhagic fever (Mysore State)
- leishmaniasis
- leprosy
- malaria
- malnutrition
- mycetoma (maduramycosis)
- poliomyelitis
- strongylodiasis
- sexually transmitted infections, including HIV/AIDS, cervical cancer, chancroid, chlamydia, gonorrhea, granuloma inguinale, lymphogranuloma venereum, syphilis
- thalassemias
- trachoma
- tuberculosis
- typhus

REFERENCES

American Psychiatric Association (2000). *Diagnostic and Statistical Manual of Mental Disorders*, 4th edn, text revision. Washington, DC: Author.

Bhatia, M. S. (2000). Compulsive spitting – a culture-bound syndrome. *Indian Journal of Medical Sciences*, **54**, 145–8.

Bhungalia, S., Kelly, T., Van De Keift, S., & Young, M. (2000). Indian health care beliefs and practices. Retrieved December 23, 2002 from http://www3.baylor.edu/~Charles_Kemp/indian_health.htm.

Chadda, R. K. & Ahuja, N. (1990). Dhat syndrome: a sex neurosis of the Indian subcontinent. *British Journal of Psychiatry*, **156**, 577–9.

Hawn, T. R. & Jung, E. C. (2003). Health screening in immigrants, refugees, and internationally adopted orphans. In *The Travel and Tropical Medicine Manual*, 3rd edn., ed. E. C. Jong and R. McMullen, pp. 255–65. Philadelphia, PA: W. B. Saunders.

Jilek, W. G. & Jilek-Aall, L. (1985). The metamorphosis of 'culture-bound' syndromes, *Social Science and Medicine*, **21**, 205–10.

Johnstone, P. & Mandryk, J. (2001). *Operation World: 21st century edn*. Waynesboro, GA: Paternoster USA.

Kemp, C. E. (2002). *Infectious Diseases*. Retrieved April 12, 2003 from http://www3.baylor. edu/~Charles_Kemp/Infectious_Disease.htm.

Kemp, C. & Bhungalia, S. (2002). Culture and the end of life: (Asian) Indian health beliefs and practices. *Journal of Hospice and Palliative Nursing*, **4**, 54–8.

Krause, I. B. (1989). Sinking heart: a Punjabi communication of distress. *Social Science and Medicine*, **29**, 563–75.

Kua, E. H., Sim, L. P. & Chee, K. T. (1986). A cross-cultural study of the possession-trance in Singapore. *Australian and New Zealand Journal of Psychiatry*, **20**, 361–4.

Morinis, A. (1985). Sanctified madness: the God-intoxicated saints of Bengal. *Social Science and Medicine, 21*, 211–20.

Population Reference Bureau (2002). *2002 World Population Data Sheet*. Retrieved May 12, 2003 from http://www.prb.org/pdf/WorldPopulationDS02_Eng.pdf.

Rajwani, R. (1996). South Asians. In *Culture and Nursing Care: A Pocket Guide*, ed. J. G. Lipson, S. L. Dibble, and P. A. Minarik. San Francisco: UCSF Nursing Press.

Roberts, J. M. (1993). *History of the World*. New York: Oxford University Press.

Rundle, A., Carvalho, M., & Robinson, M. (1999). *Cultural Competence in Health Care*. San in Francisco: Jossey-Bass.

Stein, C. E., Birmingham, M., Kurian, M., Duclos, P., & Strebel, P. (2003). The global burden of measles in the year 2000 – a model that uses country-specific indicators. *Journal of Infectious Diseases*, **187** *(Suppl. 1)*, S8–S14.

World Health Organization (2001). *HIV/AIDS in the Asia Pacific Region*. Retrieved April 12, 2003 from http://www.wpro.who.int/pdf/sti/aids2001/part2_grp2_a.pdf.

(2002a). *World Health Report*. Retrieved June 5, 2003 from http://www.who.int/whr/2002/en/.

(2002b). *Global Polio Status 2002*. Retrieved May 9, 2003 from http://www.polioeradication. org/all/global/.

(2003). *Global TB Control Report 2003*. Retrieved June 1, 2003 from http://www.who.int/gtb/ publications/globrep/index.html.

20

Iran

Introduction

Iran, known as Persia until 1935, became an Islamic republic in 1979 after the Islamic Revolution forced the ruling Shah into exile. Since the Revolution, Iran has experienced significant social upheaval. Conservative religious forces have attempted to stamp out all Western influences, including in 1979 the seizure of the US Embassy in Tehran. During 1980–88, Iran fought a bloody and costly war with Iraq over disputed territory. The war, as well as internal conflict, created massive population displacements, both internally and through emigration. Current issues affecting the country include reconciliation between clerical control of the ruling party and popular government participation, widespread demands for reform, and international tension between Iran and Iraq, and Iran and Israel (Central Intelligence Agency (CIA), 2003).

History of immigration

In the recent history of Iran, the 1979 Islamic Revolution, which ended the predominantly secular and Western-oriented Shah monarchy of decades in favor of Shiite Islamic political structure and law, is pivotal. The new political elite that emerged was made up of Moslem clerics and poorly educated middle-class bureaucrats. As there was great value placed on Western education during the period of the Shah, the vast majority of Iranians in the USA and abroad came as students, and many did not return after the Revolution. Similarly, there were many professionals who were already in the West and remained after Iran was restructured. Many were able to transfer their educational degrees and their wealth, and some have gone on to become citizens, especially in the USA. In fact, the largest population of Iranians in the Western world is in the USA (Bozorgmehr, 1996).

Refugee and Immigrant Health: A Handbook for Health Professionals, Charles Kemp and Lance A. Rasbridge. Published by Cambridge University Press. © C. Kemp and L. A. Rasbridge 2004.

However, on the whole, Iranian immigrants are surprisingly unassimiliated (Bozorgmehr, 1996). This is due, at least in part, to the nature of the more recent influx of Iranian exiles to the West, particularly religious minorities persecuted since the time of the Islamic revolution (e.g. Baha'is, Jews, Armenian Christians); and a smaller group of political dissidents. Thus this second wave of Iranians differs somewhat in demographics from the professionals and students arriving decades earlier. Through 2002, 35 218 Iranian refugees have resettled in the USA (Immigration and Refugee Services of America (IRSA), 2002), adding to a population of several hundred thousand earlier emigres. Iranian–Americans, immigrants and refugees alike, tend to be urban and educated; the largest concentration is found in southern California, particularly in Los Angeles (Sabagh & Bozorgmehr, 1987). Of all the refugees from Iran, members of the Baha'i faith are the vast majority. At least 10 000 Iranian Baha'is have found religious refuge in the USA since the Iranian Revolution (Baha'i Communications International (BCI), 2003), some forming their own communities but mostly blending into existing American Baha'i communities.

Culture and social relations

In Iranian culture, the ties to family, both nuclear and extended, supersede any other kinds of political or social alignments. The family's integrity is always more important than the individual's desires. Family ties form the basis of business as well as social relationships. Class distinctions tend to be delineated by access to political power, at least in the time of the Shah, and are quite rigid. But as mentioned, the Western population of Iranian immigrants tends to be secularized, Western educated, and upper or middle class. Elder respect is a commonality throughout all the cultural groups of Iran, regardless of kinship ties. It is considered one's sacred duty to take care of elders in times of illness.

Iranian society tends to be patriarchic. Traditionally, the male household head was in charge of all decision-making in relationship to the outside world, whereas the wife maintained considerable control over the household. Even though there has been, and continues to be, substantial reform in the area of women's rights outside of Iran, intrafamily stress still results from the perceived or real loss of status and control by men upon relocation to Western society (Hafizi, 1996).

In the West, marriage is more frequently by mutual choice rather than arranged, although there is still a marked preference toward marriage within one's own kin group, preferably second cousin or even first cousin marriage. For immigrants, a study in Los Angeles showed very little intermarriage between Iranians and the larger population: 90% of married Iranian-born females were married to another Iranian, either locally or in the homeland (Bozorgmehr, 1996). In Iran, polygamy is permissible under Islamic law, although the practice is not widespread. Divorce is permitted but is generally much more difficult for the woman than the man to initiate.

Communications

Iran has a markedly heterogeneous population based on ethnic heritage. Farsi (Persian) is the national language of Iran, but at least one-third of the population speaks a different primary language, such as Turkish, Armenian, Kurdish, Luri, and Baluchi, reflective of the sizeable minority communities. Most of these speakers are bilingual in Farsi, however, as it is typically the only language taught in schools. English is understood by a significant proportion of the Iranian community in the USA, particularly among the earlier immigrant waves of students and professionals (Bozorgmehr, 1996).

Although Farsi is derived from Arabic, the two spoken languages are not mutually intelligible. The written form of Farsi is based on Arabic script, read right to left, but it contains extra characters not found in Arabic. Farsi readers can generally read Arabic, at least for overall content. The Farsi language has never been Romanized, such that personal names are transliterated to Western characters with a great deal of inconsistency, and are usually phoneticized following French pronunciation.

Religion

Shiite Islam is followed by about 90% of the population in Iran. Within this group is some variation in religious adherence, with younger, educated and professional Iranians tending to be less conservative. Among the more fervent believers is the predominant belief in God's will (*tagdir*), as determinant of all things in life and death – an etiology of individual passivity in healthcare-seeking behavior (Hafizi, 1996).

Of all the different religious minority groups in Iran, including Sunni Muslims, Christians, Zoroastrians, and Jews, the Baha'is have been particularly oppressed by the Shiite majority. Muslims believe that the prophet Mohammed is "the seal of prophecy" and there cannot be succeeding prophets. Alternatively, the Baha'i faith, which originated some 1200 years after Mohammed, holds that "Divine Revelation is continuous and that all great religions, including Islam, are valid and represent successive stages in the spiritual evolution of human society" (BCI, 2003). This (and other beliefs) lead Islamists to regard Baha'is as infidels, subject to persecution and death under Islamic law. In Iran, hundreds of Baha'is have been executed, thousands jailed and tortured, and tens of thousands denied educational and economic opportunities under the intolerant regime since 1979 (BCI, 2003). Due to intense international pressure on the Iranian government, persecution of Baha'is is less severe in more recent years but the practice of Baha'i remains outlawed under the current regime.

Similar to the Iranian Baha'i immigrants, many of the other religious minorities such as Jews and Christian Armenians have melded into existing coreligious communities in the West and, in the case of Jews, in Israel.

Healthcare beliefs and practices

While the biomedical model of health and illness is understood by the majority of the Iranians in the West, and many in Iran, some aspects of folk causation may be expressed by the more traditional. For example, some Iranians view certain illnesses as a result of an imbalance in the body humors, a common folk etiology throughout the world.

Illness may result from eating disproportionately excessive "hot," (*gamay*) or "cold," (*sardy*) foods, culturally defined categories not necessarily referring to inherent temperature characteristics but rather the perceived effects on the body. In general, foods (or illnesses themselves) perceived to produce nausea, are classified as "cold." Watermelon, eggplant, and some animal organs are examples of "cold" foods. Or, the imbalance in homeostasis can result in a state of predisposition to other illness, including biomedically defined agents, e.g. germs. In a survey on health beliefs of Iranian immigrants, there was nearly universal agreement that diet had a great bearing on health, through humoral balance, and also, the consumption of fresh, unprocessed foods was necessary for good health (Lipson, 1992). Commonly, when the symptoms of illness are first perceived, the initial inquiry of causation is whether a person "ate something that did not agree with his *mezaj* (the individual's humoral temperament)" (Hafizi, 1996, p. 177).

Another folk belief held by some involves the power in the "evil eye" as a malevolent force in which certain people, especially those who covet one's wealth, good fortune, or health, are believed to be capable of casting an illness-causing spell. Many elderly Iranian immigrants are familiar with this concept, but few follow rituals thought to be protective against the evil eye (Lipson, 1992). In addition to using amulets and talismans, the burning of a seed known as *esfand* is also practiced to ward off malicious spirits (Lipson and Meleis, 1983). Here the incense-like smoke is allowed to fill the room, or in some cases, the soot is even rubbed on the skin. It should be noted that many less traditional Iranians, and Baha'is in particular, claim to not believe in the evil eye but simply enjoy the pleasant smell of the *esfand* in their homes.

Perhaps more common are the folk illnesses known as *ghalbam gerefteh* ("distress of the heart"), *saram sada meekoneh* ("pounding in one's head"), *narahati* ("sadness"), and *kam khun* ("blood deficiency") (Lipson, 1992; Pliskin, 1992).

"Distress of the heart," which can range in severity from tachycardia and palpitations to a heart attack, is commonly attributed to psychological stressors such as sadness, being homesick, or having insoluble problems (Lipson, 1992). It is an expression especially evoked in times of stress, from menial annoyances to life-threatening events. The second folk illness, "pounding in one's head," is attributed to general anxiety. And finally, *kam khun* is symptomatically analogous to anemia (e.g., weakness), though of a more psychosomatic nature, and is treated with iron-rich foods such as lentils, liver, and spinach (Pliskin, 1992). Literally translated complaints of these disorders may mislead healthcare providers.

Depression (*narahati*) is common among Iranian immigrants, because of adjustment difficulties and loss of homeland issues, and may manifest in somatic symptomotology. Iranian culture is replete with folk healers and traditional medical specialists (*hakim*); one survey in a small region in Iran found practitioners using herbal remedies, bone-setting (*shekasteband*), massage therapy with plant oils, cupping (*badkesh*), and leech therapy (Asefzadeh & Sameefar, 2001). The use of herbal and natural cures in Iran is a tradition extending over thousands of years.

Ibn Sina, an ancient Persian scientist, is credited as the founder of much of Islamic medicine. He discovered many medicinal cures, including a successful treatment of meningitis. However, more importantly, he developed a philosophy for medicine incorporating physical and psychological factors; and drugs and diet (Religion of Islam, 1999). Ibn Sina's influence is seen in the holistic approach of Iranian traditional medicine particularly, and Islamic medicine in general.

Some of the more common herbs and medicines are imported and are available in *atary* markets, Iranian medicine "pharmacies." Among the more common herbal treatments (Lipson, 1992; Pliskin, 1992) are the following.

- Mint tea and coriander are used for the promotion of relaxation and sleep.
- Quince seeds are sucked for relief of sore throat irritation.
- A tea made from foxglove (digitalis) called *gole gov zabon* is taken as an anxiolytic and strength tonic.
- *Khakshir* seeds from the plant Sisymbium Sophia are consumed and passed whole through the gastrointestinal tract as an "abrasive" to cleanse poisons.
- *Nabat* (rock candy) is made by boiling brown sugar, which is then cooled and allowed to coagulate around a string or object inserted in the pot. Chunks are broken off and added to hot tea, sometimes together with saffron or lemon. Believed to possess *gamay* (hot) humoral qualities, this tea is used for numerous conditions, ranging from lack of energy, "weak heart" or palpitations, to relief of menstrual cramps – or simply enjoyed as a sweet drink.

Finally, many older Iranians complain of joint pains consistent with the biomedical diagnosis of rheumatism. The folk etiology includes "catching a wind" from long-term exposure to cold and damp environments, or the symptoms may result from humoral imbalance in the diet (Pliskin, 1992).

When Iranians enter the Western medical care system, the expectation of being provided pharmaceuticals, ranging from "natural" medicines to injections, is common. Differing expectations of the provider/patient roles may lead to misunderstandings. For example, Lipson notes that some Iranian immigrants interviewed believe the relative tentativeness in diagnosing on the part of Western physicians, in comparison to Iranian practitioners, and the reliance on diagnostic tests in the Western care setting, are signs of incompetence or the lack of expertise (1992). "Doctor shopping" may be the end result.

Pregnancy and childbirth

Throughout the Middle East, and particularly for Muslims, pregnancy is perhaps the event that most marks the status of, and provides self-esteem to, women (Meleis & Sorrell, 1981). Giving birth to males demarcates a new level of social acceptance for women in many Middle Eastern cultures. In fact, the sex of the child can sometimes be of more concern than even the health of the newborn (Meleis & Sorrell, 1981). Pregnancy cravings (*viar*) are immediately supplicated, so as not to upset the mother's temperament. Throughout pregnancy, and concerning all issues of reproduction, modesty is culturally prescribed, even for non-Muslims.

In Iran, most births are assisted by a midwife in the home, but it is likely that Iranian immigrants will be familiar with hospital-based birthing and will request it. Except in the most assimilated families, fathers will not be actively involved in the birthing process or even in attendance. Except for Christian groups, circumcision for males is performed, usually in the first few days after birth and is replete with much ceremony.

Postpartum dietary prescriptions and proscriptions, especially as pertaining to humoral balance, are observed by some Iranians for a period of 40 days. Breast-feeding is the norm, for up to a year, with solids being introduced at 4–6 months of age. Traditionally, colostrum was considered "impure," and puppies were allowed to suckle until the colostrum disappeared! The more traditional, and/or Muslim women may be on guard from the "evil eye" and interpret praise towards the newborn as envy. Contraception may not be accepted by the more traditional Muslims, who may view it is potentially challenging to "God's will" (Meleis & Sorrell, 1981).

End of life

Many Iranians prefer that terminal prognosis be discussed with the male household head and concealed from the patient (Geissler, 1998). Extended family usually desire to be present at the bedside of a dying patient, preferably away from an institutional setting. In Iran as well as in other Middle Eastern cultures, to die without being surrounded by kin is considered the worst of fates, and children are expected to care for ailing parents regardless of circumstances (Lipson & Meleis, 1983).

Before death, open grieving is not practiced, but upon death mourning is quite pronounced among both men and women relatives and friends. Ripping at clothes, scratching, and even smearing the face with mud or ash are some of the common behaviors in grieving. Iranian immigrants frequently express puzzlement why other Americans appear so stoic in grieving – "Do they not love their families?"

Hafizi notes that most Muslim Iranians favor a Do Not Resuscitate order, as "death is seen as a beginning, not end, in which the mortal life gives way to spiritual existence" (1996, p. 175). Parenteral nutrition can be seen as insulting, as feeding is the responsibility of one's family. After death, the body is washed by same-sex relatives and/or an Imam or other holy person at the mosque or at home. The body is then clothed in white and buried, usually immediately. Cremation is not performed, and organ donation or autopsy are viewed dimly as well (Hafizi, 1996). Because Shiites believe that the holy Imams can intercede for the dead as well as for the living, cemeteries traditionally have been located adjacent to the most important shrines in both Iran and Shiite areas of Iraq. The expression of condolences through visiting surviving family members' households is culturally mandated for an extended period.

Health problems and Screening

The healthy life expectancy or HALE in Iran is 56.7 years and the full life expectancy is 69 years (Population Reference Bureau, 2002; World Health Organization (WHO), 2002). Infectious diseases are the leading causes of death and disability in rural Iran, while chronic non-infectious diseases are leading causes of death and disability in urban areas. Health risks for new Iranian immigrants or refugees (Hawn & Jung, 2003; Kemp, 2002; WHO, 2002) include:

- amebiasis
- anthrax
- boutonneuse fever
- brucellosis or undulant fever
- cholera
- Crimean–Congo hemorrhagic fever
- cysticercosis (tapeworm)
- dracunculiasis (Guinea worm disease)
- familial Mediterranean fever (Mediterranean area, primarily among persons of Sephardic Jewish, Armenian, and Arab ancestry)
- giardia
- helminthiasis (ascariasis, echinococcosis/hydatid disease, schistosomiasis)

- hepatitis
- hookworm
- leishmaniasis
- malaria (including chloroquine-resistant *Plasmodium falciparum*)
- plague
- sickle cell disease or sickle cell hemoglobulinopathies (occurs primarily in people of African lineage, but also to a lesser extent among people from the Mediterranean area, Arabs, and Indians)
- thalassemias
- toxocariasis
- trachoma
- trematodes (liver-dwelling: clonorchiasis and opisthorchiasis; blood-dwelling: schistosomiasis or bilharzias; intestine-dwelling; and lung-dwelling: paragonimiasis trichinosis (trichinella)
- tuberculosis (including multi-drug resistant strains)
- typhus

Acknowledgements

Dr. Farid Taie and Pedram Moghen

REFERENCES

Asefzadeh, S. & Sameefar, F. (2001). Traditional healers in the Qazvin region of the Islamic Republic of Iran: a qualitative study. *Eastern Mediterranean Health Journal*, 7, 544–50.

Baha'i Communications International (BCI) (2003). *Religious Persecution of Iranian Baha'is*. Retrieved January 27, 2003 from http://bci.org/boise/persecut.htm.

Bozorgmehr, M. (1996). Iranians. In *Refugees in America in the 1990s: A Reference Handbook* ed. D. Haines, pp. 213–31. Westport, CT: Greenwood Press.

Central Intelligence Agency (2002). Iran. *World Factbook* (updated 2003). Washington, DC Central Intelligence Agency. Retrieved May 1, 2003 from http://www.cia.gov/cia/publications/factbook/geos/ir.html.

Geissler, E. (1998). *Cultural Assessment*, 2nd edn. St. Louis: Mosby.

Hafizi, H. (1996). Iranians. In *Culture and Nursing Care: A Pocket Guide* ed. J. Lipson, S. Dibble, and P. Minarik, pp. 169–79. San Francisco: UCSF Nursing Press.

Hawn, T. R. & Jung, E. C. (2003). Health screening in immigrants, refugees, and internationally adopted orphans. In *The Travel and Tropical Medicine Manual*, 3rd edn., ed. E. C. Jong and R. McMullen, pp. 255–65). Philadelphia, PA: W. B. Saunders.

Kemp, C. E. (2002). *Infectious Diseases*. Retrieved April 12, 2003 from http://www3.baylor.edu/~Charles_Kemp/Infectious_Disease.htm.

Immigration and Refugee Services of America. (2002). *Refugee Reports, 23*, Retrieved January 29, 2003 from www.refugees.org.

Lipson, J. G. (1992). The health and adjustment of Iranian immigrants. *Western Journal of Nursing Research*, **14**, 10–24.

Lipson, J. G. & Meleis, A. I. (1983). Issues in the health care of Middle Eastern patients. *Western Journal of Medicine*, **139**, 854–61.

Meleis, A. & Sorrell, L. (1981). Arab American women and their birth experiences. *American Journal of Maternal and Child Nursing*, **6**, 171.

Pliskin, K. L. (1992). Dysphoria and somatization in Iranian culture. *The Western Journal of Medicine*, **157**, 295–301.

Population Reference Bureau (2002). *2002 World Population Data Sheet*. Retrieved May 12, 2003 form http://www.prb.org/pdf/WorldPopulationDSO2_Eng.pdf.

Religion of Islam (1999). *Introduction to Islam*. Retrieved May 12, 2003 from http://www.iad.org/Islam/medicine.html.

Sabagh, G. & Bozorgmehr, M (1987). Are the characteristics of exiles different from immigrants? The case of Iranians in Los Angeles. *Sociology and Social Research*, **71**, 77–83.

World Health Organization (2002). *World Health Report*. Retrieved June 5, 2003 from http://www.who.int/whr/2002/en/.

21

Iraq

Introduction

While the country of Iraq holds great oil wealth, the vast majority of Iraqis have benefited little from this potential. When Saddam Hussein rose to power in 1979, the country plunged into incessant war and internal strife. First came the disastrous 1980–88 Iran–Iraq war (a million killed at a cost of 100 billion dollars), then the *Anfal* or campaign to destroy Kurdish culture, followed by the Gulf War upon Saddam's invasion of Kuwait in 1990, and most recently the United States-led war of 2003 (Central Intelligence Agency (CIA), 2003; Glover, 1999). This chapter details historical and cultural factors for Iraqi refugees who fled during the Gulf War and its aftermath, through 2002. From the outset a distinction is made between Iraqi refugees and Kurdish refugees fleeing from northern Iraq ("Iraqi Kurdistan"). For this discussion, then, Iraqi refugees consist of two main groups:

- Iraqi political dissidents and surrendering or deserting members of Saddam Hussein's national army.
- Shiite Muslims, some of whom are the so-called "Marsh Arabs" from southern Iraq and a small number of whom are of Iranian descent.

There is also a third, smaller group of Iraqi "Turkomens" or Iraqis of Turkish descent.

Following the 1991 Gulf War, Shiite Muslims rebelled against the Iraqi regime. With the collapse of their rebellion in March of 1991, at least 100 000 Iraqi Shiites fled into neighboring Iran, Saudi Arabia, and the US-occupied zone along the Iraq–Kuwait border. Fearful of retribution against these refugees on the withdrawal of US troops from the region, the USA brokered a deal with the Saudi government for the establishment of a Saudi-maintained refugee camp near Rafha, and another camp called Al Artawea. Many refugees report that conditions in the Al Artawea camp were poor, especially for Arabs (as opposed to Kurds who also were

Refugee and Immigrant Health: A Handbook for Health Professionals, Charles Kemp and Lance A. Rasbridge. Published by Cambridge University Press. © C. Kemp and L. A. Rasbridge 2004.

housed there). Eventually, Al Artawea was closed, and all the refugees were sent to Rafha. Rafha camp was divided between the former members of the Iraqi army, overwhelmingly composed of single men, and the Iraqi families, most of whom were Shiites.

History of immigration

In the mid-1990s, it had became clear that Saddam Hussein's regime had not weakened, and repatriation for the tens of thousands of Iraqi refugees in neighboring countries meant certain retribution, especially for the former members of the Iraqi army and dissidents in Saudi Arabia. With pressure from the Saudi government, the USA agreed to resettle the Rafha group *en masse*, beginning in 1994. The USA government's decision met with considerable opposition, especially from veteran's groups, who argued that the resettled former members of the Iraqi army had been potential adversaries to Allied troops during the war. Furthermore, the existing resettled Kurdish populations also were distrustful of these potential "agents of Saddam." Nonetheless, over 32 000 Iraqi refugees were resettled in the United States through 2002, adding to the population of non-refugee Iraqi immigrants, for a total of about 90 000 foreign-born Iraqis (Grieco, 2003). The largest populations are in Detroit, Chicago, and San Diego.

Culture and social relations

Iraqi society on the whole can be viewed as having three classes: the political elite, the military and merchant class, and finally, peasants and laborers (Cultural Orientation, 2003). However, class differences aside, allegiance to the extended family and tribe is stronger than allegiance to a central government. Throughout the Arab world, loyalty to the family and tribe forms the basis of much of culture, with nepotism in employment common and individual behavior frequently tempered against the potential for shame to the larger family (Cultural Orientation, 2003).

It is not uncommon for girls to be involved in arranged marriages at a young age, as young as 12 or 13 years, with preference given to first-cousin marriage. To Iraqis, especially Shiites, the Islamic marriage is not only sacred, but also serves as a bond between families. However, this tradition of early marriage has flown in the face of United States law and there have been several widely publicized cases of arrests of men involved in unions with girls younger than 16. According to Islam, men may have up to four wives, but this not common among Shiites. At marriage, women come to live with the husband's family and married sons usually stay within the household. Children are to be the caretakers of their parents when they are elderly.

Iraqi households are very private and are sometimes segregated according to gender. Women in general are subservient to male authority, although it should be noted that Iraqi women on the whole enjoy more rights than other women from the Arabian peninsula (Cultural Orientation, 2003). Especially among Iraqi Sunnis, there are many educated and professional women. The husband controls the household finances, but women exert considerable influence over the children, including grown sons. Male relatives show concern over the treatment of their female kin after marriage.

Communications

Arabic is the universal language of Iraq. While there are over 15 dialects of spoken Arabic throughout the world, defined by geographical and rural/urban differences (Cultural Orientation, 2003), Iraqi refugees appear to have little difficulty in comprehending any Arabic speaker. However, literacy in Arabic is rather low in Iraq, at an estimated 58% (CIA, 2003). Even though Iraq experienced significant British political influence earlier in this century, English language fluency is rare among resettled Iraqis.

It is never acceptable for a man to shake the hand of a Shiite woman. Sunni women, on the other hand, are less restricted. Touching, and even full embracing, is quite common within (but not between) the sexes, especially when greeting. When greeting, deference is always given first to males.

Religion

Most Iraqis are Shiite Muslims, but the political elite, the military and merchant classes, and those living around the capital area of Baghdad in general are Sunni. In general, Shiites are more orthodox and strict in religious practices, food proscriptions, and especially, treatment of women. Shiite Muslim women, especially older women and widows, dress typically in black, in full "*hijab*" (purdah), covering their bodies and faces. At all public events, and even within the household, women are segregated from men.

Both Sunnis and Shiites adhere to *halal* laws regarding food. Any meat consumed by a Muslim must come from an animal slaughtered by another Muslim in a prescribed way, or it is considered impure, *haram*. This ritual involves asking God for forgiveness for taking the life of the animal. Furthermore, pork and alcohol are especially *haram* and should never be consumed. Even in the West, most Iraqis do not buy meat or chicken in a grocery store but prefer to go to farms to buy the meat fresh, or from a few trusted *halal* markets. Islam is discussed in greater detail in Chapter 5.

Health beliefs and practices

Islam and related cultural practices are important influences on health beliefs and practices. Both women and men are modest and either may resist or refuse examination or treatment by a person of the opposite gender. Dietary proscriptions and fasting requirements also influence health. During Ramadan, for example, more conservative Muslims may refuse medications or medically indicated foods during daylight hours.

The peoples of Iraq have a long tradition of complementary and alternative medical practices, although there is much variation between tribes and across geographical areas. The following discussion describes some of the more common, but by no means universal, traditional medicine beliefs and practices (Rasbridge, 2001).

- Fever is sometimes treated with cumin and egg yolk heated in water and dipped onto a rag and put over the forehead.
- Conjunctivitis may be treated by laying a cloth boiled in tea over the eye.
- Dental pain may be treated with ground cumin, ninia seed, and shabak seed, mixed together as a powder and put on the gum.
- Tonsillitis is sometimes treated by certain elderly women who insert their fingers into the mouth of the child to manipulate the tonsils by pushing from side to side or squeezing to relieve the inflammation.
- Respiratory distress is sometimes treated with honey and lemon juice or lemon and orange juice together (for cough). A sort of steam tent is made for upper respiratory infections. Anise seed, boiled in water is used for sore throat or laryngitis.
- Gastrointestinal distress may be treated in one of several ways. Abdominal pain may be treated with cumin powder dissolved in water or with green tea. *Karawya* herb, boiled in water, is also given for abdominal pain, diarrhea and constipation, especially for children. Lemon juice and plain rice are also given for diarrhea. A heated brick is sometimes used for diarrhea, where the brick is covered with a cloth and sat upon.
- Flank pain may be treated with handel, a type of bitter fruit, which is cut, boiled, and drunk as a tea.
- Infertility is sometimes addressed by placing a placenta on the threshold of the infertile couple's house.
- Joint dislocation may be treated with ninia and churned butter mixed together as a salve and applied at the site of dislocation.
- Burns are sometimes treated with barley mixed with butter, and applied as a poultice on the burn for 48 hours.
- Cysts, splinters, and pimples may be treated with a dough of flour and sugar applied to the affected area.

Henna dye is considered to have magical healing properties, and is quite commonly seen, especially on Iraqi women. For example, it can be used for treatment of migraine headaches, where the hair is dyed. Henna can also be painted on the hands and feet, not just for decoration but for pain relief and also for protection from evil spirits and "evil eye." Tattoos can also serve the same purpose. For example, Islamic holy words can be written on the hand, such as "Allah" on the front, and "Ali" on the back. Circular tattoos over the temples are common for treatment of migraine headaches.

Among the most conservative Iraqi Muslims, typically the elderly, Western preventive health concepts may conflict with the belief that God has determined one's lifespan from birth which cannot (and should not) be altered by human intervention.

Pregnancy and childbirth

In pregnancy, other female household members relieve the pregnant woman from household tasks, and in general, pregnant women receive more attention and care than usual. Some Iraqis believe that sonograms to determine the sex of a developing fetus is against God's will and should not be performed. In Iraq, midwives provide minimal prenatal care and most deliveries are at home.

After delivery, the placenta may be thrown in water, in a folk belief to encourage milk production. Circumcision of boys usually occurs within the first few days, accompanied by a ceremony and feast. Commonly, a barber performs the circumcision; crushed onions, sumaq seed, and other acidic foods are placed over the circumcision and the umbilicus for a few days to promote healing. During the circumcision, the person who holds the child is perceived to establish a very significant bond with the child. Females have their ears pierced at 1 week. Breastfeeding is the norm, a least for 1 year, for both sexes. Rice soup, potatoes, and bread are common weaning foods, as is *leban*, a yogurt-based drink.

Birth control is virtually non-existent in Iraq, as limiting births or interfering with conception in any way is thought by many to be against the laws of Islam as life is considered a gift from God. Likewise, abortion in any form is out of the question. In the West, Iraqi women are beginning to use oral contraceptives, depo-provera, IUDs, and even tubal ligation. Even among husbands support for birth control is growing. There is an acceptance, or at least a rationalization, that limiting births is a means for adaptation and economic sufficiency in the West.

End of life

Expression of pain is usually a private matter, except during labor and delivery (Geissler, 1998). On hospitalization in the West, the family will stay with the patient and often will bring food, not trusting the hospital diet to be *halal*. The eldest male present will act as family spokesman and should be included in discussions whenever possible. There are differences of opinion among Muslim clerics about whether organ donations or autopsies are acceptable (Al-Mousawi *et al.*, 1997; Geissler, 1998). Life-support measures would be acceptable to most Iraqis.

At death, the body is taken to the mosque, where family, friends, and the Imam (clergy) take turns reading from the *Qur'an*. White sheets are wrapped around the body, after ritualistic washing, and burial takes place as soon as possible, usually the same day. Traditionally, the body is wrapped in cloth (not put in a casket) and carried to the cemetery on a litter during a funeral procession. The ritualized recitation from the *Qur'an* (sometimes a tape recording may be substituted) continues until the following Friday evening prayers, asking God to forgive the deceased for past sins. Black clothes are worn during mourning. A widowed wife may remarry 6 months after the husband's death, sometimes to the husband's brother. An exception is made in cases where a husband is missing in war, in which case she may remarry only after 7 years. Cremation is not permitted by Islam (Geissler, 1998).

There is a spiritual-healing ceremony centered around the gravesite of a sheikh or very holy or powerful person. People with mental problems or infertility (almost always assumed to be the woman), are taken to the grave marker. An animal is sacrificed, and food is given to the poor. Through prayer, as the participants hold hands around the gravesite, the deceased person's spirit is called upon to ask God to intervene on the sick person's behalf. Similarly, people can have a bad spirit or *jinn* (*jinn* refers to any spirit) exorcised through this ceremony. Commonly, a certain green material is hung around the gravesite, like a curtain. Many Arabs, especially Shiites, cut scraps of the material and pin it to themselves as a sort of charm for protection against evil spirits.

Health problems and screening

As this is written, it is unclear what changes, if any, in the health status of the Iraqi people will occur after the 2003 war to overthrow the Saddam Hussein regime. Before the war, Iraqis overall had healthy life expectancies (HALE) of 50.5 years and overall life expectancies of 58 years (Population Reference Bureau, 2002; World Health Organization (WHO), 2002). If the population were studied according to ethnicity (Arabs vs. Kurds) and religion (Sunni vs. Shiite), a different picture would likely emerge, with Arabs and non-Kurd Sunnis having greater HALEs and overall life expectancies than Kurds or Shiites. Health risks in refugees and immigrants from Iraq (Hawn & Jung, 2003; Kemp, 2002; WHO, 2002) include:

- amebiasis
- anthrax

- boutonneuse fever
- brucellosis or undulant fever
- cholera
- Crimean–Congo hemorrhagic fever
- cysticercosis (tapeworm)
- dracunculiasis (Guinea worm disease)
- familial Mediterranean fever (Mediterranean area, primarily among persons of Sephardic Jewish, Armenian, and Arab ancestry)
- giardia
- helminthiasis (ascariasis, echinococcosis/hydatid disease, schistosomiasis)
- hepatitis B (13% carriage rate)
- hookworm
- leishmaniasis
- malaria
- plague
- sickle cell disease or sickle cell hemoglobulinopathies (occurs primarily in people of African lineage, but also to a lesser extent Arabs and others)
- thalassemias
- toxocariasis
- trachoma
- trematodes (liver-dwelling: clonorchiasis and opisthorchiasis; blood-dwelling: schistosomiasis or bilharzias; intestine-dwelling; and lung-dwelling: paragonimiasis)
- trichinosis (trichinella)
- tuberculosis
- typhus
- post-traumatic stress disorder
- nutritional deficits

Acknowledgements

Adil Abdullah and Mervat Moussa

REFERENCES

Al-Mousawi, M., Hamed, T., & Al-Matouk, H. (1997). Views of Muslim scholars on organ donation and brain death. *Transplantation Proceedings*, **29**, 3217.
Central Intelligence Agency (2003). *World Factbook*. Retrieved April 10, 2003 from www.cia.gov/cia/publications/factbook.

Cultural Orientation (2003). *Iraqis: Their History and Culture.* Retrieved April 10, 2003 from http://www.culturalorientation.net.

Geissler, E. M. (1998). *Cultural Assessment,* 2nd edn. Mosby: St. Louis.

Glover, J. (1999). *Humanity: A Moral History of the Twentieth Century.* New Haven: Yale University Press.

Grieco, E. (2003). *Iraqi Immigrants in the United States.* Migration Information Source. Retrieved April 10, 2003 from http://www.migrationinformation.org.

Hawn, T. R. & Jung, E. C. (2003). Health screening in immigrants, refugees, and internationally adopted orphans. In *The Travel and Tropical Medicine Manual,* 3rd edn. ed. E. C. Jong and R. McMullen, pp. 255–65. Philadelphia, PA: W. B. Saunders.

Kemp, C. E. (2002). *Infectious Diseases.* Retrieved April 12, 2003 from http://www3.baylor.edu/~Charles_Kemp/Infectious_Disease.htm.

Population Reference Bureau (2002). *2002 World Population Data Sheet.* Retrieved May 12, 2003 from http://www.prb.org/pdf/WorldPopulationDS02_Eng.pdf.

Rasbridge, L. A. (2001). *Iraqi Refugees.* Retrieved April 4, 2002 from www.baylor.edu/~Charles_Kemp/refugee_health.htm.

World Health Organization (2002). *World Health Report.* Retrieved June 5, 2003 from http://www.who.int/whr/2002/en/.

22

Japan

Introduction

The healthcare beliefs and practices of immigrants from Japan will vary widely from the traditional to the more Western oriented, dependent in large part to the degree of acculturation, and to some extent, the social background in Japan. Of course, acculturation of immigrants in general has much to do with the generation of the individual since immigration. However, even among Japanese immigrants of several generations, many core cultural values remain. This chapter focuses on these more traditional values, with the caveat that they are not universally held by all Japanese immigrants.

History of immigration

While most of the immigration from Japan to the USA occurred a century or more ago, at first to Hawaii as contract laborers, there have been more recent waves as well. The 2000 US Census showed nearly 800 000 individuals identifying their race as Japanese (Tanabe, n.d.). However, while earlier generations of Japanese Americans married other Japanese, one study in California showed almost 80% of Japanese Americans marrying individuals of another ethnicity; hence the number of individuals self-identifying as Japanese or Japanese Americans is expected to decline in the next generation (Pacbell, 2001). Similarly, in 1970, Japanese were the largest group of Asians in California, but by 1990 the population ranked fourth among peoples of Asian decent, following Chinese, Vietnamese, and Korean (Pacbell, 2001).

Japanese Americans are frequently categorized, and refer to themselves, in terms of the number of generations of their families since arrival. The following terms are commonly employed:

Refugee and Immigrant Health: A Handbook for Health Professionals, Charles Kemp and Lance A. Rasbridge. Published by Cambridge University Press. © C. Kemp and L. A. Rasbridge 2004.

- *Issei*, the generation that was born in Japan;
- *Nisei*, the first generation born overseas;
- *Sansei*, the children of first generation born overseas; and
- *Yonsei*, children of the *sansei*.

Note that these terms do not necessarily reflect age of the individual but solely the number of generations of ancestors in the USA.

Culture and social relations

Traditionally, Japanese society is rather patriarchal, with every family member's position delineated in reference to the male head of household. Japanese women are more passive and exert power primarily in the domestic arena, although of course this pattern is changing, particularly among immigrants. Respect for, and observance of, social rank is pervasive in Japanese interaction, with elders receiving profound respect.

Conversely, many Japanese immigrants made tremendous sacrifices in order for their children to have a better life. Hence through Confucianism and filial piety (see Religion below) there is both an element of expectation from parents in addition to obligations towards them (Levine & Rhodes, 1981; Tanabe, n.d.).

Family size in contemporary times is quite small. Divorce is uncommon for Japanese Americans, at fewer than 2% of those ever married. Peer and communal pressures, avoidance of shame, and the "self-consciousness of this small minority who come from a strong, extended family structure" all contribute to marital stability (Levine & Rhodes, 1981, p. 55).

Level of acculturation needs to be assessed and understood when interacting with a Japanese American patient. For example, as with many immigrant groups, the third generation may not speak their ancestor's language and may appear to be quite Westernized. Moreover, recent immigrants are likely to have either graduate educations or be very successful in business. However, despite the outward symbols, their decision-making in the health care arena (and elsewhere) may still be profoundly influenced by the more core Japanese values (McLaughlin & Braun, 1998).

In traditional Japanese families, four principles guide decision-making in the healthcare setting or otherwise (adapted from Hattori *et al.*, 1991; McLaughlin & Braun, 1998).

- Collective family interests take precedent over those of the individual.
- Harmony must be maintained at all costs.
- The family is responsible for elder care.
- All the members of the family are interdependent.

The importance of the family and roles within the family is seen in the culture-bound syndrome known as "selfish mother," in which the mother seeks personal fulfilment rather than living *kodomo ga ikigai* (my child is my reason for living) or as *ryosai kenbo* (good wife and wise mother). The "selfish mother" is thought to have a negative impact on her family, especially the mental and physical health of her children (1upinfo, 1994; Leong, 2003).

Communications

The Japanese language reflects the hierarchical nature of Japanese society. For example, Japanese is filled with honorific/humble terms, verb endings expressing relationships of superiority/inferiority, and male/female vocabulary and pronouns – all of which reflect the important degrees of politeness when addressing people of differing social statuses. Communication is often indirect – with the listener expected to understand the point of the conversation without being told the point (Murashima, 2003). Confrontation is avoided, especially with those considered in a higher status, such as physicians. Refusal is usually through polite affirmation followed by inaction rather than outright denial (1upinfo, 1994). Sustained attempts at clarifying an issue are thus likely to lead to anxiety rather than understanding.

On greeting, handshakes between men are appropriate, but embracing or even innocent touching is considered too personal. More commonly, Japanese greet by bowing the head, and the more exaggerated, the more respect shown. Direct eye contact with an individual of higher status is considered rude.

Compared to other Asian Americans, Japanese Americans, even the elderly, are relatively proficient in English (Levine & Rhodes, 1981). English as a second language is emphasized in Japan.

Religion

To understand the religious life, and moreover, the world view of people from Japan, one must take into account the three major religions (Shintoism, Buddhism, and Confucianism) that have influenced Japan throughout its history.

In Shintoism, which is indigenous to Japan, the natural world is seen to be composed of spirits, *kami*, which must be propitiated for inner and worldly harmony to be achieved. There is much emphasis on ritual meant to purify the mind and the body.

With origins in China, Confucianism as a philosophy has been very influential on the Japanese. A main tenet of Confucianism is the concept of filial piety, which is profoundly embedded in the Japanese culture. Here, respect and responsibility to parents and family in general takes precedence over all other social interactions. It is one's solemn duty to attend to the needs of one's parents in their senescence, for example. And one's good actions and deeds in life bring honor to parents and to the family on the whole.

Buddhism, introduced from Korea in the Sixth Century, teaches the cyclical nature of life, death and rebirth. Through adherence to the prescribed Eightfold Path of righteous behavior, one accumulates merit (*karma*) which in turn bears on one's position in the next life. Japanese in the homeland and among the immigrant population largely accept both Shinto and Buddhist precepts. Tanabe (n.d.) notes that birth and marriage rites are often Shinto rituals while end of life beliefs and practices follow a more Buddhist approach. Of course, there are Christian converts in the Japanese immigrant community as well, with 35% in a sample of over 2000 Japanese Americans professing Christianity (Levine and Rhodes, 1981). Overall, Japanese religious thought and practice "emphasizes the maintenance of harmonious relations with others (both spiritual beings and other humans) and the fulfilment of social obligations as a member of a family and a community" (1upinfo, 1994).

Healthcare beliefs and practices

Within Japanese culture there are several paths to deal with illness. Overall, the utilization of cosmopolitan medical services is dominant among in Japan and among Japanese immigrants. However, traditional medical practices, *kampo*, can be employed as a first resort, or sometime in conjunction with more Western care. The traditional Japanese model of health as the balanced flow of energy through the body is derived from the Chinese model. Restoration of flow can be achieved through the ingestion of herbal remedies. Similarly, shiatsu massage, hot springs baths, acupuncture and acupressure, and moxibustion may also be performed to restore the energy flow. Fever may be treated by "sweating it out" through hot drinks and warm clothing and blankets (Geissler, 1998; Tanabe, n.d.).

Also, an ill person may visit a Shinto or Buddhist shrine (or even send a family member in their stead) to venerate the spirits and seek their intervention (1upinfo, 1994). Shinto priests and Buddhist monks may be called upon to exorcise negative spirits or provide blessings of health and good luck, and the like.

Mental illness is stigmatized in Japan and is kept hidden because it is believed to bring shame on a family. For traditional Japanese, mental and emotional problems are attributable to genetics, bad karma, or poor guidance from the family (Shon & Ja, 1982). While these notions are changing, service utilization of mental health facilities is still low both in the West and in Japan.

Relationships between the patient, family, and healthcare team are consistent with the previously noted hierarchical relationships among Japanese: the physician is clearly in charge. It is unusual for patients or others to question the physician and second opinions are uncommon. The physician decides what the patient is told about her or his health problem; it is not uncommon for patients and families to not be told essential or accurate information such as diagnosis or prognosis (Murashima, 2003).

Culture-bound syndromes found among Japanese include the previously noted "selfish mother" syndrome and the following disorders (American Psychiatric Association, 2000; Matsunaga *et al.*, 2001).

- *Taijin kyofusho* or anthropophobia is an intense social anxiety characterized by fear of offending others and social withdrawal.
- *Imu* (more commonly known by the Malaysian term, *latah*) is hypersensitivity to sudden fright, with attending dissociative or trancelike behaviors.

Pregnancy and childbirth

Just as in Japan, the number of children per Japanese–American woman is very low, at less than 1.2, accounting for the lowest birthrate of all American groups (Pacbell, 2001). Abortion was common in Japan, but the use of oral contraceptives is now widespread both in Japan and among Japanese immigrants.

Traditionally, after the fifth month of pregnancy, the woman's family presents her with a special *obi* which is worn about the waist for good luck and health. About 1 month before the anticipated birth a pregnant mother leaves the household of the husband to return to the care of her parents. She remains there for the birth and for about 1 month postpartum. Breastfeeding incidence is high, but only half of babies are breastfed at 1 month, and colostrum is not fed to the newborn (Geissler, 1998).

Naming is traditionally done during a ceremony of "seventh night," when the child is officially introduced to the world. On the first birthday of the child, various tools are placed in front of the crawling child to help predict his future. The child's choice of tools is significant in determining his future profession (University of Hawaii, n.d.)

End of life

As mentioned earlier, institutionalization of the sick and dying is in conflict with Confucian values and would be avoided by the most traditional. However, among the more acculturated immigrants, acceptance of nursing homes is on the rise, especially for those facilities designed to be ethnically appropriate (McCormick *et al.*, 1996; Kendis, 1980). Dementia in particular is the illness that Japanese immigrants cite as necessitating facility-based healthcare (McCormick *et al.*, 1996).

Discussion of terminal prognosis is a delicate matter and more traditional Japanese are likely to prefer that such discussion be with the eldest male family member. Older people may defer all decision-making entirely to the eldest son. In Shinto tradition, death is considered "impure" in the sense that it should not be dwelt upon. However, at least traditionally, many embrace Buddhism later in life, wherein death is not to be feared but rather accepted and even anticipated as the natural order of the cycle of rebirth (Tanabe, n.d.).

Active euthanasia is universally viewed as contradictory to Buddhism's precept against killing. However, a more passive approach, such as allowing the patient to die through disconnection of life support, for example, may be more accepted (Braun & Nichols, 1997).

At death, grieving by family and friends is usually a private and somewhat subdued affair, as public displays of extreme emotion of any sort is normally considered inappropriate. Traditional Buddhists will request a monk to the bedside to lead the "pillow sutra," a chant to bring peace and gratitude to the deceased's spirit (Braun & Nichols, 1997). Organ donation and autopsy may not be viewed well, "because of the importance of dying intact." Similarly, the body is viewed as a gift from the ancestors and should not be defaced (Braun & Nichols, 1997; Tanabe, n.d.).

White is the color of mourning in Japanese (and most Asian) cultures. Cremation rather than burial is preferred. Seven days after the funeral another memorial service is held, and sometimes subsequent memorial services, such as at 100 days, and certain yearly anniversaries of the death. Also, Japanese culture, like many Asian cultures, celebrates the lives of all the deceased at yearly holidays, known as *Obon* season in Japanese (Braun & Nichols, 1997). Even the more acculturated Japanese immigrants frequently have a shrine or memorial (*butsudan*) in their homes, containing pictures and names of deceased relatives, where the spirits of the ancestors (*hotoke*) are remembered through prayers and symbolic offerings (Kendis, 1980).

Health problems and screening

The healthy life expectancy or HALE in Japan is 73.6 years (longest HALE in the world) and the full life expectancy is 81 years (Population Reference Bureau, 2002; World Health Organization (WHO), 2002). Chronic non-infectious diseases are the leading causes of death and disability, and health risks for new Japanese immigrants are primarily cardiac disease, cancer, diabetes, and other chronic noninfectious diseases.

Most cancer rates are lower in the Japanese immigrant population than in most other US populations, particularly breast, ovarian and prostate cancers. However, stomach cancer is twice as common in Japanese Americans than in most other US groups, perhaps due to a preference for foods high in nitrites and salts, like cured meats (Tanabe, n.d.). More than 50% of Japanese men smoke cigarettes, thus increasing risk for lung cancer, cardiac disease, and COPD (Murashima, 2003). Another disease of higher than average prevalence is Type II diabetes. A study of Nisei men between 45 and 74 in Seattle found 20% to have diabetes (half of which undiagnosed) and 56% with abnormal glucose tolerance tests, rates twice as high as the general population (Fujimoto *et al.*, 1987). Those with diabetes were found to have high fat and animal protein diets. Finally, lactose intolerance is common in Japanese and Japanese immigrants (Tanabe, n.d.). Health risks (Hawn & Jung, 2003; Kemp, 2002; WHO, 2002) include:

- anisakiasis
- arbovirus encephalitis
- hemorrhagic fever with renal syndrome
- scrub typhus: (louse-borne typhus)
- chronic non-infectious diseases such as cardiac disease and related, cancer, diabetes, COPD.

REFERENCES

1upinfo (1994). *Country Study and Guide: Japan.* Retrieved June 20, 2003 from http://www.1upinfo.com/country-guide-study/japan.

Braun, K. L. & Nichols, R. (1997). Death and dying in four Asian American cultures: a descriptive study. *Death Studies*, **21**, 327–59.

Fujimoto, W. Y., Leonetti, J. L., Kinyoun, J. L. *et al.* (1987). Prevalence of diabetes mellitus and impaired glucose tolerance among second-generation Japanese American men. *Diabetes*, **36**, 721–9.

Geissler, E. M. (1998). *Cultural Assessment*, 2nd edn. St. Louis, MO: Mosby.

Hattori, H., Salzberg, S. M., Kiang, W. P., Fujimiya, T., Tejima, Y., & Furuno, J. (1991). The patient's right to information in Japan: legal rules and doctor's opinions. *Social Science and Medicine*, **32**, 1007–16.

Hawn, T. R. & Jung, E. C. (2003). Health screening in immigrants, refugees, and internationally adopted orphans. In *The Travel and Tropical Medicine Manual*, 3rd edn., E. C. Jong and R. McMullen, pp. 255–65. Philadelphia, PA: W. B. Saunders.

Kemp, C. (2002). *Infectious Diseases.* Retrieved April 22, 2003 from http://www3.baylor.edu/~Charles_Kemp/Infectious_Disease.htm.

Kendis, R. J. (1980). The Elderly Japanese in America: An Analysis of their Adaptation to Aging. Ph.D. Dissertation, University of Pittsburgh. Ann Arbor, MI: University Microfilms International.

Leong, Y. M. (2003). Japanese. In P. St. Hill, J. G. Lipson, & A. I. Meleis (Eds.), *Caring for women cross-culturally.* Philadelphia: F. A. Davis.

Levine, G. N. and C. Rhodes (1981). *The Japanese American community: A three-generation study.* New York: Praeger.

McCormick, W. C., Uomoto, J., Young, H. *et al.* (1996). Attitudes toward the use of nursing homes and home care in older Japanese-Americans. *Journal of the American Geriatrics Society*, **44**, 769–77.

McLaughlin, L. A. & Braun, K. (1998). Asian and Pacific Islander cultural values: considerations for health care decision making. *Health and Social Work*, **23**, 116–27.

Matsunaga, H., Kiriike, N., Matsui, T., Iwasaki, Y. & Stein, D. (2001). Taijin kyofusho: A form of social anxiety disorder that responds to serotonin reuptake inhibitors? *International Journal of Neuropsychopharmacology*, **4**, 231–237.

Murashima, S. (2003). Japan. In *Cultural Health Assessment*, 3rd edn., ed. C. E. D'Avanzo and E. M. Geissler, pp. 398–403. St. Louis, MI: Mosby.

Pacbell (2001). *Japanese Americans – A Declining Population*. Retrieved June 25, 2003 from http://home.pacbell.net/cnet/japaneseamericans.html.

Population Reference Bureau (2002). *2002 World Population Data Sheet*. Retrieved May 12, 2003 from http://www.prb.org/pdf/WorldPopulationDS02_Eng.pdf.

Shon, S. P. & Ja, D. A. (1982). Asian families. In *Ethnicity and Family Therapy*, ed. M. McGoldrick, J. K. Pearche and J. Giordano, pp. 208–28. New York: Guilford.

Tanabe, K. G. (n.d.). *Health and Health Care of Japanese–American Elders*. Retrieved June 15, 2003 from http://www.stanford.edu/group/ethnoger/japanese.html.

University of Hawaii (n.d.). *Traditional Japanese Beliefs and Practices*. Retrieved June 25, 2003 from http://www.hawcc.hawaii.edu/nursing/tradjapan2.htm.

World Health Organization (2002). *World Health Report*. Retrieved June 5, 2003 from http://www.who.int/whr/2002/en/.

23

Korea

Manja Lee

Note: Although traditional Korean culture is the same across North and South Korea, this chapter addresses conditions only among immigrants from South Korea.

Introduction

The Korean peninsula, while historically and culturally dominated by China, was militarily occupied by Japan from 1910–1945. Following World War II the peninsula was divided into a southern republic (the Republic of Korea or more commonly, South Korea) and the communist Democratic People's Republic of Korea, commonly called North Korea. The Korean War was fought from 1950–1953, after which an armistice divided the peninsula at a demilitarized zone along the 38th parallel. Since then, South Korea has enjoyed rapid technological and economic growth, while North Korea has retreated into a xenophobic police state which has experienced terrible famine (1994–present) and essentially no growth except militarily (Central Intelligence Agency (CIA), 2003; Hassan, 1998; Johnstone & Mandryk, 2001).

History of immigration

Except for laborers being taken, often by force, to China or Japan, there was very little outmigration from Korea until after World War II. Since then, Koreans have immigrated primarily to the USA. The first large wave of Koreans came to the USA between 1953 and 1965. Following easing of immigration laws in 1965, a larger wave came from 1976 to 1990. Since 1988 the number of Korean immigrants has decreased, probably because of steadily improving economic conditions in

Refugee and Immigrant Health: A Handbook for Health Professionals, Charles Kemp and Lance A. Rasbridge. Published by Cambridge University Press. © C. Kemp and L. A. Rasbridge 2004.

South Korea (Columbia University, n.d.). There were slightly more than 1.1 million Koreans living in the USA in 2000 (Barnes & Bennett, 2002). Except to the People's Republic of China, there is virtually no outmigration from North Korea.

Culture and social relations

South Korea (hereafter, Korea) is an industrialized and technological country, albeit one with rural roots and a culture that is very strongly family oriented. The home life of most Koreans is based on Confucianism, including the concept of filial piety that attaches great importance to the structure of family relationships, especially the father–son relationship. The relative status of individuals within the family and in society is rigid, with older superior to younger, parents superior to children, and men superior to women. The place of individuals in the family extends to the deceased, with respect paid to ancestors on a daily basis at the family altar, as well as at holidays, especially during the Harvest Moon celebration (Im *et al.*, 2002; Purnell & Kim, 2003).

Traditionally, marriage in Korea is arranged by the parents according to Confucian precepts. Marriage is considered to secure the succession of lineage and the prosperity of the family rather than individual happiness. The parental arrangement remains relatively common, even in the West, though the final decision is usually up to the individuals involved. Korean women do not change their maiden names even after their marriage because the maiden name represents their family blood line.

Though a taboo subject outside of the family, violence toward both women and children is relatively common in Korean families (50% prevalence in some studies), both in Korea and in the West, and especially in tradition-oriented families. The violence tends to be severe and may include injury to the victim (Kim *et al.*, 2000; Purnell & Kim, 2003).

Both tradition and the exigencies of life as an immigrant lead to enormous pressure on the young to excel in school. Failure to excel shames the family and has high potential to lead to corporal punishment. As with many other traditional cultures, the perceived shame of an individual is as much or even more the shame of the family (Hassan, 1998; Purnell & Kim, 2003).

All Koreans have three names: the family name (surname) placed first, a name identifying the generation, ordinarily the same between brother and sister, and an individual given name. In the West, however, many take a Western first name.

Religion

Religion and philosophy were introduced in Korea via China with the teachings of Confucianism and Buddhism. The teachings of the West were introduced to Korea first by Jesuit missionaries and later by Protestants. There is wide variability in estimates of percentages of people practicing particular religions, but most references agree that many Koreans – 35% or more – are non-religious. Approximately 30% are Christian, 20% Buddhist, and 8% practitioners of indigenous or "new" religions. Christian churches, especially Protestant, experienced enormous growth in the last decades of the 20th century, with the number of churches doubling from 1984 to 2000 (Chang, 2003; Johnstone & Mandryk, 2001).

As Korea opened to the expanding world in the latter half of the 19th century, an indigenous religious movement arose, in part, in response to Western religions (Catholicism was known as "Western Learning" in Korea). The first of the new religions was called *Donghak*, which means "Eastern Learning." *Donghak*, later called *Chondogyo*, the Religion of the Heavenly Way, includes elements of Confucianism, Buddhism, shamanism, Taoism, and Catholicism. Other new religions (Chang, 2003) include the following.

- *Taejonggyo* is the worship of the legendary founder of Korea.
- *Chungsanggyo* focuses on magico-religious practice.
- *Wonbulgo*, is a form of Buddhism that includes social reform.

See Chapter 5 for a discussion of major world religions.

Communication

The official and universally used language is Korean, a distinct language whose alphabet is called *hangul*. Literacy is high, even in rural areas, and among immigrants to the West, literacy is close to 100%, the exceptions being a small number of the aged (Chang, 2003).

Communication tends to be relatively direct and business-like. Small-talk is not valued, nor are effusive greetings or hearty or loud communications. At the same time, however, the concept of *kibun*, which is akin to harmony or a peaceful environment, is active in interactions and relationships. In all cases, persons of lesser social status are expected to show respect and defer to persons of higher status. Personal space between people tends to be rather close, except that (public) affectionate touching, even casual contact such as back-patting, is certainly resisted (Hassan, 1998; Purnell & Kim, 2003).

Health beliefs and practices

Korean health practices are based on a complex mix of traditional and modern beliefs including the concept of the body possessing a life energy (called *ki* or in Chinese, *chi*), the need for balance (expressed as *um* (negative, cold, female) and *yang* (positive, warm, male) or in Chinese, yin and yang), religious beliefs, and biomedical beliefs (Chang, 2003; Hong, 2001; Son, 1998). Traditional Korean medicine is based on traditional Chinese medicine and is called *hanbang* and its practitioners are known as *hanuisas*. Holistic approaches to health and illness such as *hanbang* are universal in traditional Asian culture, but among Koreans the holistic approach and thus decision-making is apparently more complex than among other Asian populations (Choi *et al.*, 2003). Moreover, the development of modern medicine in Korea has not included marginalization of traditional practices as is common in other countries and cultures, so that both systems are well regarded and freely used (Hong, 2001; Son, 1998).

Um or "cold" illnesses or conditions include depression, hypoactivity, hypothermia, abdominal cramps, colds and indigestion. Yang or "hot" illnesses or conditions include hyperactivity, hyperthermia, stroke, dehydration, fever, tension and seizures. Treatment of hot/cold conditions is through the use of substances with properties of the opposite force to achieve balance. For example, the common cold is treated with hot soup made from bean sprouts and congestion is cleared by adding dried anchovies, hot spices and garlic to the soup.

Traditional treatment methods include acupuncture, herbs and moxibustion – the latter being the burning of a soft material at a specified spot corresponding to internal energy channels on the skin to restore one's *ki*. *Hanyak* is a traditional health modality similar to Chinese herbal therapies and is widely accepted among Koreans. Korean–Americans may alternate between traditional Korean therapies and Western medicine, with elders preferring *hanyak*. In large Korean communities in the USA, there are *hanyak bang* (herbal shops) where *hanui* (herbalists) prescribe appropriate *hanyak* for different illnesses according to symptoms. Traditional medical treatment is based upon physical assessment and observation of behavior.

In general, the Korean diet is high in grains and vegetables, moderate in animal and vegetable protein, moderate in calories, low in fat and sugar, but high in salt. Rice is the staple starch, but is always milled, and hence less nutritious. High incomes and the availability of high calorie, high fat, high sodium foods in the West and South Korea lead to increased chronic disease such as hypertension, cardiovascular disease, and Type II diabetes.

Culture-bound syndromes known to occur among Koreans (American Psychiatric Association, 2000; Park *et al.*, 2002) include the following.

- *Hwa-byung* translates from Korean to English literally as "anger syndrome" and is thought to arise from suppressed anger or emotions, usually stemming from conflicts with the family or others. Symptoms include anxiety, feelings of impending doom, headache, decreased appetite, insomnia, decreased energy, and the feeling that there is an epigastric mass. *Hwa-byung* is seen as fate, and treatment is symptomatic.

- *Shin-byung* begins with anxiety, weakness, dizziness, fear, anorexia, insomnia, and gastrointestinal symptoms. These progress to dissociation and the perception of possession by ancestral spirits.

Pregnancy and childbirth

The traditional (and in most cases, modern) view of pregnancy is as a blessing from ancestors or higher power. A unique Korean practice during pregnancy is *Tae Kyo*, rules for "teaching" the unborn child and molding his/her intellectual development and personality. Pregnant women traditionally are advised to enjoy fine art and literature and to avoid touching unclean things, killing living creatures, eating certain foods, and exhibiting other negative behaviors. The rate of prenatal care among Korean–Americans is lower than most major Asian–American groups (Yu *et al.*, 2001)

Traditional practice was for the woman to give a birth at home with her mother's help. Pregnancy is seen as a yang condition and the postpartum period is seen as *um*, hence a new mother should avoid cold drinks or cold food and consume hot drinks or *miyuck gook* (seaweed soup) to restore equilibrium. Traditionally, only the mother was allowed to see the birth and no visitors were allowed to visit the mother and infant for three weeks after the birth. On the 100th day after the birth of a baby, an elaborate celebration is held with invited guests. While isolating the mother and infant has decreased in practice in Korea and is impossible in the West, privacy still remains desirable. *Dol* is the first birthday celebration, and includes a banquet with invited guests.

End of life

The family is central to the process of dying, both in decision-making and in providing care. Discussion of terminal status directly with the patient is resisted by most Korean families in fear of causing added stress to the patient or hastening death. As noted earlier, the welfare of the family is paramount in health decisions and interactions, and most Korean families see no benefit in discussion about end-of-life issues. Traditionally, the family provides much of the personal care for ill or hospitalized family members.

Koreans are usually – but not always – stoical and tend not to complain of pain or other problems of disease or the care provided by staff. Do-not-resuscitate (DNR) orders are accepted, but because of the respect given to doctor's opinions, it is important to carefully clarify that DNR is the patient and family's freely given choice (Purnell & Kim, 2003). In most cases the family will attend the patient's last days and the expression of grief and emotion at the time of death may be open and intense. Organ donation and transplantation are commonly viewed as violations in the integrity of the body, hence are frowned upon.

Burial is preferred over cremation. Modern funeral ceremonies last 3 days or less. Traditionally, the period of mourning ranges from 3 months to 3 years according to the degree of the relationship. For a father and a mother the mourning lasted 3 years, but if the mother died before the father, then the mourning lasted 1 year for the mother. These customs are based on the fundamental idea of strong kinship values and family ties from Confucianism.

Health problems and screening

The healthy life expectancy or HALE in Korea is 67.4 years and the full life expectancy is 76 years (Population Reference Bureau, 2002; World Health Organization (WHO), 2002). Chronic non-infectious diseases are the leading causes of death and disability, and health risks for new Korean immigrants are primarily cardiac disease, cancer, diabetes, and other chronic non-infectious diseases. The rate of alcoholism among older men is high (>16%) (Kim *et al.*, 2002), and presumably is high among younger men as well. However, in the unlikely event that North Korean refugees arrive in the West, infectious diseases and nutritional deficits would become more important health considerations. Health risks (Chang, 2003; Hawn & Jung, 2003; Kemp, 2002; WHO, 2002) include:
- cardiac disease and related, cancer, diabetes, and other chronic non-infectious diseases
- amebiasis
- arbovirus encephalitis
- dengue fever
- filariasis (Bancroftian filariasis and Malayan filariasis)
- gnathostomiasis (possibly)
- hemorrhagic fever with renal syndrome
- hepatitis
- histoplasmosis
- hookworm
- lyme disease
- malaria
- malnutrition (North Korea only)
- sexually transmitted infections, including HIV/AIDS, cervical cancer, chancroid, chlamydia, gonorrhea, syphilis (low prevalences)

- trematodes (liver-dwelling – clonorchiasis; lung-dwelling – paragonimiasis; intestine-dwelling)
- tuberculosis.

REFERENCES

American Psychiatric Association (2000). *Diagnostic and Staistical Manual of Mental disorders*, 4th edn, text revision. Washington, DC: Author.

Barnes, J. S. & Bennett, C. E. (2002). *The Asian Population 2000*. Washington, DC: US Census Bureau. Retrieved August 17, 2003 from http://www.census.gov/prod/2002pubs/c2kbr01-16.pdf.

Central Intelligence Agency (2003). *World Factbook* (updated 3/2003). Retrieved July 11, 2003 from http://www.cia.gov/cia/publications/factbook/geos/ks.html.

Chang, S. O. (2003). Korea, South, Republic of. In *Cultural Health Assessment*, 3rd edn., ed. C. E. D'Avanzo and E. M. Geissler, pp. 422–6. St. Louis, MO: Mosby.

Choi, I., Dalal, R., Kim-Prieto, C., & Park, H. (2003). Culture and judgment of causal relevance. *Journal of Personality and Social Psychology*, **84**, 46–59.

Columbia University (n.d.). *Coming to America*. Retrieved August 13, 2003 from http://www.columbia.edu/itc/sipa/U6210/ik105/ history.html.

Hassan, F. (1998). South Korea. In *Cultural Profiles Project*, ed. C. Lee. Toronto: University of Toronto. Retrieved July 19, 2003 from http://www.settlement.org/cp/english/skorea/SkoreaEN.pdf.

Hawn, T. R. & Jung, E. C. (2003). Health screening in immigrants, refugees, and internationally adopted orphans. In *The Travel and Tropical Medicine Manual*, 3rd edn., ed E. C. Jong and R. McMullen, pp. 255–65). Philadelphia, PA: W. B. Saunders.

Hong, C. D. (2001). Complementary and alternative medicine in Korea: current status and future prospects. *Journal of Alternative and Complementary Medicine*, **7**, *Suppl. 1*, S33–40.

Im, E. O., Lee, E. O., & Park, Y. S. (2002). Korean women's breast cancer experience. *Western Journal of Nursing Research*, **24**, 751–65.

Johnstone, P. & Mandryk, J. (2001). *Operation World: 21st century edn*. Waynesboro, GA: Paternoster USA.

Kemp, C. (2002). *Infectious Diseases*. Retrieved April 12, 2003 from http://www3.baylor.edu/~Charles_Kemp/Infectious_Disease.htm.

Kim, D. H., Kim, K. I., Park, Y. C., Zhang, L. D., Lu, M. K., & Li, D. (2000). Children's experience of violence in China and Korea: a transcultural study. *Child Abuse and Neglect*, **24**, 1163–73.

Kim, J. M., Shin, I. S., Stewart, R., & Yoon, J. S. (2002). Alcoholism in older Korean men: prevalence, aetiology, and comorbidity with cognitive impairment and dementia in urban and rural communities. *International Journal of Geriatric Psychiatry*, **17**, 821–7.

Park, Y. J., Kim, H. S., Schwartz-Barcott, D., & Kim, J. W. (2002). The conceptual structure of *hwa-byung* in middle-aged Korean women. *Health Care for Women International*, **23**, 389–97.

Population Reference Bureau (2002). *2002 World Population Data Sheet*. Retrieved May 12, 2003 from http://www.prb.org/pdf/WorldPopulationDS02_Eng.pdf.

Purnell, L. D. & Kim, S. (2003). People of Korean heritage. In *Transcultural Health Care: A Culturally Competent Approach*, 2nd edn., ed. L. D. Purnell and B. J. Paulanka, pp. 249–63. Philadelphia PA: F. A. Davis.

Son, A. H. (1998). Modernisation of the system of traditional Korean medicine (1876–1990). *Health Policy*, **44**, 261–81.

Yu, S. M., Alexander, G. R., Schwalberg, R., & Kogan, M. D. (2001). Prenatal care use among selected Asian American groups. *American Journal of Public Health*, **91**, 1865–8.

World Health Organization (2002). *World Health Report*. Retrieved June 5, 2003 from http://www.who.int/whr/2002/en/.

24

Kosovo (Albania)

Tracey Mackling and Charles Kemp

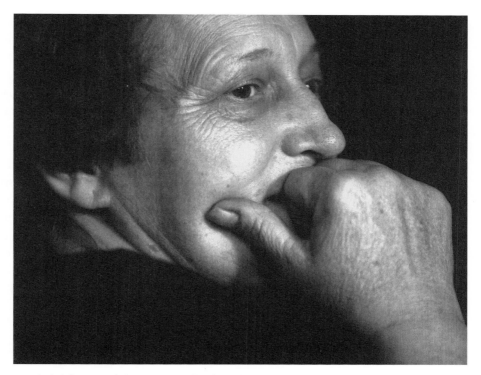

Worried. (Photograph by courtesy of Judy Walgren.)

Refugee and Immigrant Health: A Handbook for Health Professionals, Charles Kemp and Lance A. Rasbridge.
Published by Cambridge University Press. © C. Kemp and L. A. Rasbridge 2004.

Introduction

Albania and the adjoining Kosovo are in the Balkan mountains of Eastern Europe, and are bordered by Serbia, Macedonia, and Greece to the East; Montenegro to the North; and the Adriatic Sea to the West. Although Kosovo is considered a special region of Yugoslavia, about 90% of the population of Kosovo is Albanian, hence Kosovars are included here in this discussion of Albanians (Johnstone & Mandryk, 2001).

Albania was a feudal country until the end of World War II, when the communist totalitarian dictator, Enver Hoxha took power. Under Hoxha, Albania was modernized to some extent, but at the same time, was almost completely (self) isolated from the rest of Europe. Landowners, clan leaders, and clerics were imprisoned, executed, or exiled; private property was confiscated by the state; and all churches, mosques, and other religious institutions were closed. A multiparty democracy was established in 1990, and although great progress has been made toward modernizing and engaging Albania with the rest of the world, a number of problems have hampered the growth of Albania. Political/social problems in Albania today include government corruption, high unemployment, dilapidated infrastructure, gangsterism, and ongoing internal strife (Albanian.com, n.d.; Central Intelligence Agency [CIA], 2003).

Kosovo was an autonomous federal unit of Yugoslavia until 1989, when the Serbian government revoked the basic rights of the Albanians in Kosovo and suspended the Kosovo parliament. Serbian claims to Kosovo were based on Serbs living in Kosovo since the 6th century AD and the presence of Serbian cultural monuments. When peaceful attempts at resistance were deemed ineffective, a guerrilla movement called the Kosovo Liberation Army (KLA) was formed. In 1998, the Serbian (former Yugoslavian) government began a campaign of violence ("ethnic cleansing") against civilians, including women and children (Albanian.com, n.d.; CIA, 2003).

History of immigration

For many years, there has been a steady outmigration from Albania and Kosovo to other European countries. Over the past several decades, Albanians from Yugoslavia, Greece, and Macedonia migrated into Kosovo. The 1998 ethnic cleansing campaign resulted in hundreds of thousands of Kosovars leaving their homes. It is estimated that approximately three-quarters of a million Kosovo refugees fled to Macedonia, Albania, Montenegro, Bosnia, and other countries abroad. After several months of allied bombing of Yugoslavia, the Serbian government accepted a resolution to the Kosovo crisis and by June 20, Serb forces had left Kosovo. Over 715 000 refugees returned to Kosovo from neighboring countries and 30 000 from abroad.

The number of Albanians and Kosovars living abroad is large, but not known. Most are immigrants as opposed to refugees.

Culture and social relations

The extended family is the basic social unit among Albanians and Kosovars. Traditionally, families are patriarchal and although there has been progression toward equality since 1990, men remain as primary decision-makers in health and other matters. Family support during illness or infirmity is expected and, at least in Albania and Kosovo, essential to recovery (Van Hook *et al.*, 2003).

Communications

The Albanian language (*Tosk*) is one of the original nine Indo-European languages and is not derived from any other language. Almost all Albanians and around 90% of Kosovars speak Albanian. There are two primary dialects, which are mutually intelligible: Gheg in the North and Tosk in the South. Since 1974, citizens of Kosovo and Macedonia speak varieties of eastern Gheg (Albanian.com, n.d.). Physical affection is openly expressed between members of the same sex, but is more restrained between members of the opposite sex. In general, Albanians and Kosovars are warm and expressive in their interpersonal relations. Eye contact is held between social equals, but rural women may not be comfortable looking men in the eye (Van Hook *et al.*, 2003).

Religion

Despite Hoxha's efforts to eradicate all religion, about 75% of Albanians profess a belief in God. Approximately 41% of Albanians are Christian (most Orthodox or Catholic) and 39% are Sunni Muslim (Johnstone & Mandryk, 2001). Note, however, that other sources, e.g., Central Intelligence Agency (2003) put the percentages at 70% Muslim, 20% Albanian Orthodox, and 10% Catholic. Kosovo has a similar breakdown of faiths. There is not a significant presence of Islamists or other Islamic radicals in either Albania or Kosovo (Albanian.com, n.d.).

Health beliefs and practices

Although modern biomedical theories are held throughout the region, concurrent beliefs in magic and religious causation and cure are pervasive. Folk healers, including faith healers and herbalists, are common in Albania and Kosovo, but are probably less common among *émigrés*. Among people from rural or less educated backgrounds, folk illnesses may include the "evil eye." Herbal treatments are generally innocuous, e.g., teas made from various non-toxic herbs such as rosemary and oregano (Van Hook, Haxhiymeri, & Gjermeni, 2003).

The primary sources of health care in the region are government clinics and hospitals, which, although not fully equipped to Western European standards, are able to deliver health care of adequate quality as evidenced by life expectancy rates given below. Health care is focused almost exclusively on acute care, and prevention is not generally a priority. It is likely that acute-oriented attitudes toward health and health care are held by Albanians living elsewhere in the world.

Pregnancy and childbirth

Pregnancy is considered a time of vulnerability, and pregnant women thus receive special attention from the family. Most births are attended by physicians, but nurses and midwives attend at slightly less than half. The use of midwives is most common in rural areas. Among Albanians living elsewhere, medical attendance is universal. A period of 40 days postpartum is thought to be a period of great vulnerability, and mother and child may stay inside the home and avoid conflict.

On the average, Albanian women give birth to 2.3 children. Contraceptive use is widely accepted (but not necessarily available) among Albanians and Kosovars, as is abortion. The abortion rate in Albania in 1999 was 344/1000 live births (CIA, 2003; Van Hook *et al.*, 2003).

End of life

In the homeland, the family is deeply involved at the end of life. In other countries, family involvement will be less for the simple reason that there are far fewer family members available. The body is buried within 24 hours of death. If the deceased is a young person, she or he is dressed as if being married. If the deceased is a child born less than 40 days before death, there is no ceremony. Mourners dress in black, and grief is openly expressed. The initial period of mourning is 40 days, and there are ceremonies at 6 months and 1 year after death (Van Hook *et al.*, 2003).

Health problems and screening

Current statistics are not available for Kosovo *per se*, so the following is based on statistics from Albania only. The healthy life expectancy (HALE) is 58.7 years and the full life expectancy is 74 years (Population Reference Bureau, 2002; World Health Organization (WHO), 2002). Chronic non-infectious diseases are the leading causes of death and disability, and health risks for new Kosovar immigrants are primarily cardiac disease and related, cancer, respiratory illness, diabetes, and other chronic non-infectious diseases. Health risks (Kemp, 2002; Van Hook *et al.*, 2003; WHO, 2002) include:

- babesiosis (rare)
- boutonneuse fever
- encephalitis (most likely tick-borne)
- hemorrhagic fevers (HFs) (HF with renal syndrome and tick-borne HFs)
- lyme disease
- sexually transmitted infections, including HIV/AIDS, cervical cancer, chancroid, chlamydia, gonorrhea, syphilis
- trematode infection (opisthorchiasis)
- chronic illnesses as noted above
- among refugees, post-traumatic stress disorder and depression are risks.

REFERENCES

Albanian.com (n.d.). Retrieved July 10, 2003 from http://www.albanian.com/information/countries/albania/general/factbook.html.

Central Intelligence Agency (2003). *World Factbook* (updated 3/2003). Retrieved July 11, 2003 from http://www.cia.gov/cia/publications/factbook/geos/al.html.

Johnstone, P. & Mandryk, J. (2001). *Operation World: 21st century edn.* Waynesboro, GA: Paternoster USA.

Kemp, C. E. (2002). *Infectious Diseases.* Retrieved April 12, 2003 from http://www3.baylor.edu/~Charles_Kemp/Infectious_Disease.htm.

Population Reference Bureau (2002). *2002 World Population Data Sheet.* Retrieved May 12, 2003 from http://www.prb.org/pdf/WorldPopulationDS02_Eng.pdf.

Van Hook, M.P, Haxhiymeri, E., & Gjermeni, E. (2003). Albania. In *Cultural Assessment,* 3rd edn., ed. C. D'Avanzo and E. M. Geissler. St. Louis, MO: Mosby.

World Health Organization (2002). *World Health Report.* Retrieved June 5, 2003 from http://www.who.int/whr/2002/en/.

25

Kurds (from Iraq)

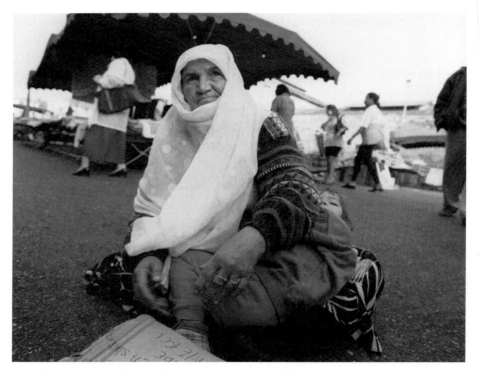

Struggling in a new culture. (Photograph by courtesy of Judy Walgren.)

Introduction

The Kurds are a diverse ethnic group of an estimated 22 million living in the homeland known as Kurdistan, encompassing parts of the countries of Turkey, Iran, Iraq, Syria, as well as provinces of the former Soviet Union. Their struggle

Refugee and Immigrant Health: A Handbook for Health Professionals, Charles Kemp and Lance A. Rasbridge. Published by Cambridge University Press. © C. Kemp and L. A. Rasbridge 2004.

for independence has waged for centuries, but political and ethnic divisions within the populations have prevented them from achieving unity. Hence they remain minorities, frequently persecuted, within the countries they live.

History of immigration

The Kurds of Iraq have a long history of persecution under the Baghdad regimes. In the mid-1970s a failed Kurdish revolution resulted in thousands of Kurds of the Kurdish Democratic Party fleeing to Iran, and they were eventually resettled to the USA and abroad.

Similarly, after the defeat of Iraqi forces in the Iran–Iraq War of 1988, Kurds in northern Iraq were particularly targeted for annihilation, and biological and chemical weapons ostensibly maintained for use against the Iranians were turned against them. A systematic plan, the *Anfal*, to destroy villages controlled by Kurdish resistors, known as *peshmerga* (literally, freedom fighters), was launched by Saddam Hussein in 1988. The worst of these attacks came on the Kurdish settlement of Halabja (Human Rights Watch, 1995). This campaign resulted in thousands of casualties and forced some 60 000 refugees to flee to the Turkish border (Human Rights Watch, 1995).

At the Turkish border, these refugees were forcibly routed by the Turkish authorities to four primary refugee camps set up inside Turkey: Diyarbakir, Silopi, Mardin, and Mush. Here they remained for an average of 2 years or more, some up to 5 years, under variable but frequently severe conditions until the international community selected some for resettlement. Many others were pushed back to Iraq.

A third, larger wave of Iraqi Kurds fled Iraq to Turkey and Iran immediately after the failed Kurdish uprising during the Gulf War, in early 1991. This group of an estimated 1.5 million refugees in the mountains of the Turkish border evoked a large humanitarian relief effort, culminating in the resettlement of some to the West beginning in the Spring of 1993.

A fourth, most recent wave of Iraqi Kurds were evacuated by United States forces from Arbil following an Iraqi army incursion and internal political strife in northern Iraq in the Fall of 1996. These refugees were airlifted directly to Guam, where they received a few months of orientation prior to their resettlement in the USA.

Culture and social relations

Historically, the Kurds come from mountainous regions where they practiced pastoralism of sheep and goats and tended small farms, growing mostly wheat, rice, and fruit. While many of the Kurds had rural origins, the cities like Dohuk, Arbil, Suleimania, and Kirkuk are growing from refugees displaced from their villages due to warfare. There are also sizeable oil reserves in Kurdistan, representing potential wealth, which adds to the political infighting in the region. Many of the adult men have been involved in the fighting as *peshmerga*.

Kurds tend to be strongly clannish in their social organization, organized around a male descendent. This is especially true of those descended from important political figures; overall there is much reverence paid to ancestors. Villages are often identified along extended family lines. To protect clan resources, intravillage marriage is preferred; in fact, first cousin marriage is common. Polygamy of up to four wives is allowed by Islamic as well as cultural mores, but is not common. Marriages were frequently arranged in the past, although this custom is beginning to wane. However, family agreement is mandatory, and the exchange of goods, including bride-price, and other ceremonial visits are still practiced according to tradition. "Exchange" marriages are also common in poorer families to save the expenses: a son and daughter from one family marry a daughter and son in another family. After marriage, the woman comes to live with the groom's family. Women retain their names at marriage, but children are named after the male line. Specifically, children traditionally receive as a last name the paternal grandfather's given name. It should be noted that some resettled refugees are now adopting American-styled naming at marriage and birth; some are even involved in legal name-changing.

There is a strong emphasis on large families, and a preference toward males, at least in Kurdistan. Traditional Kurds consider birth control immoral according to Islam (however, see Kridli, 2002), and having a large number of offspring guarantees the family line and provides workers for the homestead. However, this view is changing in the resettled population (see below).

There are several important holidays in Kurdish culture. For one, the birth of a child is celebrated by a feast given by the parents and their family. Newborn boys are typically circumcised within the first month or two. Birthdays are not widely observed, except perhaps for US-born children. The most important holiday is Kurdish New Year (*Newroz*), on March 21, celebrating an ancient Kurdish legend marking the independence of Kurds. Kurds also observe the religious period of Ramadan, although the strictness of adherence to the rules on fasting vary considerably according to their orthodoxy.

Politically, Kurds are fractionated into several political parties. In Iraq, the Kurdish Democratic Party, headed by Masoud Barzani, rivals the Patriotic Union of Kurdistan of Jalal Talabani and many other smaller political groups. These political factions have been engaged in bitter civil war in Iraq, and these divisions can carry over even to the country of resettlement. In Turkey, the main political party of Kurds is known as the Worker's Party or PKK, which is considered a terrorist group by Turkey because of its fiercely pro-independence stance.

Before the uprising of Kurds in Iraq in 1990–91, people in cities and some from the countryside could access regional Government hospitals in Northern Iraq or even Baghdad. However, more recently, with political events in Iraq, even the modern hospitals suffer chronic shortages of medicines and supplies. In villages, Western health care continues to be rudimentary at best; for example, children from these areas rarely receive childhood immunizations.

Elders in general are afforded great respect in Kurdish culture. In Islam, one is directed to afford the same care to one's aged parents as they gave in childhood. There is an Islamic expression that says, "If the parents do not forgive you, Allah will not forgive you." There is a Kurdish tradition that family gathers around a dying parent to ask for forgiveness.

Communications

While there are cultural similarities which all Kurds share, especially historical factors, there are also many differences among Kurds. For one, there are two dialects of the Kurdish language: *Sorani* and *Kurmanji* (*Bardini*), which are mostly mutually intelligible. Most Iraqi and Iranian Kurds speak *Sorani*; *Kurmanji* is the dialect of Dohuk Province in Iraq (where most US-resettled Kurds originated) as well as most of Turkey, Syria, and former Soviet Union. Most Kurds are also bilingual in the *lingua franca* of the country in which they live, for example, Arabic in Iraq, Turkish in Turkey, and Farsi in Iran. Most Kurds are literate in their own language, but only those with more advanced education, restricted generally to males, can read and write Arabic, Turkish, or Farsi.

It is appropriate to make eye contact when speaking with Kurds. When greeting, handshakes are usually appropriate between and within the sexes, and a two-handed handshake is considered especially warm and polite. The exception here is that it is inappropriate for a man to shake the hand of an elderly women. In Kurdistan, and between very close friends or relatives in the USA, men may greet each other with a kiss to both cheeks. For the most devout Muslims, especially men, one is not to be touched by anyone, including a spouse, after one has ritually purified oneself prior to the daily prayers.

In addition to linguistic traits, Kurds have also adopted (or were forced to adopt) over the years other cultural traits from the surrounding dominant cultures where they live. For example, Kurds in Turkey primarily wear the style of dress of Turks.

Religion

In terms of religion, most Kurds adhere to the Sunni tradition of Islam, which is widely practiced throughout Iraq and Turkey. A few Kurds in Iran practice

Shiite Islam. In general, Kurdish women are afforded more rights and opportunities than Iraqis and most other Muslims. Women are usually not veiled (except sometimes for the elderly), are more free to associate with men, and they may even occupy political offices. In addition to Islam, there are also converts to Judaism and Christianity throughout Kurdistan. Islam is discussed in the chapter on religions.

Health beliefs and practices

In terms of non-Western or traditional remedies in Kurdistan, there are shops that sell different herbs, with the proprietors knowledgeable of treatments. However, there are only a few herbal treatments, for such conditions as stomach problems and kidney stones. For the latter, there are certain tree leaves that are made into tea and taken on an empty stomach before breakfast. For fainting and seizures, which some believe to be brought on by possession of a *jinn* spirit, a raw onion is held under the nose, and also black ash may be applied to the forehead and cheeks. There are some leaves that grow wild, which people put on wounds, described as a thick leaf with liquid inside. One can also put snow on the wounded area to stop bleeding and pain.

We learned of very few folk treatments for children. For fever, for example, only cold wet towels are used, together with a hand fan. In general, for treatment of diarrhea one gives soup or rice water, but withholds fats, meat and cheese, tomatoes, and grapes. Raisins and yogurt, mixed with crushed ice or snow are also given for diarrhea.

There is a type of folk illness in adults and children, with the symptoms of severe abdominal pain, decreased appetite, and back inflexibility. The belief is that umbilicus "falls down" into the abdomen. Certain women have the ability to cure this illness in children by holding the child upside-down and slapping the bottom of the feet. A similar hernia-like condition can affect adults, where the umbilicus is believed to be "dislocated" from lifting heavy objects or other strenuous work. A specialist can right the problem by walking on the abdomen or vigorously massaging the abdomen by hand. This treatment is not considered a cure, however, as the condition returns. One other illness that some specialists know how to cure is a broken or dislocated coccyx, described as "bent," which can be straightened through rectal digital manipulation.

Some more traditional Kurds may hide a pretty baby, to protect it from an "evil eye," which was described as like "electricity" that comes from the eye of someone who covets one's belongings. Even a car or horse may be hidden for this reason. When a child or adult is believed to be suffering from the cast of "evil eye," a Kurdish Imam can be called for a blessing.

While there do not appear to be any traditional healers in Kurdish culture (except for those specific treatments noted above), the ranking Islamic figure, the Imam, is seen to have curative power through his spirituality through prayer. For example, if a child goes out at night and is frightened by evil spirits, the Imam can rid the child of fear through a blessing. Also, there is a charm, a quarter-sized piece of lead, on which the Imam writes or scratches, something short like "Muhammad," and on the other side "Allah." This is only for babies and children, to provide protection from evil spirits.

Similarly, the Imam is particularly sought after for a certain childhood affliction, *alamk* or "fright" from evil spirits, which is detected by rapid pulse in the neck and legs, headache, decreased appetite, and pallor. The Imam (or other knowledgeable laypersons) checks the pulse, recites appropriate verses from the Koran, and then blows air on the patient.

There is also a type of amulet for children and adults. The Imam writes verses from the Koran, especially verses dealing with spirits, folds the long strip of paper into a triangle, and puts it in a blue envelope (black for adults). It is not opened but rather hung from a string around the neck. Or, for headache treatment, it can be worn under the scarf, called *nevished*. These amulets are very commonly worn by people with mental problems, in which case it is worn under the clothing. The Imam receives payment for these amulets, although sometimes he says God will pay him in the other world.

There is also a larger version, *basband*, which provides protection from bullets and other dangerous things. It is put in leather for protection from water and sweat. *Basband* may be used to protect travelers going through unknown areas or places with bad spirits at night. Furthermore, its properties last indefinitely.

Pregnancy and childbirth

We learned of no food prescriptions or proscriptions for pregnancy. There is a generalized Islamic taboo against the sexing of a child ("only God should know"), but some old women say that a more rounded abdomen in pregnancy means a female baby.

Traditionally, a midwife assists with the birth and cuts the umbilical cord, the stump of which is then tied with a string. Until it falls off, the stump is kept clean with a crushed sumac seed mixture (sometimes also mixed with onions), that the mother changes several times a day. In the postpartum, after 40 days, there is a special bath, in which molten lead mixed in water is poured over the woman to relieve her from bad spirits. There is a postpartum sexual taboo until that time.

While birth control was considered in violation of Islamic law in Kurdistan, this view is changing as some younger married Kurdish women are accepting birth control, especially the IUD and the pill, and we know of tubal ligations being requested by some women. Alternatively, infertility is a growing concern for young couples in the West, as a high social value is placed on having children. To this extent, we know of several young couples who are attending an infertility clinic.

According to one Kurdish informant, infertility treatments that involve laboratory conception are acceptable. Pregnancy outside of wedlock is still strictly taboo at this point. Abortion is considered in extreme violation of Islamic law and Kurdish culture.

In Kurdistan villages, most babies were delivered by midwives; in the USA, midwives are known among the community, but provide little more than comfort to the pregnant women. Husbands here commonly accompany their wives to the delivery room. Virtually all newborns were breastfed in Kurdistan, for at least 1 year and sometimes longer. Weaning would always occur at subsequent conception, the belief being the milk in pregnancy is not healthy for the nursing child. Here breastfeeding is still common for Kurdish women, but mixed feeding with formula and bottles is becoming common among those women who work. Women breastfeeding in public typically cover themselves with a scarf. Manual expression of milk is not considered appropriate. For childrearing, since there is an emphasis on large families, much of the responsibility for toddlers lies with older sisters and grandmothers. Older boys are not typically involved in childcare. In general, female children are much more supervised than males.

End of life

At death, the body is ritually washed by an Imam (for a male) or a devout older woman for females (who works under the direction of an Imam, reciting the correct Koranic verses, and the like) and covered with a white sheet, fitted to the body. This is typically done at a mosque but can be performed at a funeral home here. The body is then buried as soon as possible, typically the same day. The body is placed in the grave so that the head faces Mecca. At burial, family and friends gather, and the Imam recites from the Koran. Others read from the Koran as well, in the name of the deceased. In Kurdistan, a tape of certain verses from the Koran would be played continuously over loudspeakers. The funeral party then returns to the house of the deceased for prayers and a feast.

For at least 3 days to 1 week, the family stays at home to accept visitors. After 7 days, the family prepares another feast for friends and villagers in order again to ask forgiveness for the deceased's past transgressions. This is followed by weekly graveyard visit to show respect and love, and a picture of the deceased is hung in the home. The holiday of *Eid* is also a time to visit the grave.

Health problems and screening

As this is written, it is unclear what changes, if any, in the health status of the Kurds in the Iraq region have occurred since the 2003 war to overthrow the Saddam Hussein regime. Before the war, Iraqis overall had healthy life expectancies (HALE) of 50.5 years and overall life expectancies of 58 years (Population Reference Bureau, 2002; World Health Organization (WHO), 2002). If the population were studied according to ethnicity (Arabs vs. Kurds) and religion (Sunni vs. Shiite), a different picture would likely emerge, with Arabs and non-Kurd Sunnis having greater HALEs and overall life expectancies. Health risks in Kurdish refugees and immigrants from the Iraq region (Hawn & Jung, 2003; Kemp, 2002; WHO, 2002) include:

- amebiasis
- anthrax
- boutonneuse fever
- brucellosis or undulant fever
- cholera
- Crimean–Congo hemorrhagic fever
- cysticercosis (tapeworm)
- dracunculiasis (Guinea worm disease)
- familial Mediterranean fever (Mediterranean area, primarily among persons of Sephardic Jewish, Armenian, and Arab ancestry)
- giardia
- helminthiasis (ascariasis, echinococcosis/hydatid disease, schistosomiasis)
- hepatitis B (13% carriage rate)
- hookworm
- leishmaniasis
- malaria
- plague
- sickle cell disease or sickle cell hemoglobulinopathies (occurs primarily in people of African lineage, but also to a lesser extent among people from the Mediterranean area, Arabs, and Indians)
- thalassemias
- toxocariasis
- trachoma
- trematodes (liver-dwelling: clonorchiasis and opisthorchiasis; blood-dwelling: schistosomiasis or bilharzias; intestine-dwelling; and lung-dwelling: paragonimiasis)
- trichinosis (trichinella)
- tuberculosis
- typhus

- post-traumatic stress disorder
- physical sequelae of war, e.g., old, untreated gunshot or shrapnel wounds
- nutritional deficits

Acknowledgement

This chapter is based on original work by L. Rasbridge.
Acknowledgement is given to Adil Abdullah and Pat Maloof.

REFERENCES

Hawn, T. R. & Jung, E. C. (2003). Health screening in immigrants, refugees, and internationally adopted orphans. In *The Travel and Tropical Medicine Manual*, 3rd edn., ed. E. C. Jong and R. McMullen, pp. 255–65. Philadelphia, PA: W. B. Saunders.

Human Rights Watch. (1995). *Iraq's Crime of Genocide: The Anfal Campaign Against the Kurds.* New Haven: Yale University Press.

Kemp, C. (2002). *Infectious Diseases.* Retrieved April 12, 2003 from http://www3.baylor.edu/~Charles_Kemp/Infectious_Disease.htm.

Kridli, S. O. & Fakhouri, H. (2002). Health needs of Arab-American women in Michigan. *Michigan Nurse*, **76**, 9, 14.

Population Reference Bureau (2002). *2002 World Population Data Sheet.* Retrieved May 12, 2003 from http://www.prb.org/pdf/WorldPopulationDS02_Eng.pdf.

World Health Organization (2002). *World Health Report.* Retrieved June 5, 2003 from http://www.who.int/whr/2002/en/.

FURTHER READING

Cultural Orientation (2003). *Iraqis: Their History and Culture.* Retrieved April 10, 2003 from http://www.culturalorientation.net.

Geissler, E. M. (1998). *Cultural Assessment*, 2nd edn., pp. 129–31. Mosby: St. Louis.

Grieco, E. (2003). *Iraqi Immigrants in the United States.* Migration Information Source. Retrieved April 10, 2003 from http://www.migrationinformation.org.

Rasbridge, L. A. (2000). *Iraqi Refugees.* Retrieved April 4, 2002 from www.baylor.edu/~Charles_Kemp/refugee_health.htm.

26

Laos (*Lao Lum*)

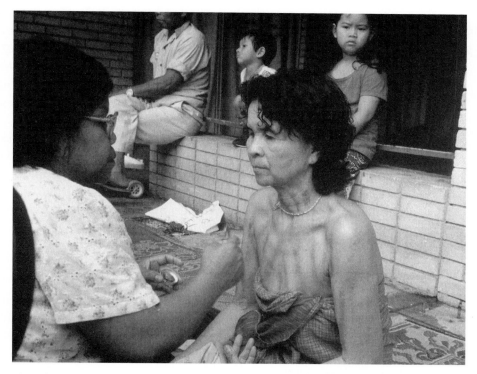

Khout lom or coining is a common traditional healing practice in Southeast Asia. (Photograph by courtesy of Lance A. Rasbridge.)

Introduction

Although this work focuses on lowland Lao (*Lao Lum*), readers should note that there are other ethnic and cultural groups from Laos living in the West, including the Hmong, Bru, Mien, Tai Dam, and ethnic Chinese from Laos. Laos is a landlocked

Refugee and Immigrant Health: A Handbook for Health Professionals, Charles Kemp and Lance A. Rasbridge. Published by Cambridge University Press. © C. Kemp and L. A. Rasbridge 2004.

country surrounded by China, Vietnam, Cambodia, and Thailand. From its beginnings in the sixth century AD, Laos has been ruled by competing kings and foreign powers (including Thailand, Japan, France). Full independence was achieved in 1954 with the end of France's colonial rule of Indochina. Years of conflict ensued and in 1975, the communist Pathet Lao emerged in control of the country.

History of immigration

When the Pathet Lao took control of Laos, both lowland Lao and indigenous people (Hmong, Bru, etc.) began fleeing to Thailand: in all, an estimated 300 000 people (Ethnomed, 1996). Laotians were resettled primarily to the United States, France, Britain, Australia, Canada and New Zealand, with about 50% going to the USA (DeVoe, 1996; Immigration and Refugee Services of America (IRSA), 2002). Similar to refugees from Vietnam, the first wave of Laotians, arriving in the West in late 1975, consisted of small numbers of high-ranking military or government officials, followed by much larger numbers of soldiers, agriculturalists, and professionals beginning in 1979 and winding down by the mid-1980s.

Laotians have tended to live in tightly knit communities to a greater extent than most other refugees from Southeast Asia. In several areas there are now rural or semi-rural communities in which Laotians live in a traditional mutually assisting social structure. Many of the adults work in nearby towns or cities, while elders live more or less traditional lives. As with other first generation refugees or immigrants, assimilation has been difficult for many older Laotians.

Culture and social relations

Traditionally, the extended family, sometimes four generations, is the central social unit within the community. Home and family are headed by the husband or oldest man, but females play a great role both economically and domestically. In Laos, married couples live in the woman's family compound, and was traced through female lines. As family structure has broken down somewhat through the refugee and resettlement experiences, some women face a greater gender inequality than that in Laos (DeVoe, 1996). Nonetheless, elders of both sexes are afforded great respect. Elder respect and other status markers are demonstrated through the Laotian language as well as body language. For example, it is considered rude to carry oneself in such a way that one's head is in an elevated position relative to an elder or other person of greater status.

Most decision-making, including health care, is done by the household elders – and may include decisions made for adults. Decision-making among the more traditional can be influenced by Laotian astrology (Geissler, 1998).

The head is the highest (literally and figuratively) and thus one should not touch another's head or shoulders. It is also impolite to point one's foot at another or sit with one leg crossed over the other so that the bottom of the foot or toe is pointed toward another (or toward an image of the Buddha). It is generally understood that it is necessary to touch a person's head during the course of some physical examinations. Modesty is highly valued, especially in women from waist to knees – and most especially in younger women.

Communications

The Laotian language is based primarily on *Pali* and *Sanskrit*, ancient languages of Buddhism and India, respectively. Spoken Laotian is replete with status markers in pronouns, verbs, and vocabulary in general.

The traditional means of salutation (coming or going) is called *wai*, which involves placing one's hands together as if praying and inclining the head. The height at which the hands are held depends on the social or spiritual status of the person being greeted, with the hands held higher for persons of greater status. Western greetings are well accepted, except that many women are not comfortable shaking hands with men.

Laotians tend to be reserved in most interactions with outsiders (and in all health care interactions). Effusiveness and expression of strong feelings, including strong positive feelings, is not valued, nor is fussing over or complimenting children or infants. In the case of infants, praise and compliments may bring ill fortune, and with children, result in self-centeredness. Children are expected to remain quiet and respectful in interactions with elders, including visitors. As much as possible, healthcare providers should not use children to translate for adults. Doing so puts both parties in an untenable social situation of the child showing superiority to the adult.

Religion

Most Laotians practice Theravada Buddhism. There are regional variations in Laotian Buddhism, generally according to the area of Laos from which a person originated. Northern Laotian Buddhism is influenced by Burmese Buddhism, while central and southern Laotian Buddhism is influenced by Khmer Buddhism. Many Laotians also practice a mix of Buddhism and Brahmanism or *Phram*. The practice of both, as well as belief in spirits is seen in the relatively common approach to shrines: inside the home is reserved for the Buddhist shrine, while outside may be found a spirit (*Phi*) house (small house or shrine on top of a pole or column). Offerings of food are to spirits, while offerings of flowers are to *Phram*. In any case, what a person does in life rather than his or her beliefs is the central canon. There are also strong elements of animism found among many Laotians. It is of little use to try to determine exactly what beliefs or combination of beliefs a Laotian might hold. The beliefs and symbolism of the traditions and faiths are combined and adapted to one another with no conflict whatsoever.

Overall, however, the basic tenets of Buddhism guide at least most traditional Laotians. To follow this path to enlightenment, it is necessary to become and remain a member of the *sangha*, i.e., the monkhood. Realistically, few are able to effectively follow this path, hence there is a focus on rebirth to a better state based on merit or karma (in *Pali, kamma*), especially related to fulfilling responsibilities to society. The ethic of Buddhism is centered around the four "Palaces of Brahma" or virtuous attitudes: loving-kindness, compassion, sympathetic joy, and equanimity.

Evangelical churches and the Church of Jesus Christ of Latter Day Saints (Mormon) are active in the Laotian communities, beginning from the time in the refugee camps in Thailand through the early days of resettlement. It is common for Laotians in the West to attend both Christian churches and Buddhist temples, the latter especially during cultural holidays (DeVoe, 1996).

Health beliefs and practices

Healthcare beliefs and practices are significantly related to Brahmanistic and animistic beliefs. Illness may be attributed to the loss of one of the 32 spirits (or souls) thought to inhabit the body and maintain health. Much health behavior centers around the prevention of "soul loss," or, in the case of a sick person, calling the bodily spirits back. The loss of a spirit may be due to being startled when walking alone, having an accident, after travel, or other causes. As with other Southeast Asians, "winds" also play a role in health and illness and bringing the winds into balance restores health or well-being (DeVoe, 1996; Keovilay *et al.*, 2000).

As among other Southeast Asians, the concept of balance and humoral theory are important in understanding health and illness. Balance is most commonly expressed as balance between "hot" and "cold" properties of illness, medicine, food, and other aspects of life. The "winds" that are thought to cause illness are also related to the idea of balance. Humoral theory includes balance in that the humors (blood, phlegm, yellow bile, and black bile) need to be in balance with respect to one another.

Laotian views of physical and mental wellness are also tied to a person's ability to sleep and eat without difficulty. Some traditional or popular commercial medicines are intended to increase both appetite and sleep. With respect to types and amounts of foods consumed, there are often important educational issues to address with Laotian patients, especially as lifespan is extended among Laotians living in the Western world.

In general, persons who are sick will look first to the family and/or community for understanding of the problem and treatment (Rynearson, 1999). Traditional treatments may be tried first; or, if the loss of spirit is thought to be the problem, a ceremony performed by a family member, elder, or, if possible, an *acharn* or teacher/healer (also known as *maw ya*). The purpose of the ceremony is to call the spirit back to the body. Another route of treatment is to go to the temple, where prayer and lustral water will be used to address the problem. Usually, the last resource is to seek treatment at a clinic or hospital. Note that traditional practices are often continued while utilizing western medicine.

Travel seems to bring increased vulnerability, hence spirits are called to the body before and after traveling. A family member may perform the ceremony before travel, but an *acharn* is preferred for the ceremony after travel as there is thought to be a high likelihood of spirits staying behind. In general, benevolent spirits, *chao thin chao than*, may be beckoned to bless or protect an individual.

Mental illness will in many cases be ascribed to spirit loss, hence to seek care from a Western source for mental or emotional distress indicates the likelihood of an ongoing and very difficult problem. The issues that affect most other health problems are magnified in the case of mental illness (Keovilay *et al.*, 2000).

Traditional treatments or indigenous practices related to health and illness include the following.

- *Khout lom* or coining is the use of a coin and mentholated medicine to rub the chest, back, upper arms, or neck in one direction with resulting ecchymosis. This is thought to release the "wind" that may be causing the illness.
- Pinching in a prescribed manner (rubbing the temples, pulling forward to the eyebrow and nose, and pinching the nose) is used to relieve headache.
- Cupping is performed by fixing a piece of cotton in the bottom of a glass, lighting the cotton on fire, and placing the open mouth of the glass on the sick person's back (or less commonly, the forehead). This creates a vacuum and thus draws the wind from the body. In one session, the procedure is carried out three to four times bilaterally down the back on either side of the spine with six to eight circular contusions resulting.
- Massage and manipulation is performed by elders and others with knowledge of healing techniques.
- Some traditional Lao medicines are available in the West, with some of these found or grown locally. Most are classified as "cool" as opposed to western medicines which are usually classified as "hot." Gathering such substances includes prayer

and other prescribed means of respectfully taking them from the earth or elsewhere. Most such medicines are imported from Thailand, Laos, or elsewhere in Southeast Asia.

- Chinese medicine is widely available from both stores and individuals. In some cases, the medicine or combinations of medicines are soaked or dissolved in vodka (called "wine") and thence consumed in small quantities. Commercial preparations from Asia and elsewhere are also used by many Laotians.

It will by now be obvious to readers that Laotian views of health, illness, and healing are complex and multidimensional, and encompass to a very strong degree, spiritual components. Spiritual or spirit-based practices are related to *Phram* beliefs rather than Buddhism, but many of these practices will occur in the context of Buddhism. Evidence of the spiritual or spirit components is seen in several phenomena (Kemp & Keovilay, 1999; Keovilay *et al.*, 2000).

- The involvement of monks and *acharn*, as well as family in spirit-based practices is seen throughout illness and health-related aspects of life from birth through death.
- Some Laotians wear *katha* (or *katout*), which is a string passed through a small cylinder or cylinders of gold or brass. The metal is inscribed with Pali prayers called *To Dham*. These are not viewed as decorative jewelry, but as potent and sacred talismans which are made by monks or holy men.
- *Yarn* refers to the magical protective tattoos found on the chest, back, and arms of some men; or to pictures and words on fabric which may be carried or put over a door. Buddha or boddhisatva images may be worn on a chain around the neck.
- One will sometimes encounter Laotians with one or more pieces of string tied around the wrist. This also has spiritual and protective meaning and derives from a practice in Laos of wearing around the wrist twisted palm leaf on which is written *To Dham*. These are thought to prevent loss of spirits.
- A small bag worn on a string around the neck is called *haksa*. The *haksa* is given by parents or grandparents and affords protection to the wearer.

Health histories may be incomplete for several reasons, the most basic of which is a reluctance to volunteer information. Such reluctance has its origin in a cultural value of privacy in personal matters, especially related to family, sexual, and illness (vulnerability) issues. Trust or its lack is a major issue. With trust based on relationships, one might assume that the history will evolve over time, rather than be completed in one or two interviews.

Some Laotians value the relating of symptoms more than the health history. Explaining links between questions or problems will help in eliciting information. Falling back on the relationship may also help. One might say, "Remember as much as possible. Help me." Regardless of what techniques are used, remember that the history will evolve over time as the relationship (hopefully) evolves.

Pregnancy and childbirth

Traditionally, the father was significantly involved in the birthing process, by supporting his wife's shoulders, catching the baby, cutting the cord, and performing the ritual burial of the placenta (D'Avanzo, 1992). Lao men are thus typically involved in, or at least present at, hospital-based births in the West. Prenatal services are widely utilized by Lao women in the West, although they frequently enter the system at 5–6 months into the pregnancy and as late as 8 months.

Pregnancy is considered a "hot" condition, and the rapid loss of heat at parturition (e.g. blood and placental loss) places the woman in extreme risk for cold illness. To correct this imbalance, numerous herbs and tonics are consumed, and other warming practices like steam baths, are sometimes performed. The mother is often kept in the home and relieved of household tasks during this vulnerable period, at least 30 days postpartum. Severe arthritis and other illnesses are believed to occur later in life if these postpartum practices are not observed.

Breastfeeding is the norm, up to 2 years, and a mashed rice mixture may be introduced to the infant as early as 2 months (Ethnomed, 1996). Colostrum is considered poisonous and usually expressed, with rice paste or boiled sugar water given instead (Geissler, 1998). Breastfeeding mothers avoid overly spicy and salty foods to prevent diarrhea in the infant.

Abortion is utilized by some Lao in the West, even though the practice is antithetical to Buddhism. Birth control, particularly oral contraceptives, is widely used among resettled Lao but may be opposed by the more traditional for fear of potential side effects, particularly cancer.

More traditional Laotians believe that illness can be brought about by past sins in this or even past lives, especially concerning birth defects and chronic illness in infants (Ethnomed, 1996). Fat infants are considered healthy (Geissler, 1998). Invasive procedures like nasal oxygen and scalp vein intravenous drips are frightening to the newborn's family because the soul or spirit may escape through these points (D'Avanzo, 1992).

End of life

"*Nobody can control when a woman delivers a baby. Nobody can control when a monk disrobes (leaves the* sangha). *And nobody can control when a person dies.*"
Laotian proverb

Illness and especially the end of life is a family affair in Laotian culture (from Keovilay *et al.*, 2000). The family stays with the patient through illness and increasingly so in the final days. In most cases, and especially in intact extended families, the family will wish to control information given to the patient with open discussion of terminal status is resisted by most Laotian families.

The traditional practice after death is for family members to wash the body and dress it with at least some clothing on backward (to confuse the spirit that might return to disturb the living) and/or torn (to discourage robbers in the spirit world from stealing the spirit). A coin may be placed in the mouth, as may an engraving which contains answers to riddles likely to be asked by spirit guardians of cardinal directions. Failure to correctly answer these riddles results in the soul wandering. The 32 spirits of the body are believed to separate from the body at death and to recombine in reincarnation. Spirits from those who died violent deaths, in childbirth, and in accidents are believed to wander the earth inflicting suffering on others (Oberg & Deinard, 1984).

Ideally, there is a day-long ceremony (3 days in Laos) conducted by monks in the home, with the body present. Central to the ceremony is chanting in *Pali*. Some Laotians believe that the chanting is to help guide the spirit onward, while others understand that the chanting is focused more on the inevitability of suffering and the transient nature of life (Langford, 2000). As with other such ceremonies, food is shared, and in particular, food is given to the monks. At some point before cremation, a string attached to the body is held by family members and after further chanting, is cut by the monk between the body and those holding the string as a symbolic separation of the living from the dead.

Cremation is preferred both in Laos and the West. Ashes and bones are sometimes sent back to Laos for interment in an auspicious place. In some cases, ashes and bones are placed in the spirit house, found at virtually all traditional Laotian homes. Additional ceremonies are held 7 and 100 days after cremation, as well as during the New Year celebration in April and at other times.

Health problems and screening

Laos is an isolated landlocked country that still has not recovered from the Indochina wars. The healthy life expectancy or HALE in Laos is 44.2 years and the full life expectancy is 54 years (Population Reference Bureau, 2002; World Health Organization (WHO), 2002). Infectious diseases are the leading causes of death and disability in Laos. Although Laos is not one of 22 countries worldwide with a "high burden" of tuberculosis (WHO, 2003), it likely has a very high burden. Health risks for new Laotian immigrants or refugees (Hawn & Jung, 2003; Kemp, 2002; WHO, 2002) include:

- amebiasis
- angiostrongyliasis
- anthrax
- capillariasis
- chikungunya
- cholera

- cryptococcosis
- cryptosporidiosis
- cysticercosis (tapeworm)
- dengue fever
- encephalitis (Japanese)
- filariasis (Bancroftian filariasis and Malayan filariasis)
- gnathostomiasis
- helminthiasis (ascariasis, echinococcosis/hydatid disease, schistosomiasis)
- hepatitis B (15.5% carriage rate)
- hookworm
- leishmaniasis
- leprosy
- leptospirosis
- malaria, including multidrug resistant (MDR) from *Plasmodium falciparum* resistant parasites and especially from malaria re-infection.
- melioidosis
- mycetoma
- sexually transmitted infections, including HIV/AIDS, chancroid, chlamydia, gonorrhea, granuloma inguinale, lymphogranuloma venereum, syphilis
- strongylodiasis
- thalassemias
- trematodes (liver-dwelling: clonorchiasis and opisthorchiasis; blood-dwelling: schistosomiasis or bilharzias; intestine-dwelling; and lung-dwelling: paragonimiasis)
- tropical sprue
- tuberculosis
- yaws (frambesia)
- post-traumatic stress disorder
- nutritional deficits

Acknowledgements

Arouny Khounvixay, Ann Rynearson

REFERENCES

D'Avanzo, C. E. (1992). Bridging the cultural gap with Southeast Asians. *American Journal of Maternal Child Nursing*, **17**, 204–8.

DeVoe, P. A. (1996). Lao. In *Refugees in America in the 1990s: A Reference Handbook*, ed. D. Haines, pp. 259–78. Westport, CT: Greenwood Press.

Ethnomed (1996). Voices of the Lao community. In *Cross Cultural Health Care Project*. Retrieved July 1, 2003 from http://ethnomed.org/ethnomed/voices/lao.html.

Geissler, E. M. (1998). Laos. In *Cultural Assessment, 2nd edn*, pp. 158–62. St. Louis: Mosby.

Hawn, T. R. & Jung, E. C. (2003). Health screening in immigrants, refugees, and internationally adopted orphans. In *The Travel and Tropical Medicine Manual*, 3rd edn., ed. E. C. Jong and R. McMullen, pp. 255–65. Philadelphia, PA: W. B. Saunders.

Immigration and Refugee Services of America. (2002). *Refugee Reports, 23*. Retrieved June 13, 2003 from http://www.refugees.org.

Kemp, C. & Keovilay, L. (1999). Health care beliefs of Laotians living in America. In the web site, *Refugee Health~Immigrant Health*. Retrieved October 27, 2000 from http://www.baylor.edu/~Charles_Kemp/laotian_health.html.

Kemp, C. E. (2002). *Infectious Diseases*. Retrieved April 12, 2003 from http://www3.baylor.edu/~Charles_Kemp/Infectious_Disease.htm.

Keovilay, L., L. Rasbridge, & C. Kemp (2000). Cambodians and Laotians – health beliefs and practices related to the end of life. *Journal of Hospice and Palliative Nursing, 2*, 143–51.

Langford, J. M. (2000). Death and dying in ethnic America: findings in Lao Lum, Khmu, Hmong, Khmer, and Cham communities. In *Death and Dying in Ethnic America*, ed. N. R. Z. Solomon and J. M. Langford Seattle: Cross Cultural Health Care Project.

Oberg, C. N. & Deinard, A. (1984). Marasmus in a 17-month-old Laotian: impact of folk beliefs on health. *Pediatrics, 73*, 254–7.

Population Reference Bureau (2002). *2002 World Population Data Sheet*. Retrieved May 12, 2003 from http://www.prb.org/pdf/WorldPopulationDS02_Eng.pdf.

Rynearson, A. (1999). Gatekeepers and culture brokers: Refugee access to American institutions. In *Selected Papers on Refugee and Immigrants*, ed. J. Lipson and L. A. McSpadden, *Vol. VII*, pp. 131–55. Arlington, VA: American Anthropological Association.

World Health Organization (2002). *World Health Report*. Retrieved June 5, 2003 from http://www.who.int/whr/2002/en/.

(2003). *Global TB Control Report 2003*. Retrieved June 1, 2003 from http://www.who.int/gtb/publications/globrep/index.html.

27

Liberia

Doug Henry

Introduction

Liberia is located on the Atlantic coast of West Africa, and is bordered by Sierra Leone, Cote d'Ivoire, and Guinea. Although rich in natural resources, more than 20 years of atrocities and widespread corruption mean that most Liberians do not benefit from these potential riches. There are approximately 16 different ethnic groups indigenous to the country, including Mandingo, Kpelle, Bassa, Gio, Kru, Grebo, Mano, Krahn, Gola, Gbandi, Loma, Kissi, Vai, and Bella. "Americo-Liberians" (those descended from former slaves of Americans) and descendants of freed Caribbean slaves comprise about 5% of the population (D'Avanzo & Geissler, 2003).

Liberia is a diverse country, and one that has undergone rapid sociocultural change in the last 25 years. Both the many changes and the multiple ethnic groups make generalizations about Liberian culture difficult. All Liberians have, however, been touched in some way by the incredibly bloody conflict that continues to devastate their country as this is written (Faris, 2003).

History of immigration

Liberia was settled in 1822 by freed American slaves and became Africa's first independent state in 1847. The "Americo-Liberians" who founded Liberia were always a small minority and in 1980, lost power in a coup led by army sergeant Samuel Doe. Doe was overthrown in 1990 by Charles Taylor and tortured to death (on videotape) (Public Broadcasting System, 2002). Since 1990, a number of Liberians have been resettled as refugees in the USA (Immigration and Refugee Services of America (IRSA), (2002). Because of their fluency in English and relative familiarity with American culture, they have not formed visible and defined ethnic enclaves as compared to other refugees.

Refugee and Immigrant Health: A Handbook for Health Professionals, Charles Kemp and Lance A. Rasbridge. Published by Cambridge University Press. © C. Kemp and L. A. Rasbridge 2004.

Culture and social relations

Traditional families are extended and much of the culture is oriented to the tribal group of the family. In most cases, men are dominant. However, the presence of secretive women's *Sande* societies may be taken to mean that women have powers that are difficult for others to understand.

Liberian boys and girls almost universally join in the men's (*Poro*) and women's (*Sande*) societies during their adolescence, where they are formally instructed in history and genealogy, rules governing social relations, medicinal plants, agriculture, and forest survival skills. They may join voluntarily, be persuaded by family, or even be "kidnapped" by older relatives or friends (though often with the tacit approval and knowledge of their parents). Membership in these societies is likely to be less among Liberian refugees.

Communications

Even though English is the official language of Liberia, important semantic differences exist between "Liberian English" and "American English" that necessitate extreme care in communication. For instance, seemingly simple and straightforward questions like "what has your child eaten today?" may often elicit a false-negative answer. In this case it is necessary to understand the cultural context of "eating" in Liberia, in which the word "food" is often taken to mean rice. Rice is the staple food in Liberia, and "to eat" literally translates into Liberian English as "to eat rice." One researcher notes that a Liberian may consume large quantities of bread, potatoes, cassava, plantain, or yams, yet still feel underfed unless rice has also been eaten (Jarosz, 1990).

Religion

Liberia was founded as a Christian state. However, less than 40% of Liberians are Christian; almost 50% of Liberians practice indigenous religions, which include ancestor worship and secret society membership; and a further 13% are Muslim (Johnstone & Mandryk, 2001). The CIA, however, estimates the breakdown of religions practiced in Liberia to be: indigenous beliefs 40%, Christian 40%, and Muslim 20% (CIA, 2003). Yet even in areas where Christianity or Islam dominates, aspects of indigenous religions enter and become a part of modern belief systems, and individuals may combine aspects of all three systems. Even those who consider themselves to be devout Muslims or Christians may also follow indigenous practices, such as prayers or sacrifices to the ancestors, traditional prophecy or divination, or the use of charms to ward off evil spirits or witchcraft.

Health beliefs and practices

Sicknesses are generally thought to arise in one of two ways: from inanimate, natural forces in the physical environment, or as the result of the actions of some intentionally malevolent power. If the sickness is unusual or unresponsive to treatment, a religious or society person may be called upon to ask the ancestral spirits to ascertain the cause.

Most Liberians see no discrepancy in attributing the etiology of disease to both naturalistic (biological) and supernatural causes. The question of immediate cause may be commonsensical or biological, but the answer to the question of "why did this occur to me" may be seen as sorcery, taboo violation, or some form of contagion (especially from breeze, cold, water, or dreaming). Consequently, Liberians may simultaneously combine indigenous and biomedical forms of treatment. If it is suspected that indigenous medication may be interfering with a biomedical treatment, the person in charge of decision-making for the sick person (perhaps a family head) may be sensitively asked what other forms of treatment are being concurrently given, without making judgments about the efficacy of the other treatment, as this may simply result in false information being given.

The use of indigenous medicines in Liberia is common, and most individuals have some knowledge of certain plants that may be self-applied in times of sickness. Liberians also have an assortment of indigenous healers, including herbalists, Muslim clergy, society elders, bone specialists, and increasingly, faith healers. A *Zoe* is a person who has and uses (or is expected to use) supernatural powers over medicines and spirits for the good of the community. *Zoes* often become *Poro* and *Sande* (secret) society elders whose groups meet in forest clearings called "*Zoe* bushes."

Supernatural treatments are often complex rituals. For example, in one kind of treatment to set a patient's bone fracture, the leg of a live chicken may be broken at same time. The practitioner then treats both fractures: oil is rubbed over the site, and small twigs are then wrapped around the wound, which has been covered in a chalky poultice. At the time that the chicken leg is healed, the patient is believed to be healed too, and the poultice removed. It should be emphasized here that such practices do not, as far as is known, exist among refugees or immigrants to the West.

Liberians, especially those from rural areas, may have different body-imagery than the ideal lean Western type. A healthy body in Liberia is perceived as a stout one, and is also associated with wealth and prosperity. The palm oil that Liberians prefer to cook their food with is high in saturated fats. As food shortages have been critical since the beginning of the civil war in 1989, chronic malnutrition, especially in children, is quite common. Many parents believe that Western medicine's tablets and injections can reverse and cure the effects of malnutrition (Geissler, 1998).

Sexually transmitted infections are common in Liberia, due at least in part to poverty, war, and violence (Henry, 1998). The HIV prevalence rate among adults is estimated at 9%, and as many as 50% of Liberian women have been raped (Central Intelligence Agency (CIA), 2003; D'Avanzo & Geissler, 2003). In Liberia, STIs are most often treated by oneself or by non-Western or "traditional" healers, typically herbalists or Muslim clergy who use ointments or teas, though less commonly an enema or vaginal implant may be used (Green, 1992).

Female genital cutting (FGC) has been performed on about 60% of Liberian women – usually type II (removal of prepuce and clitoris together with the partial or complete excision of the labia minora) (Toubia, 1999). FGC is performed in Liberia by the older *Zoes* of the women's society. See Chapter 6 for a more extensive discussion of FGC.

Pregnancy and childbirth

In Liberia, birth is handled by experienced midwives in birthing centers. In the West, however, Liberian immigrants prefer hospital births. Women may fear a protracted labor, as this traditionally indicated some unnamed transgression she had committed before. Pregnant women may be considered particularly vulnerable to illness, particularly those arriving from cold breezes, or the "ill will" inflicted by a jealous person.

Indigenous Liberian religious systems have a strong belief in the possibility of reincarnation; a newborn baby may be considered an ancestor who has returned in the form of a child. If an infant dies, the family is encouraged to not mourn, but is assisted by an older person to ascertain why the ancestor spirit has left. A sacrifice will be made to appease the anger of the spirit. Twins are widely presumed to have special powers.

Children are highly valued, as they indicate a successful marriage. In Liberia, a newborn is traditionally first held by the mother and her closest women kin, but the father is not to hold the child until after its naming ceremony several days later. Though a Christian or Islamic name may be given in a hospital in the West, infants are customarily named several days after birth. Children are constantly carried, and are usually nursed on demand. They are expected to contribute to household chores at an early age.

For boys, circumcision customarily takes place before society initiation, between the ages of 6–10. It is primarily a family affair, although the community may become involved by giving gifts or encouragement. For girls, genital cutting is the culmination of her initiation into the women's society, and is considered crucial to her future fertility and eligibility to marry.

End of life

Death may come from many sources: natural forces, the ancestors calling an individual to them, bewitchment on the part of a malicious force, or even a witch spirit residing within the person (even if unknown) inflicting death. It should be noted that witchcraft is rarely considered to be at the root of illnesses among Liberians living in the West.

Mourning and bereavement can be quite emotional compared to conservative Western norms. Funerals are important, and can be lengthy and elaborate, often going on for days or weeks at a time. The body is traditionally prepared by first washing it, dressing it in clean clothes, then wrapping it in layers of cloth and mats. The dead person is assumed not to enter the spirit world at once; women are believed to take 3 days to join the ancestors, men 4 days.

Health problems and screening

The healthy life expectancy or HALE in Liberia is 37.5 years and the full life expectancy is 50 years (Population Reference Bureau, 2002; World Health Organization (WHO), 2002). Infectious diseases are the leading documented causes of death and disability in Liberia. War wounds, malnutrition, and the sequelae of other violence are probably also major causes of death and disability. Health risks for new Liberian immigrants or refugees (Geissler, 1998; Hawn & Jung, 2003; Kemp, 2002; WHO, 2002) include:

- amebiasis
- anthrax
- cholera
- crimean–Congo hemorrhagic fever
- dengue fever and dengue hemorrhagic fever
- dracunculiasis (Guinea worm disease) (Primarily West Africa (Nigeria) and Sudan; other areas of tropical Asia and Africa, Middle East, South America)
- Ebola hemorrhagic fever and Marburg hemorrhagic fever (not current, but possible)
- echinococcosis (Hydatid disease)
- filariasis (Bancroftian filariasis and Malayan filariasis; loiasis or loa loa (worms live in subcutaneous tissue); and onchocerciasis)
- hemorrhagic fevers (HFs) (Lassa HF, Marburg and Ebola HFs, Crimean–Congo HF, Chikungunya fever, dengue fever and dengue HF, and Rift Valley fever)

- hookworm
- leishmaniasis
- leprosy
- malaria
- malnutrition
- plague
- relapsing fevers (tick-borne)
- sexually transmitted infections, including HIV/AIDS (estimated 9% prevalence rate), cervical cancer, chancroid, chlamydia, gonorrhea, granuloma inguinale, lymphogranuloma venereum, syphilis
- sickle cell disease or sickle cell hemoglobulinopathies
- strongylodiasis
- trachoma
- trematodes (liver-dwelling: clonorchiasis and opisthorchiasis; blood-dwelling: schistosomiasis or bilharzias; intestine-dwelling; and lung-dwelling)
- trypanosomiasis (African) or African sleeping sickness
- tuberculosis
- typhoid and paratyphoid fever
- typhus
- yaws (frambesia)
- post-traumatic stress disorder

REFERENCES

Ackerman, L. K. (1997). Health problems of refugees. *Journal of the American Board of Family Practice*, **10**, 337–48.

Central Intelligence Agency (2003). *World Factbook 2002* (revised 2003). Retrieved April 29, 2003 from http://www.cia.gov/cia/publications/factbook/geos/li.html.

D'Avanzo, C. E. & Geissler, E. M. (2003). *Pocket Guide to Cultural Assessment*, 3rd edn. St. Louis: Mosby.

Ellis, S. (1995). Liberia: a study of ethnic and spiritual violence. *African Affairs*, **94**, 165–7.

Faris, S. (2003). Welcoming America with loaded arms: Liberia is a place where violence is a difficult habit to outgrow. *Time Magazine* (online). Retrieved July 17, 2003 from http://www.time.com/time/magazine/article/0,9171,1101030721-464461,00.html.

Gavagan, T. & Brodyaga, L. (1998). Medical care for immigrants and refugees. *American Family Physician*, **57**, 1061–8.

Geissler, E. (1998). *Cultural Assessment*, 2nd edn. St. Louis: Mosby.

Green, E. (1992). The anthropology of sexually transmitted disease in Liberia. *Social Science and Medicine*, **35**, 1457–68.

Henry, D. (1998). *Health, Income, and Empowerment among Sierra Leonean Refugees in Guinea*. Technical report submitted to the United Nations field office. Gueckedou, Guinea.

Hawn, T. R. & Jung, E. C. (2003). Health screening in immigrants, refugees, and internationally adopted orphans. In *The Travel and Tropical Medicine Manual*, 3rd edn., ed. E. C. Jong and R. McMullen, pp. 255–65. Philadelphia, PA: W. B. Saunders.

Immigration and Refugee Services of America. (2002). *Refugee Reports,* 23. Retrieved May 14, 2003 from www.refugees.org.

Jarosz, L. (1990). Intercultural communication in assessing dietary habits: Liberia as an example. *Journal of the American Dietetic Association,* **90**, 1094–9.

Johnstone, P. & Mandryk, J. (2001). *Operation World: 21st Century Edition,* Waynesboro, GA: Paternoster USA.

Kemp, C. (2002). *Infectious Diseases.* Retrieved April 12, 2003 from http://www3.baylor. edu/~Charles_Kemp/Infectious_Disease.htm.

Moran, M. (2001). Liberia. In *Countries and their Cultures,* ed. M. Ember and C. Ember. New Haven: Human Relations Area Files and Macmillan Reference Press.

Onishi, N. (12/7/2000). In ruined Liberia, its despoiler sits pretty. *New York Times.* Vol. CL, No. 51, 595, pp. A1, A18.

Population Reference Bureau (2002). *2002 World Population Data Sheet.* Retrieved May 12, 2003 from http://www.prb.org/pdf/WorldPopulationDS02_Eng.pdf.

Public Broadcasting System (2002). *The Lone Star: The Story of Liberia.* Retrieved July 7, 2003 from http://www.pbs.org/wgbh/globalconnections/liberia/essays/history/.

Sawyer, A. (1992). *The Emergency of Autocracy in Liberia: Tragedy and Challenge.* San Francisco: Institute for Contemporary Studies.

Swiss, S. Jennings, P. J., Aryee, G. V. *et al.* (1998). Violence against women during the Liberian civil conflict. *Journal of the American Medical Association,* **279**, 625–9.

Toubia, N. (1999). *Caring for Women with Circumcision.* New York: Rainbo Publications. Also available on-line at www.rainbo.org.

World Health Organization (2002). *World Health Report.* Retrieved June 5, 2003 from http://www.who.int/whr/2002/en/.

28

Mexico

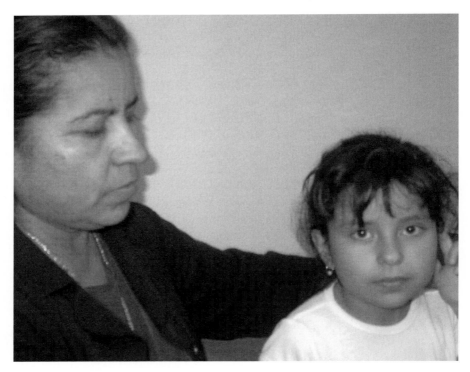

Mexican Mother and daughter in a community clinic. (Photograph by courtesy of Charles Kemp.)

Introduction

Mexico was originally populated by indigenous people or Native Americans such as the empire-building *Mexicas* (Aztecs) and Mayans, and also by the lesser-known Olmecs, Tiotihuacáns, Toltecs, and others from about 1500 BC – AD 1500. The

Refugee and Immigrant Health: A Handbook for Health Professionals, Charles Kemp and Lance A. Rasbridge. Published by Cambridge University Press. © C. Kemp and L. A. Rasbridge 2004.

Spanish arrived in central Mexico in 1519 and by 1521 had conquered the *Mexica* civilization. Spanish colonials forced the subjugated people to work in plantations, mines, and other enterprises, and in less than a century (1519–1605), the Native American population in Mexico went from 25 million to one million – "a catastrophe greater in scale than any that has occurred even in the twentieth century" (McKay *et al.*, 2000, p. 516). Mexico achieved independence from Spain in 1821 and from then until 1929, when the Institutional Revolutionary party, or PRI took power, there was a series of regimes, revolutions, and conflicts. In December 2000, the National Action Party (PAN) won power in Mexico's first free and fair elections.

The racial breakdown of people living in Mexico, and presumably Mexicans living in other countries, is 60% *Mestizo* (indigenous or Amerindian and Spanish), 30% primarily Amerindian, 9% Anglo, and 1% other (Central Intelligence Agency (CIA), 2002). The estimated population of Mexico exceeds 100 million, with between 40–66% of the population living in poverty. While the Mexican economy has grown in recent years, buying power has shrunk 80% since 1976 and inflation continues to increase at a faster rate than wages (CIA, 2002; Rangel, 1999).

History of immigration

Because of the common border between Mexico and the USA, the histories and cultures of these countries have long been intertwined. The acceleration of trade and immigration in the late 20th century increased the connections with resultant increased cultural blending as well, increasing the number and size of Mexican and other Latino enclaves in urban and rural areas throughout the USA. In 2001, Mexicans (mostly Mexican–Americans) became the largest minority population in the USA. (US Census Bureau, 2003).

There are several basic patterns of legal and illegal migration to and settlement in the USA.

- Migrant workers travel to the USA each year and follow agricultural patterns of sowing and reaping from one crop to another before returning home to Mexico.
- Others, especially men, come to the USA to work as day laborers while seeking steady employment.
- Others, especially families, come to the USA and seek employment and housing in one locale, thus establishing themselves as part of a community.
- There also are increasing numbers of Mexican migrants who are college graduates coming to the USA for professional employment.

Until the post-September 11-era, it was common for immigrants to regularly travel back and forth from the USA to Mexico. Crossing the border has always been dangerous, and multiple deaths in 2003 demonstrate the increased danger.

Culture and social relations

Familism, the valuing of family considerations over individual or community needs, is a strong value in the Mexican community (Juarez *et al.*, 1998; Lieberman *et al.*, 1997). Extended families are common, even among Mexicans outside of Mexico and it is also common for several family units to live in close proximity to one another.

The father or oldest male (direct relative) holds the greatest power in most families and may make health decisions for others in the family. Men are expected to provide for, and be in charge of, their families. Though increasing numbers of women work outside the home, home-making is the expected role. At least publicly, women are expected to manifest respect and even submission to their husbands. Privately, some women hold a greater degree of power. However, in too many marriages, the threat of physical violence is real and under-reported (De Paula *et al.*, 1996). Two specific gender roles should be noted here.

- *Machismo* or macho is stereotypically viewed as a kind of foolish male pride in which men are depicted almost as buffoons driven to folly by male hormones. To the contrary, *machismo* is a defined sense of honor that is vital to the Mexican man's sense of self, self-esteem, and manhood.
- Women are idealized in some respects and oppressed in others. Family violence is not uncommon. The woman is expected to be the primary force holding the family and home together through work and cultural wisdom.

Upward mobility, education, and other societal forces are changing the above, yet in isolated communities and among new immigrants, there is little change.

Communications

Spanish is the primary language of Mexico. There are numerous dialects and variations, but all are mutually intelligible. Among the young, it is common to use a mix of Spanish and English. Newer immigrants tend to speak only Spanish.

About 90% of Mexicans are literate (CIA, 2002) and a higher percentage of Mexicans in the USA are literate. This does not mean, however, that reading and writing are common means of communication among those from lower socio-economic backgrounds. The most commonly encountered books in many Mexican homes in the *barrio* are required schoolbooks, pictorial novelettes, and the Bible.

Verbal and nonverbal communications from Mexicans and other Hispanics usually are characterized by *respeto* (respect) and there is an element of formality in interactions, especially when older persons are involved. It is uncommon for Mexicans to be aggressive or assertive in healthcare interactions, and direct eye contact is less among Mexicans than among Anglos. Over-familiarity by strangers such as touching or casual use of first names is not appreciated early in relationships (De Paula *et al.*, 1996).

A brusque, confrontational, or loud healthcare provider may (a) not learn of significant complaints or problems and (b) find the patient unlikely to return. Despite a lack of public complaint, Mexicans tend to have an acute sense of justice and often perceive failures in communication to be due to prejudice.

Naming is an important aspect of Mexican and Central American cultures and a source of confusion where medical records are concerned. Most people have two first names, e.g., Ana María + the father's family name (*primer apellido*), e.g., Camacho + the mother's family name (*segundo apellido*), e.g., Pérez. Her full or legal name is thus Ana María Camacho Pérez, but she may also be known as Ana María Camacho. If she marries (Juan Carlos Guerrero Martinez, for example), she will take her husband's *primer apellido* as follows: Ana María Pérez de Guerrero (Guerrero being the husband's father's family name). In the USA, she will likely be known as Ana María Guerrero or perhaps Ana Guerrero or María Guerrero.

Religion

Most Mexicans are Roman Catholics, and the faith and church often are involved in day-to-day family and community life, with activities throughout the week and most of the day on Sunday. Along with Catholicism is a concurrent belief in and use of magico-religious means of dealing with life. Candles with pictures of saints are found in many homes and are often part of altars in living rooms or bedrooms. Each saint has a specialized, as well as general, religious function (Juarez *et al.*, 1998; Zapata & Shippee-Rice, 1999).

Important rites include mandatory baptism of infants, which is especially important in life-threatening situations. The Rite for Anointing the Sick (sometimes termed last rites) is required in life-threatening situations.

As in other aspects of life, the church and the people's relationship with the church is changing. One dramatic area of change is the increasing number of Catholic women who, despite clear proscriptions from the church, utilize birth control. Protestant evangelical (*Cristiana*) churches are playing an increasing role in the life of Mexican communities, offering answers to families threatened by social change, crime, gang involvement, and other such modern plagues.

Health beliefs and practices

Physical or mental illness may be attributed to an imbalance between the person and environment. Influences include emotional, spiritual, and social state, as well as physical factors such as humoral imbalance expressed as too much "hot" or "cold" (De Paula *et al.*, 1996; Spector, 1996). It is important to understand that belief in the concept of balance does not in any way obviate a concurrent belief in biomedical theories or practices (Zapata & Shippee-Rice, 1999). "Hot" and "cold" are intrinsic properties of various substances and conditions, and there are sometimes differences of opinion about what is hot, what is cold. Cold diseases/conditions commonly include menstrual cramps, rhinitis, pneumonia, and colic. "Hot" diseases/conditions include pregnancy, hypertension, diabetes, and indigestion (Neff, 1998). Cold conditions are treated with hot medications and hot with cold medications, thus bringing the individual back into balance. Problems that are primarily spiritual in nature are treated with prayer and ritual. However, few Mexicans who use folk means of treating illness are troubled by simultaneously using cosmopolitan treatments such as antibiotics, antidepressants, and so on.

Culture-bound syndromes one might encounter in a Mexican (or Central American) patient (American Psychiatric Association, 2000; De Paula *et al.*, 1996; Lieberman *et al.*, 1997; Neff, 1998; Schechter *et al.*, 2000; Spector, 1996) are as follows.

- *Antojos* are cravings in a pregnant woman. It is thought by many that failure to satisfy the cravings may lead to injury to the baby, including genetic defects.
- *Ataque de nervios* are episodic, dramatic outbursts of negative emotion – usually in response to a current stressor such as bereavement (but often related to a significant childhood stressor).
- *Barrevillos* are obsessions.
- *Bilis*, *colera*, or *muina* are thought to be bile flowing into the blood stream after a traumatic event, with the end result of nervousness and/or rage.
- *Caida de la mollera* is an illness primarily of infants and is characterized by a sunken fontanel, crying, restlessness, inability to nurse, anorexia, and diarrhea.
- *Colera* (see *bilis* above).
- *Decaiminientos* is fatigue and listlessness from a spiritual cause.
- *Dercernsos* are fainting spells.
- *Empacho* is intestinal obstruction and is characterized by abdominal pain, vomiting, constipation, anorexia, or gas and bloating. Postpartum women and infants and children are most susceptible.
- *Frio de la matriz* is coldness of the womb. Symptoms include pelvic congestion, menstrual irregularities and loss of libido, all of which may last for several years postpartum if treatment is not successful. The cause is inadequate rest after delivery.
- *Locura* refers to severe, chronic psychosis, and thus may be less a culture-bound disorder than a folk term for chronic psychosis.
- *Mal de Ojo* is the "Evil Eye" that may affect infants or women. It is caused by a person with a "strong eye" (especially green or blue) looking with admiration or

jealousy at another person. *Mal de Ojo* is avoided by touching an infant when admiring or complimenting him or her.

- *Mareos* is associated with *nerviosimo* and includes dizziness and/or vertigo.
- *Nerviosimo* (or *nervios*) is "sickness of the nerves" and is common and may be treated spiritually and/or medicinally.
- *Pasmo* is paralysis or paresis of extremities or face and is treated with massage.
- *Susto* is fright resulting in "soul loss." *Susto* may be acute or chronic and includes a variety of vague complaints. Women are affected more than men. Other terms for *susto* include *espanto*, *pasmo*, *tripa ida*, *perdida de alma*, and *chibih*.

Folk healers are utilized to varying degrees according to cultural, socioeconomic, and other factors. Folk healers found in Mexican communities (Neff, 1998; Zapata & Shippee-Rice, 1999) are as follows.

- *Yerbero is an* herbalist.
- *Sobador* is a massage therapist.
- *Partera* is a midwife who may also treat young children.
- *Cuarandero total* is a lay healer who intervenes in multiple dimensions, e.g., physical and spiritual.
- *Doctor naturalista* is "naturalist doctor."

Regardless of the source of care, the patient (and family) are likely to include faith in God as a vital component of understanding of the problem and the cure (Zapata & Shippee-Rice, 1999).

Common folk remedies from Mexico*

Remedy	Uses
Garlic (*ajo*)	*Hypertension, antibiotic, cough syrup, tripa ida*
Lead/mercury oxides (*Azarcón/Greta*)	*Empacho*, teething (remedies are heavy metal poisons)
Damiana (*Damiana*)	Aphrodisiac, *frio en la matriz*, chickenpox
Wormwood (*Estafiate*)	Aphrodisiac, *frio en la matriz*, chickenpox (remedy an intoxicant and poisonous in sufficient quantity)
Eucalyptus, e.g., Vicks Vapor Rub (*Eucalipto*)	Rhinitis, asthma, bronchitis, tuberculosis
Chaparral (*Gobernadora*)	Arthritis (poultice), tea for cancer, sexually transmitted disease, tuberculosis, cramps, *pasmo*, analgesic (remedy poisonous if taken internally in sufficient quantity)
Mullein (*Gordolobo*)	Cough suppressant, asthma, coryza, tuberculosis
Chamomile (*Manzanilla*)	Nausea, flatus, colic, anxiety; eyewash
Oregano (*Orégano*)	Rhinitis, expectorant, menstrual difficulties, worms

Passion flower (*Pasionara*)	Anxiety, hypertension
Bricklebush (*Rodigiosa*)	Adult onset diabetes, gallbladder disease
Rue (*Ruda*)	Antispasmodic, abortifacient, *empacho*, insect repellent (remedy poisonous in sufficient quantity)
Sage (*Salvia*)	Prevent hair loss, coryza, diabetes (remedy poisonous with chronic use)
Linden flower (*Tilia*)	Sedative, hypertension, diaphoretic (remedy poisonous with chronic use)
Trumpet flower (*Tronadora*)	Adult onset diabetes, gastric symptoms, chickenpox
Peppermint (*Yerba buena*)	Dyspepsia, flatus, colic, *susto*
Aloe vera (*Zábila*)	External – cuts, burns; internal – purgative, immune stimulant (remedy poisonous if taken internally in sufficient quantity)
Sapodilla (*Zapote blanco*)	Insomnia, hypertension, malaria

* Neff, 1998

Pregnancy and childbirth

Pregnancy is viewed as natural, and despite a tendency to seek prenatal care late in pregnancy or in some cases, not seeking care until delivery, birth outcome statistics for this population are good (De Paula *et al.*, 1996). When going to clinic for prenatal care, it is relatively common for a woman to be accompanied by her husband or a female relative. Female relatives tend to play a significantly supportive role throughout pregnancy and into the post-natal period or *la cuarentena*.

In most families, child-rearing is primarily the woman's responsibility. Both female and male children are encouraged to be stoic from an early age; yet paradoxically, many Mexican homes are warm and protective toward the children. Familism is a thread throughout Mexican life, including in child-rearing. Older children often have significant responsibility for younger siblings or relatives. Among Mexicans, children seem generally to be enjoyed and even treasured across generations.

End of life

The family (except for pregnant women) is often significantly involved in caring for a family member who is dying, with women doing most of the actual care and men maintaining a strong presence. In addition, many Catholic parishes have an active auxiliary, and members may be involved in caring for the person who is dying or supporting the family in the care. Pain management for Hispanics in general tends to be less adequate than for Anglos (Todd *et al.*, 2000). Autopsies and organ donations are usually resisted.

Public expression of grief is expected under some circumstances, especially among women (De Paula *et al.*, 1996), but stoicism is also valued. It is not uncommon for funeral services to include both the Catholic rosary and a sermon by a Protestant minister. Traditionally, a Catholic ritual called a *Novena* (and including a rosary) is held each day for ten days after the burial. Some Mexicans believe that children who die are angels and that crying for them will wet their wings, thus making flying more difficult. To those who have this belief, then, crying for deceased adults is more acceptable than crying for children (Munet-Vilaró, 1998).

The Day of the Dead (*El Dia de los Muertos*) provides an opportunity for Mexicans to confront mortality in a culturally supportive atmosphere. *El Dia de los Muertos* is held November 2nd, the same day as the Catholic feast of All Souls. The former is rooted in pre-Christian rituals and among some families and in some communities includes giving candy shaped like a skull to each child with the child's names written on the skull; other death symbols abound during this time. Family altars are cleaned and the spirits of dead relatives invited to share the essence of food placed on the altar or a table (Munet-Vilaró, 1998).

Health problems and screening

In Mexico, the healthy life expectancy (HALE) or "the expected number of years to be lived in what might be termed the equivalent of "full health'" is 62.6 years for men and 65 years for women; the full life expectancy is 73 years for men and 78 years for women (Population Reference Bureau, 2002; World Health Organization (WHO), 2002). Increased HALE would be expected among Mexicans living in the USA or other developed nations for extended periods. In fact, there is consistent data showing that Hispanics living in the USA tend to be characterized by adverse social characteristics (especially poverty) that typically result in poor morbidity and mortality rates. However, the mortality (but not morbidity) rates are better than non-Hispanics in the USA – the "Hispanic paradox." The reasons for this paradox are unclear, but may include supportive aspects of Hispanic cultures and other factors (Franzini *et al.*, 2001).

Health issues and problems of Mexican immigrants include difficulty in accessing and utilizing the healthcare system, Type I diabetes, obesity, late diagnosis of cancer, and substance abuse (especially of alcohol abuse among men and especially weekend binge drinking) (Alaniz, 2002; DHHS, 1998; Nielsen, 2001; Spector, 1996). Health risks for immigrants from Mexico and other areas of Latin America (Ackerman, 1997; Centers for Disease Control, 2003; Gavagan & Brodyaga, 1998; Hawn & Jung, 2003; Kemp, 2002) are noted below. Note, however, that Mexico is a large country with jungles, deserts, and temperate climates; health risks antecedent to migration vary according to climate and other factors:

- amebiasis
- angiostrongyliasis
- anisakiasis
- arbovirus encephalitis (Eastern equine encephalomyelitis (EEE))
- Chagas' disease
- cholera
- chromomycosis
- cryptococcosis
- cryptosporidiosis
- dengue fever
- dracunculiasis (Guinea worm disease)
- filariasis (Bancroftian filariasis, Malayan filariasis, and to a lesser extent, onchocerciasis)
- hepatitis B
- leishmaniasis
- leprosy
- leptospirosis
- malaria
- mucocutaneous leishmaniasis (*Espundia*)
- mycetoma
- paracoccidioidomycosis (South American blastomycosis)
- STDs, including HIV/AIDS, chancroid, chlamydia, gonorrhea, granuloma inguinale, lymphogranuloma venereum, syphilis
- strongylodiasis
- toxoplasmosis
- trichuriasis (trichocephaliasis or whipworm)
- tuberculosis (Note that having had a BCG vaccination (a) may confound the Mantoux/PPD by causing variable results and (b) does not contraindicate PPD as is sometimes thought) (Uphold & Graham, 1998).
- tungiasis
- typhoid fever
- yaws (frambesia)
- yellow fever
- chronic non-communicable diseases as discussed above

Acknowledgements

Lupe Springer and Estevan Garcia

REFERENCES

Ackerman, L. K. (1997). Health problems of refugees. *Journal of the American Board of Family Practice*, **10**, 337–48.

Alaniz, M. L. (2002). Migration, acculturation, displacement: migratory workers and "substance abuse." *Substance Use and Misuse*, **37**, 1253–7.

Centers for Disease Control (2003). *Health Information for Travelers to Mexico and Central America*. Retrieved June 11, 2003 from http://www.cdc.gov/travel/camerica.htm.

Central Intelligence Agency (2002). *World Factbook*. Retrieved January 22, 2003 from http://www.odci.gov/cia/publications/factbook/geos/mx.html.

Franzini, L., Ribble, J. C., & Keddie, A. M. (2001). Understanding the Hispanic paradox. *Ethnicity and Disease*, **11**, 496–518.

Gavagan, T. & Brodyaga, L. (1998). Medical Care for immigrants and refugees. *American Family Physician*, **57**, 1061–8.

Geissler, E. M. (1998). *Cultural Assessment*. St. Louis: Mosby.

Hawn, T. R. & Jung, E. C. (2003). Health screening in immigrants, refugees, and internationally adopted orphans. In *The Travel and Tropical Medicine Manual*, 3rd edn. ed. E. C. Jong and R. McMullen, pp. 255–65. Philadelphia, PA: W. B. Saunders.

Juarez, G., Ferrell, B., & Borneman, T. (1998). Perceptions of quality of life in Mexican patients with cancer. *Cancer Practice*, **6**, 318–24.

Kemp, C. E. (2002). Infectious diseases. Retrieved April 12, 2003 from http://www3.baylor.edu/~Charles_Kemp/Infectious_Disease.htm.

Lieberman, L. S., Stoller, E. P., & Burg, M. A. (1997). Women's health care: cross-cultural encounters within the medical system. *Journal of the Florida Medical Association*, **84**, 364–73.

McKay, J. P., Hill, B. D., Buckler, J, & Ebrey, P. B. (2000). *A History of World Societies*, 5th edn. Boston: Houghton Mifflin Company.

Munet-Vilaró, F. (1998). Grieving and death rituals of Latinos. *Oncology Nursing Forum*, **25**, 1761–3.

Neff, N. (1998). Folk medicine in Mexicans in the Southwestern United States. Retrieved September 24, 2000 from http://192.147.157.49/galaxy/Community/Health/Family-Health/Mexican-Health.html (no longer available on the internet).

Nielsen, A. L. (2001). Drinking in adulthood: Similarities and differences in effects of adult roles for Hispanic ethnic groups and Anglos. *Journal of Studies on Alcohol*, **62**, 745–9.

Population Reference Bureau (2002). *2002 World Population Data Sheet*. Retrieved May 12, 2003 from http://www.prb.org/pdf/WorldPopulationDS02_Eng.pdf.

Rangel, E. (1999, May 26). Working toward the middle. *The Dallas Morning News*, pp. D1, D10.

Schechter, D. S., Marshall, R., Salman, E., Goetz, D., Davies, S., & Liebowitz, M. R. (2000). Ataque de nervios and history of childhood trauma. *Journal of Trauma and Stress*, **13**, 529–34.

Spector, R. E. (1996). *Cultural Diversity in Health and Illness*, 4th edn. Stamford, CT: Appleton & Lange.

Todd, K. H., Deaton, C., D'Adamo, A. P., & Goe, L. (2000). Ethnicity and analgesic practice. *Annals of Emergency Medicine*.

United States Census Bureau (2003). *Population Estimates by Age, Sex, Race and Mexican Origin*. Retrieved January 25, 2003 from http://www.census.gov/Press-Release/www/2003/cb03-16.html.

United States Department of Health and Human Services (1998). *Frequently Asked Questions*. Available: http://www.4women.gov/faq/latina.htm.

Uphold, C. R. & Graham, M. V. (1998). *Clinical Guidelines in Family Practice*, 3rd edn. Gainesville, Florida: Barmarrae Books.

World Health Organization (2002). *World Health Report*. Retrieved June 5, 2003 from http://www.who.int/whr/2002/en/.

Zapata, J. & Shippee-Rice, R. (1999). The use of folk healing and healers by six Latinos living in New England. *Journal of Transcultural Nursing*, **10**, 136–42.

FURTHER READING

American Psychiatric Association (APA) (2000). *Diagnostic and Statistical Manual of Mental Disorders, 4th edn, text revision*. Washington, DC: Author.

Chavez, L. R., Hubbell, F. A., & Mishra, S. I. (1999). Ethnography and breast cancer control among Latinas and Anglo women in southern California. In *Anthropology in Public Health*, ed. R. A. Hahn, pp. 117–41. New York: Oxford University Press.

De Paula, T., Lagana, K., & Gonzalez-Ramirez, L. (1996). Mexican Americans. In *Culture and Nursing Care*, ed. J. G. Lipson, S. L. Dibble, and P. A. Minarik, pp. 203–21. San Francisco: UCSF Nursing Press.

Hargraves, J. L. (2001). *Race, Ethnicity and Preventive Services: No Gains for Hispanics*. Center for Studying Health System Change. Retrieved January 12, 2003 from http://www.hschange.com/CONTENT/287/.

Hoffner, R. J., Kilaghbian, T., Esekogwu, V. I., & Henderson, S. O. (1999). Common presentations of amebic liver abscess. *Annals of Emergency Medicine*, **34**(3), 351–5.

Hunt, L. M., Arar, N. H., & Akana, L. L. (2000). Herbs, prayer, and insulin: use of medical and alternative treatments by a group of Mexican–American diabetes patients. *Journal of Family Practice*, **49**, 216–23.

Kemp, C. (1999). *Terminal Illness: A Guide to Nursing Care*. Philadelphia, PA: Lippincott-Williams & Wilkins.

Pan American Health Organization (2002). *Mexico (Country Health Profile Updated for 2001)*. Retrieved January 22, 2003 from http://www.paho.org/English/SHA/prflMEX.htm.

29

Nigeria

Jenny Murray, Mindy Early, and Charles Kemp

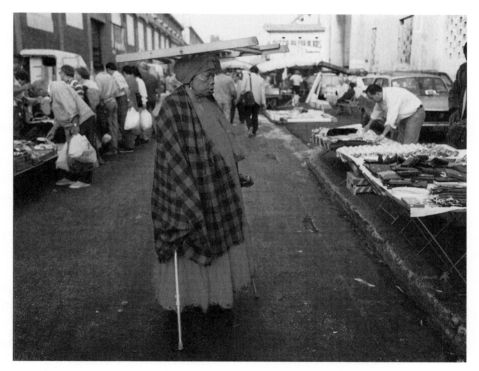

African culture meets French. (Photograph by courtesy of Judy Walgren.)

Introduction

The Federal Republic of Nigeria is in West Africa and is bounded by the Gulf of Guinea (Atlantic Ocean) in the south, Benin to the west, Niger to the north, and Cameroon to the east. With approximately 130 million people, Nigeria is the

Refugee and Immigrant Health: A Handbook for Health Professionals, Charles Kemp and Lance A. Rasbridge. Published by Cambridge University Press. © C. Kemp and L. A. Rasbridge 2004.

most populous African nation and possesses great oil reserves, mineral resources, and fertile land. Unfortunately, a culture of corruption, ethnic and tribal rivalry, religious conflict, and falling oil prices have kept this potentially rich nation mired in poverty (Johnstone & Mandryk, 2001; Population Reference Bureau (PRB), 2002).

There are more than 490 ethnic groups in Nigeria, including the Guinean (50% of the population and including the Yoruba and Igbo among the 70 Guinean peoples), the Hausa-Chadic (20% of the population and over 100 peoples), the Bantoid peoples (12% of the population and over 200 peoples), the Fulbe or Fulani (11% of the population and seven groups), and other smaller groups. The population of Nigeria is roughly 52% Christian, 41% Muslim, and 6% traditionalist (Johnstone & Mandryk, 2001).

History of immigration

Immigrants *to* Nigeria are drawn from neighboring nations by economic opportunity. In 1983 Nigeria ordered all resident aliens to leave the country, ostensibly because of economic conditions. At that time about 700 000 Ghanaians left, along with many others from African and Asian countries. Outmigration of large numbers of Nigerians to Europe and North America began about that time. In the 1990s, a few Nigerians came to Western countries as political refugees, some of whom had been tortured. Many Nigerian immigrants and refugees are well educated, but in the West are often underemployed (Early *et al.*, 2000).

Culture and social relations

With multitudinous tribes, ethnic groups, traditions, and several competing religions, it clearly is difficult or impossible to conceptualize "Nigerian culture." Still, there are beliefs, practices, and patterns that reach across most groups.

Traditionally, most Nigerian families are extended, though nuclear families are also common in urban areas and are the norm for overseas Nigerians. The importance of support from extended families and the respect given to elders may be manifested in the West by Nigerians adopting fictive older kin referred to as "uncle" or "aunty."

Males are dominant and make most of the decisions, particularly among Muslims, but also among Christians. Marriage is often at an early age – especially for women or girls, and childbearing thus also begins early. Both Muslim and Christian men may have more than one wife, and this practice is carried over to Western countries (Henry & Kemp, 2002).

Individuals are rarely the lone decision-makers during an illness. The extended family is often involved in providing advice or even diagnoses or treatment. If the patient is unable to make decisions, authority usually passes to the eldest male present from the family. If a woman is sick, her husband will usually have decision-making power, but decisions surrounding a sick husband are usually presided over by his brothers, sisters, or uncles. A woman may, however, have consideration input for healthcare decisions, especially concerning her own children or a member of her side of the family.

Communications

English is the official language of Nigeria, and is understood or spoken to at least some extent by most educated people. Although there are more than 400 other languages at use in Nigeria, 21 of these are spoken by 96% of the people. The most widely spoken language, especially in northern and central Nigeria, is Hausa. Yoruba is the primary language of the southwest, Igbo the primary language of the southeast, and pidgin English is used throughout the south (Johnstone & Mandryk, 2001). At least among immigrants and when interacting with Westerners, Nigerians usually are soft spoken. In contrast to many other refugee or immigrant groups, there is a tendency among some Nigerians to be very insistent about receiving services to which they feel entitled.

Long and effuse greetings are commonly used and are important in healthcare encounters. Elders are particularly respected regardless of gender, and consideration can be shown to them by shaking hands with the right hand while supporting the forearm with the left hand.

Religion

For many Nigerians, regardless of specific faith, religion is very important and permeates daily life. Along with the well-known world religions, traditional religious or spiritual beliefs are very much imbedded in the daily lives and even faith practices of both Christians and Muslims. Many Nigerians, for example, offer prayers or sacrifices to ancestors, practice or subscribe to traditional prophecy or divination, or use charms to ward off evil spirits or witchcraft along with Christian or Islamic worship (Henry & Kemp, 2002).

Christianity is more commonly practiced in the south, as are traditional/ethnic religions. Christian denominations include (in descending order of percentage of adherents) independent (especially Bible or Pentecostal churches), Protestant, Catholic, and Anglican. The north is dominated by Muslims (exclusively Sunni) and *shari'a* (Islamic law) has been imposed in eight northern states. Despite the previously noted geographic trends in religion, there are Christians in the north, Muslims in the south, and traditional beliefs are found throughout Nigeria. Religious conflict in Nigeria is intense and violence is common (Johnstone & Mandryk, 2001). See Chapter 5 for discussion of religions.

Although there is great variation within indigenous religions, nearly all share beliefs in (a) one supreme creator of the universe; (b) other gods and spirits present in virtually all of nature, e.g., trees, rivers, and rocks; and (c) ancestral spirits that may help individuals, providing appropriate rituals are followed (Henry & Kemp, 2002).

Health beliefs and practices

Traditionally, health and illness are seen by many Nigerians as not only physical or mental in nature, but also as influenced by the individual's relationships with family, society, and the moral order of existence. Illness then, is a social and moral problem, as well as a personal/physical one, with these realms conceptually intertwined. In Hausa, for example, the word *ciwo* is usually used to describe pain or sickness in different parts of the body, yet can also mean an offense, a drawback, or a discouragement. Likewise, *cuta* can mean a problem with bodily function, but in a related word form means an offensive act, or to deceive or cheat (Henry & Kemp, 2002).

Traditional causation beliefs include (a) illness that "just happens" as a result of natural environmental forces such as changes in temperature and (b) illness caused by a malevolent power, e.g., by witchcraft, sorcery, or evil spirits. There also is common belief in the concept of balance or humors, such as blood, water, urine, and phlegm, and also the concept of "hot" and "cold" conditions and counterbalancing treatments. Further, health is thought to be related to a balance of sweet, sour, bitter, or salty substances or foods. Culture-bound illnesses found among Nigerians (Levine & Gaw, 1995; Makanjuola, 1987) include the following.

- *Ode Ori* (literally, "hunter of the head") is a disorder featuring the sensation of an organism crawling through the head and other parts of the body, vision changes, noises in the ears, palpitations, and other somatic complaints. Anxiety and depressive symptoms are prominent.
- Brain fag is a self-descriptive disorder that includes "brain tiredness" and "too much thinking," as well as headache, pressure or tightness in the neck, difficulty concentrating, agnosia, visual complaints, and difficulty concentrating. Brain fag occurs with greatest frequency in male students.
- *Boufee Delirante* (a French term) is a transient psychotic state consisting of sudden aggressive behavior, agitation, and confusion, sometimes with paranoid ideation and auditory and/or visual hallucinations.
- Possession by spirits or supernatural beings occurs in Nigeria, as well as other areas of Africa.

Western biomedical treatments may be used concurrently with traditional treatments, or one used if the other fails. The traditional treatment (which may include pills, teas, prayers, charms, or other measures) is thought to heal the illness through restoration of balance, and thus results in health.

Several broad types of traditional healers practice in Nigeria, and to a lesser extent, among Nigerians in the West (Henry & Kemp, 2002):

- Herbalists are the most common of traditional Nigerian healers. Among Christians and adherents to traditional religions, herbalists may be male or female.
- Muslim healers use a combination of prayers, divination, and plants or herbs. Their medicines often include written passages from Islamic texts.
- Faith healers are usually Christian or followers of traditional ethnic religions along with Christianity.
- Traditional "barbers" may circumcise, tattoo, perform uvulectomy, practice cupping, and practice other invasive procedures.

Nigerians living in the West are usually well educated, hence less likely to follow traditional beliefs or utilize traditional treatments for illness. Still, illness and regression go hand in hand, and traditional explanations or treatments among Nigerians should not surprise Western healthcare providers.

Approximately 60% of adult Nigerian women have undergone female genital cutting (FGC) during infancy, usually Type I or II, although Type III is practiced in the Muslim north (Toubia, 1999). See Chapter 6 for further discussion of FGC.

Pregnancy and childbirth

In Nigeria, obstetric care is shifting from midwives or traditional birth attendants to hospitals and clinics; in the West, Nigerian women exclusively use modern obstetric care. The practice of child and adolescent marriage, common in most of Nigeria has a negative impact on maternal and child morbidity and mortality. The extent to which child and adolescent marriage is practiced in the West is not known, but there is no reason to think it does not exist. Nigeria is one of 12 countries worldwide with the life expectancy (at birth) for women being equal to or less that that of men (52 years for men and women) (PRB, 2002).

After delivery, women are expected to stay inside the home for 40 days, bathing several times/day, and in general, being attended to by women of the family. Prolonged breastfeeding is the norm. Infants are sometimes purged to rid them of what are thought to be impurities they may have swallowed while in the uterus. Uvulectomy is performed on some infants (D'Avanzo & Geissler, 2003).

Among the traditional beliefs among the Hausa-Fulani about pregnancy is the idea that "cold" or *sanyi* causes illness, especially edema. The treatment includes very hot baths called *wankan-jego* in which the water is splashed over the woman's body using bunches of twigs. It is common for women to sustain severe burns during *wankan-jego* (Mabogunje, 1990).

In most of the world, the problem of vesicovaginal fistula no longer exists. However, the practice of the *gishiri* cut, a crude local symphysiotomy along with prolonged labor results in a high incidence rate in Nigeria. Women with vesicovaginal fistula have unremitting urinary incontinence and are thus lifelong social outcasts (Wall, 2002).

End of life

Communication about terminal illness among Nigerians is commonly indirect. The informed patient may not tell the family, and the informed family may withhold the news from the patient. In general, however, the family is crucial in communicating to the patient both information about the disease and the treatment plan. Illness trajectory predictions are not well received by most Nigerians. Whether Christian or Muslim, the common belief is that "God's time is the best." In Nigeria, dying at home is almost always preferable to the hospital, but this does not necessarily hold true for those living in the West.

Burial is preferred by most Nigerians. Many, especially the Igbo from the East, will spend large sums of money to ship a body of a family member back to Nigeria for burial. Muslims are buried in Muslim cemeteries when available, with the head pointed facing the holy city of Mecca. Otherwise, men are traditionally buried facing east towards the rising sun and women are buried facing toward the west and the setting sun.

Both Muslims and Christians believe that, following death, the soul is released from the body and must be judged before God to enter Heaven. Traditional religions emphasize reincarnation, in which the deceased is often thought to return as a member of the maternal line. Depending on ethnicity, religion, and other factors, there may be complex rituals to prepare the body before burial, especially if the family decides precautions are necessary to prevent an illness suffered by the deceased from being passed on to the soul's next life. For instance, a person who was blind in one life may have special medicines placed over the eyes upon burial, to prevent blindness in the next life.

Mourning can be quite emotional, especially when compared to Western norms. Funerals are elaborate, especially for those of high social standing, and more so for men than for women or children. Additional ceremonies usually occur 7 days, and again 40 days, after death. It is often thought that the more music and dancing, the better a person's chances of beginning a successful afterlife (Henry & Kemp, 2002).

Death is often especially difficult for surviving widows, as the deceased's male relatives are entitled to the entire material belongings of the estate. The widow may then take up (conjugal) residence with one of her former husband's brothers.

Health problems and screening

The healthy life expectancy or HALE in Nigeria is 41.9 years and the full life expectancy is 52 years (PRB, 2002; World Health Organization (WHO), 2002a). Infectious diseases are leading documented causes of death and disability in Nigeria, although hypertension and related disorders are becoming significant causes of morbidity and mortality. More than 5% of Nigerians were HIV positive in 1999 (Central Intelligence Agency, 2002). Nigeria is one of 3 countries in the world with high intensity indigenous transmission of polio; one of 22 countries with a high-burden of tuberculosis; and one of 11 countries accounting for more than 66% of world deaths from measles (Stein *et al.*, 2003; WHO, 2002b; WHO, 2003). For Nigerians living in the West, health risks include cardiac and related disorders, cancer, diabetes, and COPD. Health risks for new Nigerian immigrants or refugees (Hawn & Jung, 2003; Kemp, 2002; WHO, 2002a) include:

- amebiasis
- anthrax
- cholera
- dracunculiasis (Guinea worm disease)
- Ebola hemorrhagic fever and Marburg hemorrhagic fever (not current, but possible)
- echinococcosis (Hydatid disease)
- filariasis (Bancroftian filariasis and Malayan filariasis; loiasis or loa loa (worms live in subcutaneous tissue); and onchocerciasis)
- hemorrhagic fevers (HFs) (Lassa HF, Marburg and Ebola HFs (possibly), Crimean–Congo HF, Chikungunya fever, dengue fever and dengue HF, and Rift Valley fever)
- hepatitis B
- hookworm
- leishmaniasis
- leprosy
- malaria
- malnutrition
- measles
- plague
- polio
- relapsing fevers (tick-borne)
- sexually transmitted infections, including HIV/AIDS (>5% rate), cervical cancer, chancroid, chlamydia, gonorrhea, granuloma inguinale, lymphogranuloma venereum, syphilis
- sickle cell disease or sickle cell hemoglobinopathies

- strongylodiasis
- trachoma
- trematodes (liver-dwelling: clonorchiasis and opisthorchiasis; blood-dwelling: schistosomiasis or bilharzias; intestine-dwelling; and lung-dwelling)
- trypanosomiasis (African) or African sleeping sickness
- tuberculosis
- typhoid and paratyphoid fever
- typhus
- yaws (frambesia)

Acknowledgement

Doug Henry

REFERENCES

Central Intelligence Agency (CIA) (2002). *World Factbook* (revised 2003). Retrieved June 23, 2003 from http://www.cia.gov/cia/publications/factbook/geos/ni.html.

D'Avanzo, C. E. & Geissler, E. M. (2003). *Cultural Health Assessment*. St. Louis, MO: Mosby.

Early, M., McKinney, S., & Murray, J. (2000). *Nigerian Refugees and Immigrants*. Retrieved January 18, 2003 from http://www3.baylor.edu/~Charles_Kemp/nigerian_refugees.htm.

Hawn, T. R. & Jung, E. C. (2003). Health screening in immigrants, refugees, and internationally adopted orphans. In *Travel and Tropical Medicine Manual*, 3rd edn. ed. E. C. Jong and R. McMullen, pp. 255–65. Philadelphia, PA: W. B. Saunders.

Henry, D. & Kemp, C. (2002). Culture and the end of life: Nigerians. *Journal of Hospice and Palliative Nursing*, **4**, 111–15.

Johnstone, P. & Mandryk, J. (2001). *Operation World: 21st Century Edition*. Waynesboro, GA: Paternoster USA.

Kemp, C. (2002). *Infectious Diseases*. Retrieved April 12, 2003 from http://www3.baylor.edu/~Charles_Kemp/Infectious_Disease.htm.

Levine, R. E. & Gaw, A. C. (1995). Culture-bound syndromes. *Cultural psychiatry*, **18**, 523–36.

Mabogunje, O. A. (1990). Ritual hot baths (wankan-jego) in Zaria, Nigeria. *Newsletter of The Inter-African Committee on Traditional Practices Affecting the Health of Women and Children (IAC)*, 9, 10. Retrieved November 10, 2000 from http://www.iac-ciaf.ch.

Makanjuola, R. O. A. (1987). "Ode Ori": A culture-bound disorder with prominent somatic features in Yoruba Nigerian patients. *Acta Psychiatrica Scandinavia*, **75**, 231–6.

Population Reference Bureau (2002). *2002 World Population Data Sheet*. Retrieved May 12, 2003 from http://www.prb.org/pdf/WorldPopulationDS02_Eng.pdf.

Stein, C. E., Birmingham, M., Kurian, M., Duclos, P., & Strebel, P. (2003). The global burden of measles in the year 2000-A model that uses country-specific indicators. *Journal of Infectious Diseases*. 187(Supp. 1), S8-S14.

Toubia, N. (1999). *Caring for Women with Circumcision.* New York: Rainbo Publications.

Wall, L. L. (2002). Fitsari 'dan Duniya. An African (Hausa) praise song about vesicovaginal fistulas. *Obstetrics and Gynecology,* **100,** 1328–32.

World Health Organization (2002a). *World Health Report.* Retrieved June 5, 2003 from http://www.who.int/whr/2002/en/.

   (2002b). *Global Polio Status 2002.* Retrieved May 9, 2003 from http://www.polioeradication.org/all/global/.

   (2003). *Global TB Control Report 2003.* Retrieved June 1, 2003 from http://www.who.int/gtb/publications/globrep/index.html.

30

Pakistan

Introduction

The Islamic Republic of Pakistan as a country was born in 1947 from the division of the Indian subcontinent into India and Islamic East and West Pakistan in the wake of British colonial withdrawal. Having a country divided by more than a thousand kilometers of unfriendly (Indian) territory was untenable and East Pakistan (now Bangladesh) was partitioned off in 1971 after the third war between India and Pakistan. Dispute between India and Pakistan continues at present. All of this political turmoil and restructuring has led to large population movements internally (Central Intelligence Agency (CIA), 2003).

While modern Pakistan has largely completed the transition from an overwhelmingly agricultural to an industrial economy, social development has lagged far behind. Primarily due to the very high population growth rate, poverty is widespread, and quality of life indicators like literacy rates, human rights, and access to health care are poor (CIA, 2003). Consequently immigration to the West is comparatively high.

History of immigration

Pakistani immigrants in the West are found in the largest numbers in the United Kingdom, with 476 555 enumerated in the 1991 UK Census (Shaw, 1998), and the USA, numbering 81 691 according to the 1990 US Census (Periyakoil *et al.*, n.d.). In the USA, the population of Pakistani immigrants has grown proportionately over the last several decades, increasing from 4.5 per 1000 immigrants in 1962 to 81 per 1000 in 1990 (US Dept. of Commerce 1996). In Britain Pakistanis represent the third largest ethnic community, behind Indians and Afro-Caribbeans (Shaw, 1988). In the UK the largest communities are found in London, Manchester, Birmingham, Leeds

Refugee and Immigrant Health: A Handbook for Health Professionals, Charles Kemp and Lance A. Rasbridge. Published by Cambridge University Press. © C. Kemp and L. A. Rasbridge 2004.

and Glasgow; and in the USA in New York, Chicago, Los Angeles, and Washington, DC.

There is a wide range of socioeconomic and educational backgrounds among the peoples of Pakistan, and these differences are reflected in the immigrant populations. A random sample of Pakistanis in Britain found nearly 95% coming from rural origins. A person's area of origin in Pakistan is also significant to their identity in the community. The reasons for immigration are complex, but the vast majority come to the West for economic opportunity as well as certain "push" factors like land pressure in the homeland (Shaw, 1988). With all the background diversity, Pakistanis in the West fill occupational roles ranging from taxi drivers to physicians. Most Pakistanis immigrate through legal means, but there is a sizeable population of Pakistanis who are now out of legal status, through expiration of student and tourist visas, for example. Whatever the differences between Pakistani immigrants, some of the commonalities are that many speak little English, practice at least some folk medical practices, and many are women or children (Jan & Smith, 1998).

Culture and social relations

Punjabis are the majority ethnic group in Pakistan, followed by Sindhi, Balochi, and Pashtun. There are some marked cultural differences between ethnic groups, but in social organization there are many shared values. For example, in all Pakistan, there is preferential first cousin marriage, as the bride and groom's families already know and trust each other, and because families wish to keep wealth within their kin groups. The bride resides in the home of her husband's parents, at least for a year or so. In the West, Pakistani immigrant newcomers usually stay in the apartments of extended family, often in violation of housing codes for occupancy. In Pakistan and to a large degree in the West as well, Pakistani women marry Muslim men, usually Pakistani. Alternatively, Pakistani men are permitted to marry women from Jewish or Christian backgrounds as well as Muslims. Among the more traditional, there is still a dowry system and heavy expenditures on the marriage ceremonies of girls (Kassam, 1998; Periyakoil *et al.*, n.d.).

Pakistani society is markedly patriarchal, with the oldest male member the head of the household. All decisions with the outside world are under his authority, while women retain considerable control over the households. Perhaps half of all women in Pakistan veil in public places, but significantly less so in the West. The elderly are afforded a great deal of honor and respect. Elders, especially females, may defer important decision-making to their children (Kassam, 1998; Periyakoil *et al.*, n.d.).

Communications

Although English is the official language, Urdu is the national language in Pakistan. It is related to Arabic and Iranian (Persian) and borrows many words from both. Urdu is also similar to Hindi, spoken in India. Some elders in the West, especially women, may not have other than rudimentary English skills.

Traditionally, there is no system of surnames for Pakistani Muslims; a woman at marriage retains her given birth name, and offspring do not necessarily receive their father's second name (Shaw, 1988). To abide by Western custom, immigrant Pakistanis frequently adopt a "family name" which usually refers to their tribal or caste affiliation (Shaw, 1988).

Religion

In Pakistan, more than 97% of the population is Muslim, about three quarters of whom are Sunni, and the minority Shiite (Kassam, 1998; Parviz, 2003). Jan and Smith (1998) note that family health patterns may be integrated into the daily practices of Islam. In the West, the vast majority of Pakistanis retain their Islamic faith. In some cases the practice of faith is nominal and in other cases, very conservative. See Chapter 5 for a discussion of Islam and its influences on health beliefs and practices.

Health beliefs and practices

The more traditional believe that illness can be direct punishment from God for not following Islamic precepts; therefore, maintaining health is integrally associated with leading the proper life spiritually (Periyakoil *et al.*, n.d.). Some may view illness as a test from God to be accepted without complaint, as atonement for past sins.

There is much reliance on Islamic amulets, known as *taawiz*, often containing quotes from the Koran or otherwise blessed by an Imam. They may even be personalized by containing the bearer's name and father's name. These religious symbols when worn, carried, or pinned on clothing can cure existing maladies and moreover prevent illness inflicted through the evil eye or spirits (*jinn*). This practice is very popular even among the more acculturated immigrants. Similarly, but less common in the West, is the practice known as *chasht*, where a piece of paper bearing a Koranic verse is dissolved in water and consumed (Hunte & Sultana, 1992). In Pakistan, certain religious shrines and tombs were believed to possess innate healing powers and were frequently visited by the infirm. While these shrines do not exist in the West, there is a brisk market in religious icons and amulets from the homeland, through Western-based publications and even over the internet (S. Qureshi, personal communication, June 28, 2003).

Another very common illness etiology is the evil eye (*nazar*), covetous glances or spells cast by certain individuals. *Nazar* can cause such conditions as weakness and fatigue, diarrhea, and anorexia (Hunte & Sultana, 1992). Even the more acculturated display a vestige of recognition of the evil eye, as compliments are often immediately followed by the exclamation *mashallah*, "thanks be to God." Spirits can also cause various illnesses, purportedly by casting their shadow on a person (Jan & Smith, 1998).

According to Muslim cosmology, Allah created men, angels, and spirits (*jinn*) (Shaw, 2000). Religious specialists known as *pirs* are sought out to exorcise these widely believed-in *jinn*, in addition to reversing the effects of *nazar*. Some *pir* from Pakistan make travelling circuits through Western immigrant communities (Shaw, 2000). There is no government certification of these practitioners, and many may prey upon the more traditional and gullible Pakistanis (S. Qureshi, personal communication, June 28, 2003).

Pakistanis in their health beliefs and practices also draw from the vast knowledge base of Islamic medicine, known as *Unani* or *Hikmat*, derived in part on Greek humoral theory. Here, illness is viewed as the imbalance or obstruction of the vital forces in the body and therapy revolves around restoration of equilibrium. According to this theory, food, medicines, and even physiological states and illnesses are categorized according to opposing qualities, like "hot" (*garm*) and "cold" (*thand*). Some of the more common illnesses can be managed at home through diet management and remedies available at medicine shops, *pansari*. For example, toothache, stomach distress, and skin rashes are all considered to be signs of excess "heat" (*garm*) erupting from the body; reducing "hot" foods such as meats, tea, and sugar, and/or increasing consumption of "cold" foods (e.g. fresh fruits, rose petals and certain medicinal herbs) can correct the perceived imbalance (Hunte & Sultana, 1992; Shaw, 2000). Typically, illness diagnosis and treatment is initially under the domain of the female household elders, but traditional medical specialists, *hakim*, may be consulted if symptoms worsen. *Hakim* utilize a vast array of medicines, from herbs and plants to elaborate concoctions of minerals, some even containing toxic elements (Shaw, 2000).

In the West, it is more likely that biomedical care will be sought when symptoms cannot be relieved by home remedies. Not only are traditional *hakim* scarce, but the decision to use *hakim* was frequently economic, as they were less expensive than Western-trained providers. We have heard of *hakim* disparaged by the more Westernized Pakistanis – "They just check your pulse and diagnose you, sometimes without even looking at you." The use of Western (cosmopolitan) medicine is common even in rural Pakistan, and pharmaceuticals, particularly injectible antibiotics, are coveted. However, cosmopolitan medicines are frequently used simultaneously with more traditional remedies, in a quest for immediate relief of symptoms, and

multiple doctor usage (doctor shopping) is common, so incompatible drug interactions may result (Hunte & Sultana, 1992).

Pregnancy and childbirth

Premarital sex is rare, at least in Pakistan, and abortion rarer still, as it is specifically
proscribed by Islam. Traditionally, early pregnancies were frequent in girls and large
families the norm. Great importance was placed on male children, and women were
under considerable stress, and could even be divorced, if males were not produced.
Birth control was considered against Islam, not only as potentially defiant to God's
will, but also in that it obstructed the production of future spreaders of Islam. In
the West, smaller families are understood as an economic necessity, and the use of
various birth control measures is increasingly common (Shaw, 2000).

After birth, money, sweets, and practical gifts are presented to the mother and
child by friends and relatives. Money notes are first placed among the infant blankets
for good luck (Shaw, 1988). In Pakistan, the birth was celebrated with the slaughter
of a goat or sheep (two or more for birth of males), in a ceremony known as
aqeeqa (Shaw, 1988). Circumcision of boys occurs in the hospital, or rarely in the
traditional manner by a barber, at the time of the shaving of the first hair on the
head (about 1 week after birth). A black thread tied around the infant's wrist, or
black soot dabbed on the head (to make the infant appear unattractive), protects
the newborn from the evil eye. Swaddling was common traditionally, to protect the
child from being scared (startle reflex) by *jinn* (Mull *et al.*, 1990; Shaw, 1988).

Infants are breastfed, for at least 9 months. In rural areas of Pakistan, colostrum
is regarded as "polluted" and is discarded; similarly, a woman frightened during
breastfeeding would consider the milk polluted and discard it (Mull *et al.*, 1990).
More traditional mothers also believe that breastfeeding in cool outside air, or while
contacting water, such as when laundering, may cause diarrhea in the child (Mull &
Mull, 1988). During breastfeeding, the mother increases her consumption of dairy
products for breast milk production.

Traditionally, the expectant mother moves into her mother's household about
6 weeks before birth and remains 6 weeks afterward, with much ceremony at the
time of return to her husband. While immigrant women may not have this opportunity, avoidance of heavy exertion before delivery and observance of certain taboos,
such as food avoidances and even sex, are still practiced by some. Shaw (2000)
reports the postpartum sexual taboo to be 60 days (others report 40 days), during
which time the woman is considered polluted, similar to a menstruating woman.
According to the principles of *Unani*, pregnancy is a humorally "hot" condition
and parturition marks a dangerous loss of "heat" which must be regained in the
postpartum, e.g. through diet and traditional medicines. A specially prepared sweet
mixture containing honey, flour, sugar, and pistachio is particularly common for

Pakistanis in England (Shaw, 2000). Fathers were typically not present at births in Pakistan but are becoming more involved in the West.

End of life

Advanced directives and end of life planning are not comfortable concepts to Pakistani elderly, the most traditional of whom believe that talking of the subject may cause it to happen (Periyakoil, n.d.). "Destiny" and God's will" are key expressions in discussing a poor prognosis. Same sex providers are usually preferred, especially in extended care, and even more so, in the preparation of the deceased's body. According to Muslim ritual, the body should be washed by family and a holy person, the latter leading prayer recitation, *yaseen*. When death is imminent, and at burial, the body should be oriented facing Mecca. Common to all Islamic cultures, cremation is not allowed, and autopsy is disapproved of by the more conservative. Also, burial is not in a casket in Pakistan. However, Western laws will be followed, if reluctantly, by Pakistani immigrants. For Pakistanis in Britain, most of the deceased are shipped back to Pakistan for burial in a Muslim cemetery (Shaw, 1988).

Organ donation is usually opposed on religious grounds. Apart from the importance of "wholeness" of the body in the afterlife, Islam says that on Judgement Day, all one's organs are summoned to testify on one's life; thus one could not trust the organs of another. In reality, in Pakistan, those in need of organ transplants are said to travel to India for the operation. According to Periyakoil *et al.* (n.d.), withholding of food is forbidden, and this fact may affect decisions involving withdrawal of parenteral nutritional systems.

Health problems and screening

The healthy life expectancy or HALE in Pakistan is 50.9 years and the full life expectancy is 63 years (Population Reference Bureau, 2002; World Health Organization (WHO), 2002a). Infectious diseases are the leading causes of death and disability in Pakistan. Pakistan is one of three countries in the world with high intensity indigenous transmission of polio; one of 22 countries with a high-burden of tuberculosis; and one of eleven countries accounting for more than 66% of world deaths from measles (Stein *et al.*, 2003; WHO, 2002b, 2003). For Pakistanis living in the West, health risks include cardiac and related disorders, cancer, diabetes, and COPD. Health risks for new Pakistani immigrants (Hawn & Jung, 2003; Kemp, 2002; Periyakoil *et al.*, n.d.; WHO, 2002a) include:

- amebiasis
- anthrax
- boutonneuse fever
- brucellosis or undulant fever

- cholera
- Crimean–Congo hemorrhagic fever
- cysticercosis (tapeworm)
- dracunculiasis (Guinea worm disease)
- familial Mediterranean fever (Mediterranean area, primarily among persons of Sephardic Jewish, Armenian, and Arab ancestry)
- giardia
- helminthiasis (ascariasis, echinococcosis/hydatid disease, schistosomiasis)
- hepatitis B
- hookworm
- leishmaniasis
- malaria (including chloroquine-resistant *Plasmodium falciparum*)
- plague
- sickle cell disease or sickle cell hemoglobulinopathies (Occurs primarily in people of African lineage, but also to a lesser extent among people from the Mediterranean area, Arabs, and Indians)
- sub-mucosal (oral) fibrosis, related to the prevalence of chewing *paan*, a betel nut and tobacco quid
- thalassemias
- toxocariasis
- trachoma
- trematodes (liver-dwelling: clonorchiasis and opisthorchiasis; blood-dwelling: schistosomiasis or bilharzias; intestine-dwelling; and lung-dwelling: paragonimiasis trichinosis (trichinella))
- tuberculosis (including multidrug resistant strains)
- typhus

Acknowledgements

Dr. Zeba Kamal and Saeed Querishi

REFERENCES

Central Intelligence Agency (CIA) (2003). *World Factbook* (updated in 2003). Retrieved June 27, 2003 from http://www.cia.gov/cia/publications/factbook/geos/pk.html.

Hawn, T. R. & Jung, E. C. (2003). Health screening in immigrants, refugees, and internationally adopted orphans. In *The Travel and Tropical Medicine Manual*, 3rd edn., ed. E. C. Jong and R. McMullen, pp. 255–65. Philadelphia, PA: W. B. Saunders.

Hunte, P. A. & F. Sultana (1992). Health-seeking behavior and the meaning of medications in Balochistan, Pakistan. *Social Science and Medicine*, **34**, 1385–97.

Jan, R. & Smith, C. (1998). Staying healthy in immigrant Pakistani families living in the United States. *The Journal of Nursing Scholarship*, **30**, 157–9.

Kassam, M. (1998). Pakistan. In *Cultural Profiles*, ed. C. Lee. Toronto: University of Toronto. Retrieved August 14, 2003 from http://www.settlement.org/cp/english/pakistan/PakistanEN.pdf.

Kemp, C. (2002). *Infectious Diseases*. Retrieved April 12, 2003 from http://www3.baylor.edu/~Charles_Kemp/Infectious_Disease.htm.

Mull, J. D. and D. S. Mull (1988). Mother's concepts of childhood diarrhea in rural Pakistan: what ORT program planners should know. *Social Science and Medicine*, **27**, 53–67.

Mull, J. D., Anderson, J. W., & Mull, D. S. (1990). Cow dung, rock salt, and medical innovation in the Hindu Kush of Pakistan: The cultural transformation of neonatal tetanus and iodine deficiency. *Social Science and Medicine*, **30**, 675–91.

Parviz, S. (2003). Pakistan. In *Cultural Health Assessment*, 3rd edn., ed. C. E. Erickson & E. M. Geissler, pp. 603–7. St. Louis, MO: Mosby.

Periyakoil, V., Mendez, J. C., & Buttar, A. B. (n.d.). *Health and Health Care for Pakistani American Elders*. Retrieved June 20, 2003 from http://www.stanford.edu/group/ethnoger/pakistani.html.

Population Reference Bureau (2002). *2002 World Population Data Sheet*. Retrieved May 12, 2003 from http://www.prb.org/pdf/WorldPopulationDS02_Eng.pdf.

Shaw, A. (1988). *A Pakistani Community in Britain*. Oxford: Basil Blackwell.

  (2000). *Kinship and Continuity: Pakistani families in Britain*. Amsterdam: Harwood Academic Publishers.

Stein, C. E., Birmingham, M., Kurian, M., Duclos, P., & Strebel, P. (2003). The global burden of measles in the year 2000: a model that uses country-specific indicators. *Journal of Infectious Diseases*, **187** (Suppl. 1), S8–S14.

World Health Organization (2002a). *World Health Report*. Retrieved June 5, 2003 from http://www.who.int/whr/2002/en/.

  (2002b). *Global Polio Status 2002*. Retrieved May 9, 2003 from http://www.polioeradication.org/all/global/.

  (2003). *Global TB Control Report 2003*. Retrieved June 1, 2003 from http://www.who.int/gtb/publications/globrep/index.html.

31

Philippines

Timothy Benner

Introduction

The Republic of the Philippines (hereafter, the Philippines) is an archipelago of over 7000 islands off the east coast of mainland Southeast Asia. The Philippines was a Spanish colony from 1565 until 1898 when it was ceded to the United States after the Spanish–American War. The Philippines attained independence in 1946 after World War II. Since then the country has been relatively stable, except for an ongoing Muslim insurgency in the southern islands against the secular government (Central Intelligence Agency, 2002).

The Philippines is an impoverished nation: in 2000, 34% of all families lived below the poverty line (National Statistics Office, Republic of the Philippines, 2003a). Because of mass poverty, many Filipinos outmigrate in search of better economic opportunities.

History of immigration

The USA is the most significant Western destination for Filipino migrants. The Bureau of Citizenship and Immigration Services (2002) reports over 1.6 million immigrants to the USA who were born in the Philippines from the period from 1935 to 2002. The most recent of three waves of immigrants (1966–present) came after the USA liberalized immigration quotas, targeting educated, skilled individuals and supporting the reunification of families (Kitano & Daniels, 1988; Root, 1997). This dramatically increased the number of educated upper and middle-class Filipinos, especially women in the healthcare professions. Another significant aspect of Philippine immigration is the tendency for Philippine nationals to temporarily leave the Philippines for employment.

Refugee and Immigrant Health: A Handbook for Health Professionals, Charles Kemp and Lance A. Rasbridge. Published by Cambridge University Press. © C. Kemp and L. A. Rasbridge 2004.

Culture and social relations

The Philippines, because of its geographical location and makeup, is an area of great environmental and cultural diversity. The dominant cultural groups are Christianized lowland rice farming groups, but there are many ethnic minorities (usually from the more mountainous inland areas) and some Muslim groups from the southern regions of the archipelago. With over 90 distinct languages and as many separate cultural groups, it is very difficult to make generalizations about Filipinos as a whole, but there are similarities among many of the groups, especially the Christianized lowland groups from which the majority of migrants originate.

There are several significant concepts or values that may influence Filipino health behaviors (Pido, 1986; Wilson & Billones, 1994).

- *Bahala na* is the belief that one need not worry about unpleasant circumstances because such things are beyond an individual's ability to control, or even "God's will."
- *Amor proprio* (self-esteem) deals with the sense of pride that one has in one's own and one's family's accomplishments.
- *Hiya* (shame or embarrassment) deals with privacy and has both a physical and psychological/familial aspect. Physically, a high value is placed on the privacy of the physical self, including viewing or touching, especially between genders. Psychologically or regarding the family, *hiya* acts to maintain the privacy of the family. Concern about public perceptions of the community may influence health or help-seeking behavior, and concerns about confidentiality and negative stereotyping may cause individuals to not seek help to avoid a perceived negative perception within the community (Kelaher *et al.*, 2001).
- *Utang na loob* refers to a debt of gratitude and involves the right to expect something in return for a favor. It influences all personal relationships but is especially apparent between parents and children.
- *Pakikisama* (to accompany or go along with for the benefit of group harmony) governs family relationships as well as the individual's interactions with the wider community. It expresses itself most completely in the fact that most Filipinos avoid direct interpersonal conflict in order to preserve harmonious relationships within the group, especially the family. *Pakikisama* also leads to Filipinos sometimes giving verbal agreement to something with which they do not agree (and will not do).

Filipino families tend to be matrifocal or female centered despite the fact that the eldest male is acknowledged as the leader of the household and the ultimate authority in decision making. The mother in a Filipino family has the responsibility of taking care of the children and the day-to-day maintenance of the household. A common pattern of decision-making is for the wife to make most of the healthcare decisions for the family, and at the same time, to discuss them with her husband, so that he has the public face of any action.

Communications

The national language of the Philippines is Tagalog or "Pilipino" but this is only one of eight major languages and over 90 minor ethnic languages spoken in the archipelago. English is the language of higher education, government, and commerce and most Filipinos can understand and speak some English, with the well educated being quite fluent. Younger individuals and Filipinos born in the USA tend to be more fluent in English.

The Filipino culture also places a high value on wisdom acquired through life experience and thus there is a great deal of respect for elders. Typically, elders are addressed with the honorific *lolo* or *lola* (grandfather and grandmother, respectively) or by their surname. To address them by their first name alone is to disrespect their position in the family and their accumulated wisdom. Because of the respect Filipinos have for education, most elders tend to communicate with formality and reservation and will assume competence of health professionals, usually taking any information at face value and not asking questions (Wilson & Billones, 1994).

A final issue is the importance placed on maintaining eye contact while speaking to Filipinos. This is related to the folk belief that a witch "cannot stand your gaze." Therefore if one does not maintain eye contact while speaking, he/she may be perceived to harbor animosity or is otherwise untrustworthy (McKenzie & Chrisman, 1977).

Religion

From the outside, the Philippines appears to be an overwhelmingly Roman Catholic country. There is, however, a great deal of religious diversity, including a significant Muslim population in the southern islands and many non-Christian minorities scattered throughout; there is even considerable diversity within the Christian community. Regardless of which religion a particular individual may adhere to, Filipino religious thought has an immediacy based on the perceived close relationship between the supernatural and daily human life. This relationship predates both Christianity and Islam and to some degree affected how these two religions were adopted once they arrived. As a result much of the religion practiced in the Philippines now can be characterized as syncretic and is often at variance with strict interpretations of the adopted religions because of the inclusion of underlying earlier indigenous beliefs (Rodell, 2002).

Underlying the two world religions is a complex animistic belief system that blends the natural and supernatural worlds and includes beliefs in natural and ancestral spirits, witches, and other supernatural creatures. Some of the most commonly held beliefs deal with two classes of spirits – *anitos* and *asuangs*. *Anitos* are generally benign spirits who sometimes may be ancestral spirits but more commonly are nature spirits who live in special natural objects such as old trees and powerful rivers. Small sacrifices are often made to these spirits at small homemade shrines in order to gain favors or ward off any negative forces. *Asuangs* are generally malevolent spirits which may attack pregnant women, people who are out alone late at night, or the sick. These spirits are completely unpredictable and cannot be placated with sacrifice and are often used to explain confounding issues associated with illness, miscarriage, and death. However, one can beseech an *anito* for assistance against a troublesome *asuang*. Most often the spiritual world remains benign as long as spirits are appropriately satiated with the proper prayers and offerings.

Formal religious doctrine and magic are also both closely interwoven with health practices. Belief in various supernatural causes of disease is widespread. Spirits, witches, and sorcerers may all be seen as instrumental in bringing illness and misfortune and therefore spiritual practices such as prayer or the utilization of an indigenous healer or medium may be necessary to achieve a satisfactory cure (McKenzie & Chrisman, 1977). Filipino-Americans may also tend to blend the natural and the supernatural in their beliefs about health and illness in much the same way as native Filipinos. In fact even well-educated, acculturated Filipino–Americans will easily discuss the spiritual nature of illness but may do so laughingly and state the effectiveness of Western biomedical treatment. However, among elders and some of the less educated, these beliefs will be more strongly held.

Health beliefs and practices

While grounded in different cultural traditions, Filipino views about health and the management of illness are complementary to mainstream Western cultural views. The biomedical model is widespread and well known to both long-time immigrants as well as recent arrivals. Typically, overseas Filipinos can provide great detail about illness management practices and disease symptoms. However, they may tend to diminish the importance of their illness, even when serious, because of a cultural emphasis on appearing healthy and active, especially among elders (Becker *et al.*, 1998). Filipinos may also downplay the severity of pain or other symptoms and tend to suffer stoically.

Most Filipinos associate disease with the total life situation, including both biomedical and supernatural explanations and because of this they may pursue a multilinear path of treatment incorporating: home remedies such as teas and herbal preparations, massage, and lifestyle changes; spiritual remedies such as prayer, cleansing, and folk healers; and finally, Western biomedicine.

Three concepts underlie Filipino folk health practices (McKenzie & Chrisman, 1977):

- Flushing is based on the notion that the body is a container that can collect impurities and must be cleansed through a complex system to stimulate perspiration, vomiting, flatus, or menstrual bleeding. Flushing may be accomplished through massage or by drinking various herbal mixes – sometimes accompanied by religious or magic ritual.
- The balance of "hot" and "cold" is based on the idea that unhealthy bodies are thought to suffer from too much heat or too much cold. Imbalance may occur through immoderate working, drinking, or smoking. Improper eating also leads to imbalance, and the hot or cold properties of various foods are commonly used to treat health problems arising from imbalance. Ginger, for example, is considered "hot" and may be applied locally along with massage to treat sprains, dislocations, or sore muscles by applying heat.
- Protection is used as both a preventative measure and to help people who are already ill from becoming worse from negative outside influences. Protection encompasses both natural and supernatural practices to keep the body pure from outside influence. Natural ways of protection include living a healthy, virtuous life, eating well and getting enough rest, and drinking or eating substances that are thought to be strengthening. Supernatural methods of protection include prayer, wearing amulets or tokens, or wearing a small image of Christ, Mary, or a Saint on a piece of cloth next to the skin.

Folk remedies are still used among many overseas Filipinos because such measures are well known, accessible, trusted, inexpensive, and perceived as effective in dealing with everyday health issues. They are often used concurrently with biomedical treatment. Folk practitioners are active in many Filipino communities and are seen as experts in dealing with supernatural and folk remedies, and may also be adept at using massage and joint manipulation for dealing with sprains, minor breaks, and minor traumas.

The role of the family is also important in treating Filipinos (Becker *et al.*, 1998). In the Philippines, family members are expected to help their hospitalized relatives by acting as watchers, and by feeding, washing, and turning the patient (Daniel *et al.*, 2001). The concept of *hiya* is important here because some Filipinos, especially the elderly patients, may choose to do without something that they value, such as cleanliness, rather than ask a stranger to help if it violates their sense of personal privacy (Wilson & Billones, 1994). If the patient is unable to avoid *hiya*, he or she may become withdrawn and passive in order to disassociate from the experience.

Pregnancy and childbirth

Until a child is born to a new couple they are not yet considered to be an independent family and are to some extent not treated as full adults. There is a slight preference for male children but the gender of the child is not nearly as important as it is in patrilineal societies. The important thing is that there is a child which validates the marriage and expands the extended family, giving everyone expanded roles (Bigkis, n.d.).

According to Filipino folk beliefs, pregnancy is a "hot" period and heat is said to be lost when a woman gives birth. Therefore, traditional custom in the Philippines dictates that women should not bathe for about 10 days after giving birth, and during menstruation. Sponge baths, herb poultices and sitting in the smoke from an herbal fire or steam baths are used as alternatives (McKenzie & Chrisman, 1977). Additionally women were expected to rest for at least a week or up to a month in order to recover from giving birth. Parturition is believed to make women vulnerable to subsequent illness different from nonparous women. *Bughat* or *binat* (relapse) is believed to be the result of leaving a sickbed too early or returning to activity too soon after giving birth, and may recur for an indefinite time after parturition. Symptoms can be quite variable and include back or abdominal pain, vomiting, stomach upset or pain, weakness, and general malaise (Lieban, 1983).

In the Philippines, much of the responsibility of caring for newborns is initially undertaken by extended family members to allow the mother to recover and thus help avoid *bughat/binat*. Mild postpartum depression is fairly common among Filipinas and serves as a kind of catch phrase to refer to numerous physical and mental problems associated with caring for babies and small children (Kelaher *et al.*, 2001).

Filipinas, especially younger women, prefer to have female doctors, especially with pregnancy or other "female" issues such as menstruation. Embarrassment (*hiya*) is common when discussing sexual issues and anything having to do with physical functions and is intensified for women when speaking to a male doctor.

Breastfeeding on demand is common for rural Filipinas for as long as 12 to 18 months, but for a shorter period in urban areas and among overseas Filipinas. Some mothers are reluctant to feed colostrum to their newborns and some mothers believe that a mother's mood could be transmitted through breast milk; therefore they do not feed their babies if they feel sorrow or anger (Queensland Government, n.d.). Babies tend to sleep with their parents or at least in the same room until they are toddlers and most parents are reluctant to have their children sleep elsewhere unless it is with another relative. Discipline for young children is quite lenient and most adults are very tolerant and include young children in adult activities. As children get older, respect for parents and elders is stressed and they are disciplined more regularly by scolding, spanking or pinching.

End of life

Discussions about serious illnesses and the possibility of death are fairly open among Filipinos, though some elders and family may avoid talking about advance directives or dying as some believe this may bring on the event. It would be best to approach a discussion gradually and in the presence of a trusted physician, clergy, or healthcare professional who is a relative (McBride, 2000). Since the large majority of Filipinos are Catholic, the necessity to prepare for an impending death is important in terms of making confession and preparing for a funeral.

After death occurs the family will usually want to stay with the body 24 hours a day for as long as 3 days. If the death occurs in the home, the body will be washed and laid out for viewing where friends and relatives can come to pay their respects to the deceased. Filipinos are very demonstrative in their grief and crying and wailing is common, especially among women. The body can also be laid out in a chapel where it is expected that at least one relative will always be there to carry on a vigil with candles and prayers. People will get together at the deceased's house with food, music, and card games to mourn the deceased. Burial is preferred with the whole extended family accompanying the body to the cemetery to be interred. There are nightly prayers for 9 days after death and then again on the 40th day, when it is believed that the soul ascends to heaven. The death will also be commemorated on a yearly basis with prayers or a gathering.

Many Filipino-Americans feel that these traditions will be neglected if they die overseas because they would not be allowed to hold 24-hour vigils with the body or they would not be able to afford an elaborate funeral, so they make preparations to return to the Philippines in their old age or buy insurance to return their bodies to the Philippines after death (Becker, 2002). The most important factor in determining which country to die in is the presence of extended family.

Health problems and screening

The healthy life expectancy or HALE in the Philippines is 51.1 years and the full life expectancy is 68 years (Population Reference Bureau, 2002; World

Health Organization (WHO), 2002). Infectious diseases are the leading causes of death and disability in the Philippines. The Philippines is one of 22 countries worldwide with a "high burden" of tuberculosis (WHO, 2003). Health risks for new Filipino immigrants (Hawn & Jung, 2003; Kemp, 2002; WHO, 2002) include:

- amebiasis
- angiostrongyliasis
- anthrax
- capillariasis
- chikungunya
- cholera
- cryptococcosis
- cryptosporidiosis
- cysticercosis (tapeworm)
- dengue fever
- encephalitis (Japanese)
- filariasis: (Bancroftian filariasis and Malayan filariasis)
- gnathostomiasis
- helminthiasis (ascariasis, echinococcosis/hydatid disease, schistosomiasis)
- hepatitis B
- hookworm
- leishmaniasis
- leprosy
- leptospirosis
- malaria, including multi-drug resistant (MDR) from *Plasmodium falciparum* resistant parasites and especially from malaria re-infection.
- melioidosis
- mycetoma
- sexually transmitted infections, including HIV/AIDS, chancroid, chlamydia, gonorrhea, granuloma inguinale, lymphogranuloma venereum, syphilis
- strongylodiasis
- thalassemias
- trematodes (liver-dwelling: clonorchiasis and opisthorchiasis; blood-dwelling: schistosomiasis or bilharzias; intestine-dwelling; and lung-dwelling: paragonimiasis)
- tropical sprue
- tuberculosis (including multi-drug resistant)
- typhus
- yaws (frambesia)

REFERENCES

Becker, G. (2002). Dying away from home: quandaries of migration for elders in two ethnic groups. *Journal of Gerontology*, **57B**, S79–95.

Becker, G., Beyene, Y., Newsom, E. M. & Rodgers, D. V. (1998). Knowledge and care of chronic illness in three ethnic groups. *Family Medicine*, **30**, 173–178.

Bigkis (n.d.). *Childbirth or Prenatal Education for Filipinos*. Retrieved July 10, 2003, from http//www/bigkis.com.au/.

Bureau of Citizenship and Immigration Services (2002). *Statistical Yearbook of the Immigration and Naturalization Service Prior to the Fiscal Year 2002 edition*. Retrieved July 6, 2003, from http://www.immigration.gov/graphics/shared/aboutus/statistics/ IMM02yrbk/IMM2002list.htm.

Central Intelligence Agency (CIA) (2002). *World Factbook*. Author. Retrieved August 6, 2003 from http://www.cia.gov/cia/publications/factbook/geos/rp.html.

Daniel, P., Chamberlain, A., & Gordon, F. (2001). Expectations and experiences of newly recruited Filipino nurses. *British Journal of Nursing*, **10**, 254–6, 258–65.

Hawn, T. R. & Jung, E. C. (2003). Health screening in immigrants, refugees, and internationally adopted orphans. In *The Travel and Tropical Medicine Manual*, 3rd edn., ed. E. C. Jong and R. McMullen, pp. 255–65. Philadelphia, PA: W. B. Saunders.

Kelaher, M., Potts, H., & Manderson, L., (2001). Health issues among Filipino women in remote Queensland. *Australian Journal of Rural Health*, **9**, 150–7.

Kemp, C. (2002). *Infectious Diseases*. Retrieved April 12, 2003 from http://www3.baylor.edu/~Charles_Kemp/Infectious_Disease.htm.

Kitano, H. L. & Daniels, R. (1988). *Asian Americans: Emerging Minorities*. Englewood Cliffs, NJ: Prentice Hall.

Lieban, R. W. (1983). Gender aspects of illness and practitioner use among Filipinos. *Social Science and Medicine*, **17**, 853–9.

McBride, M. (2000). Health and health care of Filipino American Elders. In Core Curriculum in Ethnogeriatrics, 2nd edn., ed. G. Yeo. Stanford CA: Stanford GEC. Retrieved August 11, 2003 from http://www.stanford.edu/group/ethnoger/ebooks/filipino_american.pdf.

McKenzie, J. L. & Chrisman, N. J. (1977). Healing, herbs, gods, and magic: folk health beliefs among Filipino-Americans. *Nursing Outlook*, **25**, 326–9.

National Statistics Office, Republic of the Philippines (2003a). *2000 Family Income and Expenditure Survey (FIES) Final Release on Poverty*. Retrieved July 6, 2003, from http://www.census.gov.ph/data/sectordata/2000/ie00pftx.html.

Pido, A. (1986). *The Filipinos in America: Macro-micro Dimensions of Immigration and Integration*. Staten Island, NY: Centre for Migration Studies.

Population Reference Bureau (2002). *2002 World Population Data Sheet*. Retrieved May 12, 2003 from http://www.prb.org/pdf/WorldPopulationDS02_Eng.pdf.

Queensland Government (n.d.). *Community Health Profiles: Philippines*. Retrieved July 10, 2003, from http://www.health.qld.gov.au/hssb/cultdiv/cultdiv/philippn.htm.

Rodell, P. (2002). *Culture and Customs of the Philippines*. Westport, CT: Greenwood Press.

Root, M. P. (1997). *Filipino Americans: Transformation and Identity.* Thousand Oaks, CA: Sage Publications.

Wilson, S. & Billones, H. (1994). The Filipino elder: implications for nursing practice. *Journal of Gerontological Nursing,* August, 31–6.

World Health Organization (2002). *World Health Report.* Retrieved June 5, 2003 from http://www.who.int/whr/2002/en/.

  (2003). *Global TB Control Report 2003.* Retrieved June 1, 2003 from http://www.who.int/gtb/publications/globrep/index.html.

32

Roma (Gypsy)

Kathryn Ryczak and Charles Kemp

Note: The term Gypsy is used in the title of this chapter only to aid readers. For the most part we use the correct terms: *Romani, Roma,* or *Rom* as explained below. As with other populations, there are differences among and within groups. Much of what follows is based on *Vlax Romani* customs, but can, in many cases, be applied to other *Romani.*

Introduction

A few *Romani* terms are helpful to understanding the Roma culture. *Romani,* the adjective; *Roma,* plural noun; or *Rom,* singular noun, are the preferred terms when referring to people commonly and incorrectly known as Gypsies. Not all *Romani* people refer to themselves as *Roma,* e.g., some refer to themselves as Travelers (though not all Travelers are *Roma*). *Gadje* is the plural term referring to non-*Roma* people or customs and *gazho* is the singular term. An individual *Romani* household is known as a *familia.* Unrelated *familia* living cooperatively in a given geographical region are called a *kumpania* and the *vista* is composed of numerous *kumpania* and can span a country (Bodner & Leininger, 1992; Hancock, 1999; *Patrin Web Journal,* n.d.).

While there are differences among groups and individuals among the *Roma,* there are at least several commonalities (Bodner, 1992; Hancock, 1980; Hancock, 1999; Koupilová *et al.,* 2001; *Patrin Web Journal,* n.d.), including:

- strong social and cultural bonds to sustain the *Romani* way of life or *Romaniya*
- social isolation from mainstream society
- elaborate constructs of prohibitions and rituals
- loyalty to the family.

Many *Roma* maintain social isolation through their own conscious and asserted effort, and through prejudice from non-*Roma* (Koupilová *et al.,* 2001; Reyniers, 1995). In Western Europe and the USA, there are two primary reasons why the

Roma are so successful at remaining largely invisible. First, the large number and variety of minority groups in these areas afford the opportunity to blend into other cultures, with *Roma* sometimes presenting themselves as members of another minority. Second, misconceptions arise from folklore and media with the image of the "gypsy" based on either romanticized or pejorative fiction (Hancock, 1999; Patrin Web Journal, n.d.). As a result, little of substance or accuracy is known about the *Roma*. Elsewhere in the world, e.g., Eastern Europe, there are recognized *Romani* communities that are the subject of significant discrimination and in some cases (e.g., post-war Kosovo), outright repression (Erlanger, 2000).

Though traditionally nomadic, many *Roma* now live in established communities in houses. However, some who live in permanent housing may also travel during part of the year for purposes of working (Van Cleemput, 2000). There also remain Roma who live in traditional circumstances such as tent encampments near cities and towns (Gourgoulianis *et al.*, 2000)

Many older *Roma* are not literate. In recent years, some younger members of the *familia* have been allowed to attended *gadje* schools until about the age of ten and are thus able to read important *gadje* documents. There now are increasing numbers of college-educated *Roma* – at least in Western countries (like Canada, Western Europe, and the USA). In Eastern Europe, however, educational levels of Roma children decreased in the post-communist 1990s (Reyniers, 1995).

History of immigration

The *Roma* originated in India and migrated to Europe around AD 1000. They reached the Balkans by the 14th century and spread throughout Western Europe by the 15th century. In the 17th century, some *Roma* were brought to the American colonies as slaves and, in the 18th century, groups of *Roma* were deported to the American colonies. A wave of migration from Eastern to Western Europe occurred in the mid-19th century when *Roma* slavery was abolished in Romania. A second wave came from Yugoslavia to Western Europe in the 1960s and 1970s; and a third wave came in the 1990s with political and economic changes in Eastern Europe (Fraser, 1992; Hancock, 1999; Reyniers, 1995).

Another large group of *Roma* migrated to the USA by way of Russia and later, Argentina in the late 19th and early 20th Centuries. Current *Roma* population estimates in the USA are difficult to determine as the census does not record their cultural identity, and the *Roma* population does not record births or deaths. The national population of *Roma* in the USA is estimated to be one million (Bodner & Leininger, 1992).

In Europe, large *Roma* ghettos exist at the outskirts of many urban areas, especially in Eastern Europe. There are an estimated 8 000 000 *Roma* in Europe, with the majority in Central and Eastern Europe and there are an estimated 12 000 000 *Romani* worldwide (Liegeosis, 1994; Reyniers, 1995; Smith, 2000).

Throughout their history in the West, the *Roma* have experienced discrimination because of *gadje* folklore, *Roma* practices, and the prejudice inherent in all societies. Even the Bible has been used to justify discrimination against the *Roma*:

"Cursed be Canaan;
A servant of servants
He shall be to his brethren"
            Genesis 9:25

There is also the legend (still alive in rural Balkan countries) that the *Roma* made the nails that were used to crucify Christ and/or that they stole the fourth nail, thus making the crucifixion more painful. Gypsy hunting and other such persecutions have occurred almost from the beginning of the *Roma* presence in Europe, and continue to this day. Nazi Germany institutionalized the hatred and killing, with Gypsies treated the same as Jews in all respects. Approximately 500 000–1 500 000 Roma were murdered in the Holocaust ("the devouring" to *Roma*).

Culture and social relations

There is an extensive and complicated social structure among the *Romani* people. Generally, there are four loyalties and/or identities (nation, clan, family, and *vista*). First, *Roma* are divided into *Natsias* or nations, which is their main identity group. The four major *Roma* nations are the *Machwaya, Kalderasha, Churara,* and *Lowara*. The nations are then divided into *Kumpania* or clans. A clan is "an alliance of families united by ancestral, professional, or historical ties" (Hancock, 1980, p 442). This loyalty or group consists of extended family that travel and reside together and maintain economic control over a particular territory. Each clan has a leader and the social structure of the clans may differ. There are no "Gypsy Kings" (*Patrin Web Journal,* n.d.).

The *Roma* are ethnocentric, tending to demonstrate a sense of moral superiority and contempt toward the *gadje*. The *Roma* have a strict taboo code that classifies all outsiders as soiled or unclean. This code prevents interaction with the *gadje* and further limits acculturation. Some refuse to use the *gadje* language to record births, participate in census or other surveys, or to record deaths, though they maintain enough of a link with the outside world to meet their primary economic and cultural needs. Very few are employed by *gadje* except as contractors and then nearly always on a temporary basis (*Patrin Web Journal,* n.d.).

Important *Romani* concepts related to health care are "*wuzho*" and "*marimé*." *Wuzho* is the *Roma* word for pure while *marimé* is a broad term referring both to a state of pollution or impurity or a sentence of expulsion imposed for violation of a ritual or moral nature. Other terms for *marimé* are *moxadó, melali, mageradó, mokadi, kulaló, limaló, prastló, palecidó, pekelimé, gonimé* and *bolimé* – clearly this is an important concept!

The *Romani* culture has strict rules about anything considered polluted. Women are particularly associated with *marimé*, with any part of a woman's body above the waist being *wuzho* or pure and below the woman's waist being *marimé* or polluted – especially the genitoanal area and its secretions. To the *Roma*, failure to keep the two sections separate in everyday living may result in serious illness. Certain food or animals (birds and cats) may also be considered *marimé* (Mandell, 1999; *Patrin Web Journal*, n.d.; Sutherland, 1992).

When a young woman reaches menarche, she must begin observing the washing, dressing, cooking, eating and behavioral rules of adult women for her own protection as well as the protection of others. Her clothes must be washed separately from those of men and children, she cannot cook food for others during menstruation, and she must show respect to men by not passing in front of them, stepping over their clothes, or allowing her skirts to touch them. Pre-pubescent girls and older women have more freedom because they do not menstruate (*Patrin Web Journal*, n.d.).

Because they do not observe body separation, *gadje* are seen as a source of impurity and disease. The impure public places where *gadje* congregate are also considered potential sources of disease. These places are considered less clean than the *Romani* home or open outdoors. Some *Roma* attempt to lessen the pollution by using disposable paper cups, plates and towels (Mandell, 1999; *Patrin Web Journal*, n.d.).

Roma tend to marry young. Some clans practice arranged marriages while others allow courtship. If the marriage is arranged, the groom's father selects and pays for a *bori* or daughter-in-law through the help of a marriage arranger. Marriage in the *Romani* culture has occurred as early as age 9 but usually does not take place before the age 14. Marriage to *gadje* is considered a serious transgression in some clans and may be grounds for expulsion (Belgum, 1999; Bodner & Leininger, 1992).

Communications

The language of the *Roma* is called *Romani* and is derived primarily from *Sanskrit*, with strong influences from Persian, Greek, and Slavic languages (note that these track the *Roma* diaspora summarized above). Until recent years, *Romani* was solely a spoken language, but there is increasing use of written forms of *Romani*. There are different forms of *Romani* depending on which clan the *Rom* belongs to. Interaction between different clans is limited, and the form of *Romani* spoken is an important means of distinguishing between clans.

There also are customs in communicating with *gadje*. In the healthcare setting, only the elder males are likely to communicate with healthcare personnel. Women are not permitted to interrupt men or be alone with a man who is not her husband or relative (*Patrin Web Journal*, n.d.).

Religion

There is not a separate *Romani* religion. Since they are generally a nomadic people, they have traditionally adopted the dominant religion of the country in which they live. For example, the *Roma* and *Boyash* clans are largely Roman Catholic, while the *Romnichals* are largely Protestant. There are also Eastern Orthodox, Hindu and Muslim believers among the *Roma*.

Although the *Roma* adopt the religious practices of those around them, they also maintain several strong faith practices and beliefs in the supernatural, omens and curses. They also have female healers, called *drabarni* or *drabenhgi*, who prescribe traditional healing rituals and cures. Interestingly, the *Roma* do not believe in fortune telling. This practice is used only to earn money from the *gadje* (Mandell, 1999).

Health beliefs and practices

Many *Romani* classify illness into either *rromane nasvalimata* (natural to *Roma*, e.g., heart problems, rashes, anxiety) or *gadzikane nasvalimata* (the result of contact with non-*Roma*, e.g., sexually transmitted diseases). For *rromane nasvalimata*, a *drabarni* or traditional healer (female) may be consulted; for the non-*Roma* illnesses, mainstream healthcare is likely to be sought. Diet and health are linked – in terms of the perceived auspiciousness of foods, not their nutritional values (Hancock, 2002).

Roma who enjoy good health are believed to be blessed with good fortune, and those who are ill are said to have lost their good luck. Many *Roma* see the mainstream healthcare system as causing more harm than good, and tend to use the *gadje* healthcare system primarily in crisis situations when there is an acute and/or unresolved condition for which folk medicine has failed. Some *Romani* may request specific "famous name" physicians and demand specific treatment even if the treatment or physician is inappropriate. There also is preference for older physicians over younger ones. Sharing medications is common and *Roma* have also been known to request a specific color of medication for a specific illness (Mandell, 1999; Sutherland, 1992).

For the *Roma*, illness is not just the concern of the individual but a problem shared by the entire clan. When a clan member enters a hospital, family members are expected to remain with that person day and night to watch over, protect, and perform caring and curing rituals, except, sometimes, when the illness is *gadzikane nasvalimata* such as HIV. *Roma* are especially fearful of any surgical procedure that requires general anesthesia because of a belief that a person under general anesthesia undergoes a "little death." For the family to gather around the person coming out of the anesthesia is especially important.

Pregnancy and childbirth

Among *Roma* women, the first pregnancy tends to be at a young age, and there is a tendency to have a high birth rate (Semerdjieva *et al.*, 1999). A woman is considered to be *marimé* (polluted or unclean) during her menses, pregnancy and for 6 weeks after the birth of the child. Childbirth should not occur at the *familia's* usual home lest the home lose its purity. For this reason, there is increased acceptance of hospital births.

A new baby is immediately swaddled tightly and should only be handled by his/her mother to maintain a state of purity. When a baby is delivered in a hospital, the mother should be allowed to practice ritualistic cleansing and the father not expected to visit during this *marimé* time. There are rituals (that vary with clan) involving the formal recognition of the infant by its father (Mandell, 1999; *Patrin Web Journal*, 1999).

In the first weeks postpartum at night, no member of the family is allowed to go in and out of the mother's room, and all the windows and doors are kept shut lest the spirit of death called "the night" enter and harm the baby. If a baby dies, it is bad fortune and the parents must avoid the baby's body. Traditionally, the body is buried in a secret place by the grandparents. Another way to avoid bad luck after the death of a baby is to leave the funeral and burial to hospital authorities.

Children are a major focus of *Romani* culture and are believed to bring good luck. Child rearing is the responsibility of everyone in the family. Due to the large and complex social structure, most of the children are raised and cared for by many different people including extended family members and clan members living in the same residential area. In *Romani* culture older children act in some respects as adults. Teenagers do not experience a carefree adolescent period as with many Western cultures. They are expected to begin adult socialization and to start a trade by about 10 years of age. Separation is by gender to learn the skills of the adult.

End of life

When a *Rom* is about to die, there is an extensive ritualistic process that must initiated. Through an elaborate communications system, relatives from other geographic areas come to be with the dying, and presence at the moment of death is important. To avoid touching the body of the deceased (which is *marimé*), the imminently terminal person may be dressed in her or his best clothes. A special candle is brought into the room and at the time of death this candle is lit and a window opened. It is believed that the candle will light the way to heaven for the deceased person's soul. For 3 days, the family and others grieve by remaining in the presence of the dead. During this time they do not bathe, shave, wear jewelry, change clothes or prepare food, but alcohol may be consumed (Bodner & Leininger, 1992; *Patrin Web Journal*, n.d.).

Displays of grief may include moaning and shouting out to the deceased, scratching the face, pulling hair out and throwing themselves to the floor or into a wall. There is great fear among the survivors that the dead might return in a supernatural form to haunt the living. For this reason the name of the deceased should not be mentioned, the body not touched, and all objects belonging to the deceased destroyed (Belgum, 1999; *Patrin Web Journal*, n.d.).

After a 3-day wake, the funeral is held, followed by a death feast in honor of the deceased. For this feast, food is always prepared in units of three (three chickens, three pots of potatoes, etc.). Additional feasts are held to mark the 3 days, 9 days, 6 weeks and 1 year intervals after the death. Close relatives of the deceased wear mourning clothes for a full year. It is believed that after 1 year the soul enters heaven.

Health problems and screening

In Eastern Europe, most *Roma* have a life expectancy of under 50 years, and in Western Europe a life expectancy ranging from 62–65 years (Reyniers, 2000; Van Cleemput, 2000). Poverty, isolation, prejudice, a lack of advocates, and other factors discussed above and below contribute to these short lifespans (Koupilová *et al.*, 2001).

The *Romani* culture in itself can sometimes increase risk for health problems as follows (Gourgoulianis *et al.*, 2000; Sutherland, 1992; Van Cleemput, 2000):
- Avoidance of *gadje* may result in resistance to childhood and adult immunizations, health screening, and other health promotion activities.
- Social isolating behaviors such as refusal to register births and deaths can result in significant trends in morbidity and mortality being hidden. Isolation and tradition also lead to an increase in consanguineous marriages, and thus an increased risk for birth defects.
- Beliefs about *marimé* mean that cervical and colon cancer screening are especially difficult to promote.

- Dietary habits of high fat and sodium as well as an almost universal heavy use among men of tobacco put the Roma at increased risk several chronic illnesses, compounded by late recognition.
- Crowded living conditions lead to an increase incidence of gastrointestinal infections, respiratory infections and hepatitis.

Health risks for Eastern European *Romani* (Ackerman, 1997; Hajioff & McKee, 2000; Kalaydjieva *et al.*, 2001: Kemp, 2002) include the following:

- babesiosis (rare)
- boutonneuse fever
- encephalitis (most likely to be tick-borne)
- hemorrhagic fevers (HFs) (HF with renal syndrome and tick-borne HFs)
- hepatitis B and C
- lyme disease
- sexually transmitted infections, including HIV/AIDS, cervical cancer, chancroid, gonorrhea, granuloma inguinale, lymphogranuloma venereum, syphilis
- trematode infection (opisthorchiasis)
- tuberculosis (multidrug resistant)
- birth defects and genetic disorders
- post-traumatic stress disorder
- chronic illnesses, such as cardiovascular disease and related disorders, chronic lung disease, obesity, diabetes
- nutritional deficits

REFERENCES

Ackerman, L. J. (1997). Health problems of refugees. *Journal of the American Board of Family Practice*, **10**, 337–48.

Anerson, G. & Tighe, B. (1973). Gypsy culture and health care. *American Journal of Nursing*, **73**, 282–5.

Belgum, D. (1999). Dealing with cultural diversity: a hospital chaplain reflects on Gypsies and other such diversity. *Journal of Pastoral Care*, **53**, 175–81.

Bodner, A. & Leininger, M. (1992). Transcultural nursing care values, beliefs, and practices of American (USA) gypsies. *Journal of Transcultural Nursing*, **4**, 17–28.

Erlanger, S. (April 2, 2000). Across a new Europe, a people deemed unfit for tolerance. *New York Times*, B1, 16.

Fraser, A. (1992). *The Gypsies*. Cambridge: Blackwell.

Gourgoulianis, K. I., Tsoutsou, P., Fotiadou, N., Samaras, K., Dakis, D., & Molyvdas, P. A. (2000). Lung function in Gypsies in Greece. *Archives of Environmental Health*, **55**, 453–4.

Hajioff, S. & McKee, M. (2000). The health of the Roma people: a review of the published literature. *Journal of Epidemiological Community Health*, **54**, 864–8.

Hancock, I. F. (1980). Gypsies. In *Harvard Encyclopedia of American Ethnic Groups*, ed. S. Thernstrom, pp. 440–5. Cambridge: Harvard University Press.

(1999). The Roma: myth and reality. *Patrin Web Journal*. Retrieved December 1, 2002 from http://www.geocities.com/Paris/5121/mythandreality.htm.

(2002). *We are the Romani People*. Hertfordshire: University of Hertfordshire Press.

Kalaydjieva, L., Gresham, D., & Calafell, F. (2001). Genetic studies of the Roma (Gypsies): a review. *BMC Medical Genetics*, **2**. Retrieved December 3, 2002 from http://www.biomedcentral.com/1471-2350/2/5.

Kemp, C. (2002). *Infectious Diseases*. Retrieved April 12, 2003 from http://www3.baylor.edu/~Charles_Kemp/Infectious_Disease.htm.

Koupilová, I., Epstein, H., Holčik, J., Hajioff, S., & McKee, M. (2001). Health needs of the Roma population in the Czech and Slovak Republics. *Social Science and Medicine*, **53**, 1191–204.

Liegeosis, J.-P. (1994). *Roma, Gypsies, Travellers*. Strasbourg: Council of Europe Press.

Mandell, F. (1999). Gypsies (Roma). In *Cultural Competency in Health Care*, ed. A. Rundle, M. Carvalho, and M. Robinson, pp. 56–60. San Francisco: Jossey-Bass.

Patrin Web Journal (n.d.). *Romani Culture and History*. Retrieved September 22, 2001 from http://www.geocities.com/Paris/5121/index.html.

Reyniers, A. (1995). *Gypsy Populations and their Movements within Central and Eastern Europe and Towards some OECD Countries. Paris*: Organization for Economic Co-operation and Development. Retrieved December 4, 2002 from http://www.oecd.org/pdf/M00018000/M00018683.pdf.

(2000). *Gypsies: Trapped on the Fringes of Europe*. Retrieved December 6, 2002 from http://www.britannica.com/bcom/original/article/0,5744,8969,00.html.

Semerdjieva, M., Mateva, N., & Dimitrov, I. (1999). Influence of family traditions on reproductive behavior of Gypsy population. *Folia Medica*, **41**, 116–20.

Smith, D. (April 23, 2000). Renegade in most secretive world. *New York Times*, A15, A23.

Sutherland, A. (1992). Gypsies and health care. *Western Journal of Medicine*, **157**, 276–80.

Van Cleemput, P. (2000). Health needs of travellers. *Archives of Disease in Childhood* (online), 82. Retrieved December 4, 2002 from http://adc.bmjjournals.com/cgi/content/full/archdischild;82/1/32.

FURTHER READING

Shields, M. N. (1981). Selected issues in treating Gypsy patients. *Hospital Physician*, **17**, 85–92.

Smith, M., Erickson, G., & Campbell, J. (1996). Gypsies: health problems and nursing needs. *Journal of Multicultural Nursing and Health*, **2**, 35–42.

Thomas, J. (1985). Gypsies and American medical care. *Annals of Internal Medicine*, **102**, 842–5.

Webb, G. (1960). *Gypsies: The Secret People*. Westport: Greenwood Press Publishers.

Wetzel, R., Dean, M., & Rogers, M. (1983, November). Gypsies and acute medical intervention. *The Art of Pediatrics*, **72**, 731–5.

Wilke, W. S. (ed.). (1993, November/December). Tales of a Gypsy doc: perspectives on social care and medical aspects of care of the American Gypsy population. *Cleveland Journal of Medicine*, **60**, 427–8.

Russia

Introduction

The history of modern Russia and the former Soviet Union, from the time of the czars, is replete with tumultuous social change, but none has been more profound than the reforms initiated by Mikhail Gorbachev in the late 1980s. His introduction of *perestroika* "restructuring" and *glasnost* "openness" were efforts to modernize the communist state but resulted in a revolution. By the end of 1991, the Soviet Union broke apart into 15 independent republics. The ensuing ultranationalism unleashed waves of ethnic discrimination and heightened already existing religious and ethnic tensions that had been held in check under the communist regime. In some regions, tensions escalated to full-scale war, in particular in Chechnya and in the fighting over Nagorno-Karabakh between Armenia and Azerbaijan. The end result has been the creation of millions of refugees.

Many refugees from the former Soviet Union have not faced the extreme circumstances of war and other violence typical of the refugee experience. Still, discrimination against certain groups is common. The largest group of refugees from Russia is Jews, who have faced discrimination for hundreds of years. Beginning at least from the time of the czars, Jews have been barred from participation in government and in some cases denied access to education and other benefits. Anti-Semitism increased dramatically in the period of the collapse of the Soviet Union, especially in the Ukraine. While Israel has from its inception welcomed Soviet Jewry, many have preferred resettlement to the West, the United States in particular (Gold, 1996).

History of immigration

Refugees and immigrants from the former Soviet Union have been resettled in three broad geographical regions: North America, Western Europe, and Israel.

Refugee and Immigrant Health: A Handbook for Health Professionals, Charles Kemp and Lance A. Rasbridge. Published by Cambridge University Press. © C. Kemp and L. A. Rasbridge 2004.

In America, through 2002, 454 106 refugees were admitted from the republics of Armenia, Azerbaijan, Belarus, Georgia, Kazakhstan, Kyrgyzstan, Moldova, Russia, Tajikistan, Turkmenistan, Ukraine, and Uzbekistan (Immigration and Refugee Services of America, 2002). The majority of all former Soviet Union refugees are Jewish.

In the USA, most have been resettled by the Hebrew Immigration Aid Society (HIAS) and have enjoyed what is widely considered to be the greatest benefits in terms of indicators like per capita assistance dollars of any resettled refugee group (Gold, 1996). They have also received extensive assistance from existing synagogues and organizations in the communities of resettlement. At least half of all the Jewish refugees and immigrants live in New York and California, Los Angeles in particular. Of all major refugee groups, Soviets become naturalized citizens at the highest and fastest rates (Gold, 1996). Notably, an estimated 20% of refugees from the former Soviet Union are 65 years or older (Brod & Heurtin-Roberts, 1992).

Outside of refugees leaving the Former Soviet Union because of religious persecution, there are some refugees resettled on the basis of discrimination because of nationality. Many found themselves unwelcome in the strong nationalist waves during the break-up of the former Soviet Union, especially those with family roots from different areas, or families of mixed marriages, e.g. Armenians and Azerbaijanis. In most of these cases, the couples fled to Moscow before resettlement in the West.

Culture and social relations

Many Soviet families of three and sometimes four generations have been resettled intact. Family reunification through non-refugee processing is also common. Due to the multigenerational nature of households, and the relatively small family sizes, compared with most other resettled refugee groups, ample resources can be devoted to child-rearing. Accordingly, as mothers of small children can join the other adults in the workforce, with grandparents as child caretakers, the economic adjustment of Russian-born refugees in the United States has been relatively swift (Gold, 1996).

On the other hand, as there are proportionately more elderly than commonly found in resettled refugee groups, other problems of health and social adjustment are present in the Russian community. Intergenerational conflict inevitably results because of the far swifter rates of assimilation between school-age children and the elderly. While there is some downward economic mobility initially with Soviet immigrants, and while there is individual variation, income levels approach and even exceed national averages in a relatively short period of time. This is due in part to the high education and professional training levels of Soviets prior to emigration, including among women. Furthermore, the marriage rate for the Soviet immigrants is much higher than any other immigrant group (Gold, 1996). Clearly, family and even community cohesiveness characterize this resettled population.

Communications

Even though almost all Republics have a local language as a native tongue (e.g. Ukrainian in the Ukraine, Azeri in Azerbaijan), the Russian language is also spoken by all Russian-born refugees and immigrants. Russian language was mandatory throughout the educational system under communist rule. The Russian alphabet is written in Cyrillic characters and is not comprehensible to English readers. Gold notes that, with the exception of the elderly, Soviet refugees make rapid progress with English acquisition (1996). When greeting, handshakes and cheek kissing among family and close friends is normal. Direct eye contact when communicating is expected.

Upon marriage, the norm is for the bride to take the family name of the husband, although this is not universal. Also, children frequently bear the first name of the father as their middle name. In both cases, a suffix is added to the name to convey sex. Spoken names follow first, middle, and then last name convention. Elders are highly respected and frequently greeted with kinship terms "Aunt" or "Uncle," and the ubiquitous *babushka* (grandmother), irrespective of consanguineal relationship (Evanikoff, 1996).

Religion

Even though the majority of Soviet refugees, Jews in particular, were resettled on the basis of religious persecution claims, observers have noted that most are not particularly observant in practice in the USA (Gold, 1996). There are a few other religious minorities resettled in the West, including Muslims from Azerbaijan, Tajikistan, Kyrgystan, and Uzbekistan; Armenian Christians; Pentecostals; and Russian Orthodox. In many cases, an inter-religious marriage is the source of persecution that accounts for their status as refugees.

Health beliefs and practices

There is a wide range of spiritual healers and traditional medicine specialists both in the Republics and within resettled populations. Repressed under communist rule, many alternative medicine practitioners (*shamans* in Azeri language) now operate freely in the Republics and in the immigrant communities. In urban centers in the United States and Europe, there are now commercial outlets dedicated to herbs and other medicines imported from Russia.

There are myriad home remedies in traditional Russian culture. Among these are the following.

- Sore throat is treated with a baking soda and water gargle, and a warm milk drink.
- Sinus congestion can be treated by the application of onion juice squirted directly in the nostrils, or by drinking a baking soda/butter/milk mixture, stimulating mucous which is then spat out.
- For congestion in infants, cut raw onion is placed around the head. A topical rub of Vodka on the chest and back can also be used for coughing.
- Constipation may be treated by eating prunes and raisins two to three times a day, with infants receiving boiled prune water.
- Dental pain is treated with a salt-water rinse and analgesics.
- Fever is combated by bundling the patient in layers of blankets and even soaking the feet in a hot water bath, together with hot teas, especially black tea with honey and lemon, to decrease temperature. A cool compress of Vodka on the forehead is also used to decrease temperature.
- Nausea is treated with lemon.
- Cough and respiratory symptoms are treated by breathing in the steam from boiling potato peels. Cupping, the placing of a heated cup on the back such that a vacuum is created, is also practiced by the more traditional for treatment of cough, respiratory congestion, and other ailments. A type of pre-packaged patch impregnated with pepper is placed on the chest wall for relief of respiratory ailments.
- Pain may be treated with a commercially available pain reliever/cure-all, known as "No-Shpa."
- Abdominal pain or peptic ulcer is treated with green tea – often with other substances are added for specific health benefits.

A characteristic of the former Soviet Union system was that there was little government expenditure on persons perceived as non-productive, especially the elderly. The aged were typically cared for by their adult children, as nursing homes were rare. Consequently, when the younger generation refugees were given the possibility to emigrate, they had little choice but to bring the elders too. In fact, for Soviet Jews, this extended family emigration was sometimes mandated (Wheat *et al.*, 1983). Consequently, the older generation may not always be motivated towards Western resettlement, and their adjustment that much more stressful. And by virtue of their life experiences, with some elderly having been through the horrific battles of World War II (more than 49 million Russians killed), persecution and deprivation, and communist rule, they are at great risk for having depleted emotional, physical, and financial resources (Brod & Heurtin-Roberts, 1992; Glantz, 2002).

Medicine compliance is frequently an issue with Russian refugees. Western pharmaceuticals were in short supply and hence highly valued in the former Soviet Union. When given freely and readily here, the mystique may diminish, and the Russian patient may not comply (Wheat *et al.*, 1983). Also, it is widely believed that all Western drugs are in some ways poisonous, and are discontinued as soon as symptoms diminish (Wheat *et al.*, 1983). "Natural" medicines and treatments were far more common in the homeland, the latter including spas, sanatoriums, and the like.

Medical care in the former Soviet Union was very authoritative, and preventive medicine virtually unknown (Brod & Heurtin-Roberts, 1992). Full disclosure of diagnoses, especially for cancers, was rare (Cronkright *et al.*, 1993). Home visits for general medical care of acute problems were common in the former Soviet Union, and hospitalization for even minor problems was also the norm (Cronkright *et al.*, 1993). The preference for outpatient care in the West rather than hospitalization, together with the more frequent use of oral medications over injections, are sources of frustration for Russian immigrants (Grabbe, 2000).

Mental health services may be viewed with skepticism by immigrants for several reasons: Russian immigrants and refugees are more accustomed to seeking a "cure" from their physician for emotional problems, as opposed to talk therapies (Brod & Heurtin-Roberts, 1992). Furthermore, the psychiatric system under communism had as much to do with incarceration and abuse of political dissidents as it did with treating mental illness.

Pregnancy and childbirth

Until recently, oral contraceptives were not widely available in Russia, and abortion was the predominant means of limiting births. During pregnancy, the mother was discouraged from any heavy lifting or other exertion. In fact, miscarriage would sometimes be induced through repetitive lifting of weighty objects. Another reported abortifacient was the consumption of a full glass of vodka on an empty stomach in the first month of pregnancy. When a woman experienced constipation, especially during the first trimester, she was warned not to push too hard lest the baby be pushed out too. Under the communist regime, there was an institutionalized decree providing freedom from strenuous employment after 7 months of pregnancy. Prenatal care in the former Soviet Union was far from universal, and when available, visits were much less frequent than in the West.

The use of any Western pharmaceuticals during pregnancy was shunned by many, and a proscription against caffeine also widely observed. Even oral pain medicines and epidurals were rarely used in the home country, although this pattern may change in other locales. Russian women are said to be very patient and stoic at parturition, and rarely cry out. Castor oil or an enema were often given immediately before birth to ease the birthing process. Fathers were typically not involved in the birth (Evanikoff, 1996).

Postpartum women were often hospitalized a week or more, even after normal delivery. Separation of the mother and newborn was common in Russia. On arrival at home, mother and child were frequently sequestered, for a week or sometimes up to 40 days. This period was to promote the restoration of health in the woman; in some cases work of any sort, cold foods and drinks, and sex were proscribed during this period. Additionally, the newborn was protected from the "evil eye" of covetous visitors, with only close relatives permitted to enter the home. Similarly, baby showers or even any form of prenatal preparation for the newborn were not done, so as not to tempt fate or otherwise attract evil forces. Knocking on wood three times and spitting over the left shoulder three times were (and are still) commonly performed to ward off the evil eye. Less commonly, rubbing a pinch of salt over the infant and then burning the salt was practiced to ward off the "evil eye." Naming might not occur for a week or more after birth.

Newborns were considered sensitive to bright light and extremely sensitive to cold. Typically, babies were bundled, especially around the abdomen, and fully swaddled for up to 3 months. The belief was that swaddling would promote straight limb growth and otherwise keep a baby from fussing. The swaddled newborn was placed on his or her back or side on a firm mattress with no pillow. A certain herbal bath, believed to contain daisy flowers (pictured on the package), was also commonly used to quell a fussy baby. Circumcision was performed shortly after birth for Jewish and Muslim boys but was rarely performed for Christians.

Breastfeeding was typically the norm, for a year or more. Keeping the breasts covered and warm during the lactation period, and consuming quantities of tea mixed with warm milk, were seen as ways to promote the milk supply. These practices were thought by some to prevent breast cancer later in life. There was also a belief that breast milk can become tainted when a nursing mother is made nervous or frightened and that this first breast milk should be expelled to prevent diarrhea in the nursing infant (Evanikoff, 1996).

End of life

Cultural beliefs and practices surrounding death and dying vary considerably for immigrants and refugees from Russia based on religious background (Jewish, Muslim, Christian, or no religion), and to a lesser degree, nationality. However, in general, the terminally ill should be cared for by the family in the home as institutionalization is viewed dimly and as a last resort. Many Russians believe that a terminal prognosis should be withheld from the patient, and sometimes even spouses, for fear of causing psychological insult.

Russians hold the body, in life as well as death, as sacred; hence organ donation and autopsy are not common (Evanikoff, 1996). For virtually all groups, burial is the norm, sometimes with an elaborate procession including special music, to the burial site; cremation is not practiced due to the ensuing harm to the spirit. For Christians, viewings are common, and in many cases the elderly purchases funeral clothes ahead of time. Mourning clothes of black are worn by men and women, and mirrors are covered. Grieving continues through 9 days, at which time a feast is prepared for friends and relatives. After 40 days, another remembrance celebration is held, releasing the spirit. Remarriage is permissible after 1 year.

Health problems and screening

Heavy smoking, high alcohol intake, lack of physical fitness, poor diet, and crowded living conditions have been reported for Russian and Ukrainian immigrants in the USA (Duncan & Simmons, 1996). Specific to diet, Romero-Gwynn *et al.* note that the dietary acculturation among resettled former Soviet Union refugees, unlike many other immigrant groups, has not been significant (1997). They cite the presence of elderly in households who act as dietary "gatekeepers" as one possible explanation for this conservatism. These authors describe the immigrants' diet as high in sources of fat and sodium (due to heavy intake of salt-treated and pickled foods), and poor in fresh fruits and vegetables (Romero-Gwynn *et al.*, 1997). Concerning the latter, we have frequently heard that many fruits common in the West, such as bananas and oranges, were never even seen in the former Soviet Union.

The healthy life expectancy or HALE in Russia is 56.7 years and the full life expectancy is 65 years (Population Reference Bureau, 2002; World Health Organization (WHO), 2002). Chronic non-infectious diseases are the leading causes of death and disability; and health risks for new Russian immigrants are primarily cardiac disease, cancer, diabetes, obesity and other chronic non-infectious diseases. Russia is a vast land and conditions vary, hence health risks (Centers for Disease Control, 2003; Hawn & Jung, 2003; Kemp, 2002; WHO, 2002, 2003) as follows do not apply to all locales:

- babesiosis (rare)
- boutonneuse fever
- bovine spongiform encephalopathy ("mad cow disease")
- cholera
- diphtheria
- encephalitis (most likely to be tick-borne)

- hemorrhagic fevers (HFs) (HF with renal syndrome and tick-borne HFs)
- hepatitis
- lyme disease
- malaria (only in parts of Armenia, Azerbaijan, Georgia, Kyrgyzstan, Tajikistan, Turkmenistan, and Uzbekistan – not Russia *per se*)
- sexually transmitted infections, including HIV/AIDS, cervical cancer, chancroid, chlamydia, gonorrhea, syphilis
- trematode infection (opisthorchiasis)
- tuberculosis (Russia is one of 22 "high-burden" countries in the world)

Acknowledgement

Yana Marshalkovskaya Brown.

REFERENCES

Brod, M. & S. Heurtin-Roberts (1992). Older Russian immigrants and medical care. *Western Journal of Medicine*, **157**, 333–6.

Centers for Disease Control (CDC) (2003). *Health Information for Travelers to Eastern Europe and the Newly Independent States of the Former Soviet Union (NIS)*. Retrieved July 21, 2003 from http://www.cdc.gov/travel/easteurp.htm.

Cronkright, P. J., KeHaven, K. & Kraev, I. (1993). Issues in the provision of health care to Soviet emigrants. *Archives of Family Medicine*, **2**, 425–8.

Duncan, L. & Simmons, M. (1996). Health practices among Russian and Ukrainian immigrants. *Journal of Community Health Nursing*, **13**, 129–37.

Evanikoff, L. (1996). Russians. In *In Culture and Nursing Care: A Pocket Guide*, ed. J. Lipson, S. Dibble and P. Minarik, pp. 239–49. San Francisco: UCSF Nursing Press.

Glantz, D. M. (2002). *The Battle for Leningrad: 1941–1944*. Lawrence, Kansas: University Press of Kansas.

Gold, S. J. (1996). Soviet Jews. In *Refugees in America in the 1990s: A Reference Handbook*, ed. D. Haines, pp. 279–304. Westport, CT: Greenwood Press.

Grabbe, L. (2000). Understanding patients from the former Soviet Union. *Family Medicine*, **32**, 201–6.

Hawn, T. R. & Jung, E. C. (2003). Health screening in immigrants, refugees, and internationally adopted orphans. In *The Travel and Tropical Medicine Manual*, 3rd edn., ed. E. C. Jong and R. McMullen, pp. 255–65. Philadelphia, PA: W. B. Saunders.

Immigration and Refugee Services of America (2002). *Refugee Reports*, **23**. Retrieved June 11, 2002 from www.refugees.org.

Kemp, C. E. (2002). *Infectious Diseases*. Retrieved April 12, 2003 from http://www3.baylor.edu/~Charles_Kemp/Infectious_Disease.htm.

Population Reference Bureau (2002). *2002 World Population Data Sheet.* Retrieved May 12, 2003 from http://www.prb.org/pdf/WorldPopulationDS02_Eng.pdf.

Romero-Gwynn, E., Nicholson, Y., Gwynn, D. *et al.* (1997). Dietary practices of refugees from the former Soviet Union. *Nutrition Today,* **32**, 153–7.

Wheat, M. E., Brownstein, H. & Kvitash, V. (1983). Aspects of medical care of Soviet Jewish immigrants. *Western Journal of Medicine,* **139**, 900–4.

World Health Organization (2002). *World Health Report.* Retrieved June 5, 2003 from http://www.who.int/whr/2002/en/.

(2003). *Global TB Control Report 2003.* Retrieved June 1, 2003 from http://www.who.int/gtb/publications/globrep/index.html.

34

Somalia

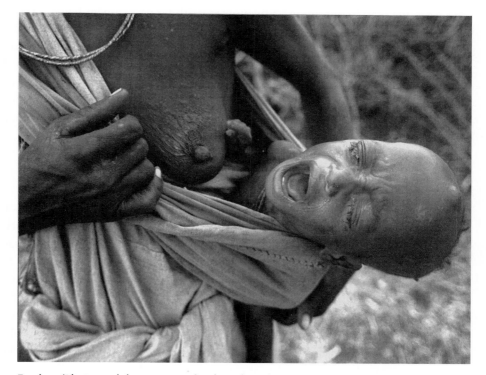

Famine. (Photograph by courtesy of Judy Walgren.)

Introduction

Like many other African countries, the area inhabited by ethnic Somalians has experienced great divisiveness since at least the mid-1800s, when the area was carved into multiple territories (Lewis, 1996; Putman & Noor, 1993). France controlled

Refugee and Immigrant Health: A Handbook for Health Professionals, Charles Kemp and Lance A. Rasbridge. Published by Cambridge University Press. © C. Kemp and L. A. Rasbridge 2004.

the north, now known as Djibouti, Britain and Italy colonized areas further south, and still other regions were under the rule of neighboring Kenya and Ethiopia. In 1960, the Italian and British areas were united into an independent Somalia, and in 1977 Djibouti became a separate nation after receiving independence from France. The regions of Kenya and Ethiopia which contain large numbers of ethnic Somalis are sources of border disputes presently.

The anti-colonial, pro-Soviet civilian government formed at independence was toppled in a coup led by General Mohammed Siad Barre in 1969. While popular at first, Barre's regime became increasing oppressive and autocratic, leading to the birth of clan-based opposition militias. In 1988, full-scale civil war broke out, leading to Barre's exile in 1991. However, up to the present, the clans have continued the bloody war amongst themselves, with no government being established. The continuous warfare, together with border clashes, has brought the Somali economy to near collapse. Mass starvation has ensued, and the level of inter-clan violence has become extreme, with rape and torture commonplace. An estimated 400 000 Somalis died during this period, and at least 45% of the population has been displaced by the fighting (Putnam & Noor, 1993). Humanitarian relief forces from the UN and the USA attempted to intervene, but by Spring of 1994 all foreign troops had been withdrawn due to the instability.

History of immigration

Beginning in 1991, at least one million Somalis fled to the neighboring countries of Djibouti, Kenya, Ethiopia, Burundi and Yemen, adding to the already overwhelming populations of refugees in the Horn of Africa. While most remain in refugee camps, some numbers have been repatriated, and several tens of thousands have been resettled to the West. The USA and UK have the largest numbers, followed by the Netherlands, Denmark, Canada, and Sweden (United Nations High Commissioner for Refugees (UNHCR), 2003). Of all the displaced Somalis, certain clan-based ethnic groups, particularly the Barawans and Benadir, have been selectively resettled *en masse*; plans to resettle Somali Bantu in 2003 are being formulated. While these groups share many cultural characteristics with mainstream Somalis, there are important differences as well, as detailed in the box below.

Culture and social relations

While Islam and the Somali language unite all of Somalia, the societal structure is markedly fractionated by membership in patrilineal clans (descent through male lines). There are a few main clans, and multiple subclans, sometimes with geographical and even social class orientation. For example, Barawans lived in the

Kismayu area, where they were predominantly fisherman and small-scale artisans like shoe cobblers. Much of the current strife in Somalia is centered around clan disputes, as allegiance to the clan far outweighs allegiance to a united Somalia. Among resettled Somalis, secondary migration for subclan reunification frequently occurs. Likewise, Somali refugees may claim fictitious family relations, such as disguising second wives as sisters or daughters, or even convenience marriages, when it is perceived to improve their acceptance for resettlement. Many of these artificial families immediately scatter to other areas to rejoin clan members upon arrival. Another concern for the resettlement providers is the common practice of corporal punishment of children, and less frequently, wives.

Benadir

The Benadir are a Somali ethnic group from the Benadir region of Somalia: the southern coastal region including Mogadishu (Mypist, 1995; USCC, 1996). Unlike most Somalis, who are nomadic, the Benadir have a long history as urbanized merchants and artisans. The Benadir exhibit strong clan allegiance, through intramarriage and self-governance. They are devout Sunni Moslems, and are well known for their peace-loving, non-violent ways. For all these reasons, the Benadirs consider themselves a different, élite, class from other Somalis; consequently, they have been the targets of jealousy and animosity for centuries.

When massive internecine warfare erupted in 1990, the unarmed and nonaligned Benadir were caught in the middle. They suffered greatly at the hands of the other Somali clans: homes and businesses were destroyed, women were raped in front of male relatives, and countless were slaughtered. Those that could fled Somalia, for Kenya, Ethiopia and Yemen, and many died on the high seas during flight. Because of their vulnerability, even among other Somali refugees, the UN established a separate Benadir refugee camp, Swaleh Nguru, in Kenya.

With the camp population exploding (approximately 22 000 in 1996), health conditions deteriorating, their homes and livelihoods destroyed, and the likelihood that they could never repatriate to Somalia without persecution, resettlement overseas became the only durable solution for the Benadir plight. Since Spring of 1996, about 3000 Benadir refugees have been resettled in about 20 sites throughout the USA. Of these thousands, there are about a dozen major clans and many more subclans; family name usually corresponds to clan membership. The elder clan leaders serve as the cornerstone of Benadir society and should be included in all decisions surrounding Benadir resettlement.

Bantu

The Somali Bantu are a minority ethnic group who fled Somalia to Kenyan refugee camps due to extreme persecution and prejudice throughout the civil unrest of the last decade (Cultural Orientation Project, 2002). Their ancestral roots are from Southeast Africa and they are primarily descendants of slaves taken from that region. Their ancestors either escaped slavery or were freed and eventually settled in farming communities along the Juba River in Somalia over a century ago. Since their original settlement, the Bantu have endured continuous marginalization in Somali society, differing in history, as well as cultural, linguistic and physical characteristics from the indigenous Somalis. For generations they have been denied political, economic, and educational opportunities and most have lived in small farming villages apart from other Somalis. As they were ruthlessly routed from Somalia by the warring factions and their farms and lands confiscated, most Somali Bantus in Kenya have no prospects to return. Thus, since 1999, the USA has designated the group of 13 000 or so Somali Bantus in UNHCR camps to be of high priority for resettlement.

Communications

Somali is the common language of Somalia, and since Islam is so widespread, Arabic is spoken by many Somalis. Additionally, educated Somalis are frequently conversant in Italian, English, and/or Russian, depending on their experiences with the former colonial powers. Some Somalis near Kenya can also speak Swahili. The Benadir have demonstrated some knowledge of English prior to resettlement due to their relatively high education levels. Alternatively, the Bantu are unlikely to have much experience with English, except among the young who may have received some education throughout the prolonged refugee camp stay. Furthermore, fluency even in Somali is not universal for Bantu, as ancestral tribal languages are sometimes spoken among some Bantu clans.

Religion

Somalis almost universally can be categorized by their strong adherence to Islam, the Sunni sect in particular. Accordingly, Islam religion shapes many aspects of Somali culture. For example, there is strict separation of the sexes, and women, including sometimes prepubescent girls, are expected to cover their bodies, including hair, when in public; facial veiling is uncommon in the USA. However, women in Somali culture do have considerable status, and many resettled refugee women are highly educated and held professional positions inside Somalia.

Handshakes are appropriate only between men or between women. The right hand is considered clean, and is used for eating, handshaking, and the like; children are taught early to use only their left hand for hygiene during toilet training. Even in the USA, Muslims prefer to wash with poured water after a bowel movement. Ritual cleaning of the body, especially before prayers, is dictated by Islam.

Devout Muslims pray five times a day to Allah; in reality, schedules in the United States do not always permit this. Many religious holidays and events are marked by the ritualized sacrifice of a goat or lamb; sometimes resettled Somalis arrange for this practice through rural farmers. Islam particularly proscribes the consumption of alcohol and pork.

Birthdays are not particularly celebrated by Somalis, and it is not uncommon for people to not know the exact date of their birth. At the time of immigration, birthdays are typically rounded off to the nearest year, e.g. 1-1-98, 12-31-62, etc. Alternatively, the anniversary of family members' deaths are observed and celebrated.

Health beliefs and practices

Herbal medicines are widely used in Somalia, especially for chest and abdominal symptoms; the herbal pharmacopia is vast, and some recipes are closely guarded (Rasbridge, 2000). A very common practice is the chewing of the *khat* herb, a mild stimulant. *Khat* is used both ceremoniously and more recreationally. There are various traditional medical practitioners in Somalia, especially herbalists, midwives, bone-setters and religious practitioners. Special healers treat psychosomatic disorders, sexually transmitted diseases, respiratory and digestive diseases, and snake and other reptile bites.

Another common traditional practice is termed "fire-burning," where a special stick is burned or a metal object heated and then applied to the skin, particularly to reduce swelling. Similar techniques of moxibustion are used to heal such ailments as stomach aches and headaches. Concepts involving spirits, such as "evil-eye," where excessive praise or attention can attract evil spirits to an infant or child, can be viewed as causing illness. Curing ceremonies involving ritualized dancing are used mostly for psychosomatic disorders, and cures based on Islamic texts and Koranic prayers may also be invoked. There is understanding about the communicability of some diseases, such as tuberculosis and leprosy, and physical isolation of infected individuals is sometimes performed.

The common practice of female genital cutting (FGC) is certain to create controversy in the areas of Somali resettlement (see Toubia, 1999). An estimated 98% of Somali girls 8–10 years of age undergo FGC, usually Type III (or infibulation), which consists of the removal of the clitoris, the adjacent labia (majora and minora), followed by the pulling of the scraped sides of the vulva across the vagina. The sides are then secured with thorns or sewn with catgut or thread. A small opening to allow passage of urine and menstrual fluid is left. An infibulated woman must be cut open to allow for intercourse on her wedding night, and the opening may then be closed again afterwards to secure fidelity to her husband. Less severe "female circumcision" is also performed, where the clitoris and part of the labia is excised, ostensibly to keep women pure and chaste. Cultural orientation programs in refugee camps warn of the illegality of these practices in the West, and Somali caseworkers are quite emphatic that FGC is not being performed among resettled communities. However, we have heard discussion that some girls would, in the future, be sent to Somalia for the procedure.

Pregnancy and childbirth

Somali families are typically large; a total of seven or eight children (or more) is considered ideal. Contraception, and similarly, abortion, are anathema to most Somalis, given the strong Muslim belief that pregnancy is a blessing from God and should not be interfered with. Even sexing of the fetus is not encouraged, as it is considered God's will and cannot be changed. Prenatal care is sought by refugee Somali women in the West, although there is a marked preference for female examiners. Most women fear Caesarean section delivery, the perceived method of choice for American women, as it is thought that the surgery may impede subsequent pregnancies and render the postpartum mother infirm. Alternatively, many women are concerned that episiotomies or even natural childbirth could damage the infibulation (see below).

There is a culturally sanctioned 40-day abstinence period, *afatanbah*, in the postpartum, when the mother remains in her household and is assisted by female relatives and neighbors. Amulets made from garlic can be worn by the mother and newborn to ward off evil spirits during this period, and incense is burned for the same purpose. There is traditionally a naming ceremony during this period, but hospital procedures requiring birth certificates have changed this practice.

Breastfeeding is the norm, in Somalia and in the refugee community here, sometimes for two years or longer. However, early supplementation with animal milk in Somalia or formula in the USA is not uncommon, and at least some women believe erroneously that colostrum is not healthy for the newborn. Infant care includes massages and warm water baths. Traditionally, an herb called *malmal* mixed into a poultice is applied to the umbilicus for a week or so; some Somalis report the availability of this herb in the USA.

End of life

In Somali culture, and Islamic culture in general, the concepts of nursing homes and hospice apart from the family are anathema. To the Somali, caring for an ailing parent or other family member is the utmost responsibility. In fact, looking after older parents is considered an honor and a privilege, indeed, an opportunity for spiritual growth as specifically referenced in the Koran. Patience and tolerance in dealing with the senile or otherwise infirm is paramount.

For Somalis, Islam is a powerful influence on all life cycle events, especially concerning dying and death. When death is imminent, rituals related to dying include the facing of the ill person toward Mecca and the recitation of specific versus from the Koran, so that God will forgive the person's sins. Ideally, a Muslim cleric, known as a sheikh, or other elder is summoned to lead the prayer, which may be spoken directly in the ear of the dying person. After death, the body is ritually cleansed by the family members of the same sex and wrapped in a white shroud.

As the deceased must be buried intact for life anew, most Muslim scholars have the opinion (fatwa) that autopsies are against the will of Allah and hence are forbidden (Sheikh, 1998) except when required by civil law. In certain cultures, sources cite that organ donation may be allowed (Al-Mousawi *et al.*, 1997); similarly, it is not uncommon for Muslim physicians to recommend transfusions as a life-saving measure. However, these practices are very controversial to most Somalis and the debate rages in Somalia and here. Many believe that organ transplantation and transfusions could put the recipient at risk of inheritance of the past sins of the unknown donor and hence are strictly forbidden. Medical products derived from animals may also be *haram*, forbidden, especially those from a pig. Technologically based life support measures may be opposed by Somalis and some other Muslims, on the belief that God has already chosen the date of death and this cannot be altered.

The funeral, in the mosque, should take place as soon as possible after death and the body buried in a Muslim cemetery, which is not always available in the West. In more traditional societies, the wrapped body is buried without a coffin, with the head oriented toward Mecca. Cremation is not permitted. Mourning lasts for several days and is a family and public community process, usually with men and women separate. Somalis and other Muslims consider the funeral observance the most important rite they can perform for their deceased family members, while also a time to reflect on the preciousness of life here on Earth. Islam teaches that there are three gifts that can help a person even at death: the charity which he had given, the knowledge which he had taught, and the prayers on his behalf by a righteous child.

Health problems and screening

The healthy life expectancy or HALE in Somalia is 35 years (decreased from 2000–2001) and the full life expectancy is 47 years (Population Reference Bureau, 2002; World Health Organization (WHO), 2002a). Infectious diseases are the leading documented causes of death and disability in Somalia. Somalia is one of 9 countries in the world with indigenous transmission (low intensity) of polio and one of 11 countries accounting for more than 66% of world deaths from measles (Stein *et al.*, 2003; WHO, 2002b, 2003). Health risks for new Somali immigrants or refugees (Hawn & Jung, 2003; Kemp, 2002; WHO, 2002a) include:

- amebiasis
- anthrax
- boutonneuse fever (African tick fever)
- chikungunya
- cholera
- dracunculiasis (Guinea worm disease)
- echinococcosis (hydatid disease)
- filariasis – Bancroftian filariasis and Malayan filariasis, loiasis or loa loa (usually found in tropical Africa, but potential exists), onchocerciasis (usually found in tropical Africa, but potential exists)
- hemorrhagic fevers (HFs): Lassa HF, Marburg and Ebola HFs (not currently, but the potential exists), Crimean–Congo HF, chikungunya fever, dengue fever and dengue HF, and Rift Valley fever
- hookworm
- leishmaniasis
- leprosy
- malaria (including multi-drug resistant)
- malnutrition
- measles
- plague
- poliomyelitis
- relapsing fevers (tick-borne)
- sexually transmitted infections, including HIV/AIDS, cervical cancer, chancroid, chlamydia, gonorrhea, granuloma inguinale, lymphogranuloma venereum, syphilis
- sickle cell disease or sickle cell hemoglobulinopathies
- strongylodiasis
- trachoma
- trematodes (liver-dwelling: clonorchiasis and opisthorchiasis; blood-dwelling: schistosomiasis or bilharzias; intestine-dwelling; and lung-dwelling)
- tuberculosis (including multi-drug resistant)
- typhoid and paratyphoid fever (sometimes termed enteric fever)
- typhus
- yaws (frambesia)
- post-traumatic stress disorder

Acknowledgements

Mohammed Farah and other anonymous reviewers from the Somali community.

REFERENCES

Al-Mousawi, M., Hamed, T., & Al-Matouk, H. (1997). Views of Muslim scholars on organ donation and brain death. *Transplantation Proceedings*, **29**, 3217.

Cultural Orientation Project (2002). *Somali Bantu–Their History and Culture*. Retrieved November 2, 2002 from www.culturalorientation.net.

Hawn, T. R. & Jung, E. C. (2003). Health Screening in immigrants, refugees, and internationally adopted orphans. In *The Travel and Tropical Medicine Manual*, 3rd edn., ed. E. C. Jong and R. McMullen, pp. 255–65. Philadelphia, PA: W. B. Saunders.

Kemp, C. (2002). *Infectious Diseases*. Retrieved April 21, 2002 from www.baylor.edu/~Charles_Kemp/Infectious_Diseases.htm.

Lewis, T. (1996). *Somali Cultural Profile*. Retrieved April 12, 2002 from http://healthlinks.washington.edu/clinical/ethnomed/somalicp.html.

Mypist, E. (1995). *Notes on Benadir Refugees*. Mombasa: United Nations High Commissioner for Refugees.

Population Reference Bureau (2002). *2002 World Population Data Sheet*. Retrieved May 12, 2003 from http://www.prb.org/pdf/WorldPopulationDS02_Eng.pdf.

Putman, D. B. & Noor, M. C. (1993). *The Somalis: Their History and Culture*. Washington: The Refugee Service Center, Center for Applied Linguistics.

Rasbridge, L. A. (2000). *Somali Refugees*. Retrieved April 4, 2001 from www.baylor.edu/~Charles_Kemp/refugee_health.htm.

Sheikh, A. (1998). Death and dying – a Muslim perspective. *Journal of the Royal Society of Medicine*, **9**, 138–40.

Stein, C. E., Birmingham, M., Kurian, M., Duclos, P., & Strebel, P. (2003). The global burden of measles in the year 2000 – a model that uses country-specific indicators. *Journal of Infectious Diseases*. **187** *(Supplement 1)*, S8–S14.

Toubia, N. (1999). *Caring for Women with Circumcision*. New York: Rainbo Publications.

United Nations High Commissioner for Refugees (2003). *2002 Annual Statistical Report: Somalia*. Accessed August 20, 2003 at http://www.unhcr.ch.

United States Catholic Conference. (1996). *Benadir Refugees from Somalia*. Washington: Refugee Information Series, Migration and Refugee Services.

World Health Organization (2002a). *World Health Report*. Retrieved June 5, 2003 from http://www.who.int/whr/2002/en/.

(2002b). *Global Polio Status 2002*. Retrieved May 9, 2003 from http://www.polioeradication.org/all/global/.

(2003). *Somalia*. Retrieved from http://www.who.int/country/som/en/.

FURTHER READING

Ackerman, L. K. (1997). Health problems of refugees. *Journal of the American Board of Family Practice*, **10**, 337–48.

Gavagan, T. & Brodyaga, L. (1998). Medical care for immigrants and refugees. *American Family Physician*, **57**, 1061–8.

35

Sudan

Introduction

Sudan, the largest country in Africa, is in Northwest Africa and is bordered on the north by Egypt; on the east by the Red Sea, Eritrea, and Ethiopia; in the south by Kenya, Uganda, and Congo; and in the west by the Central African Republic, Chad, and Libya.

The people of Sudan have endured great persecution and strife for generations: endemic political and religious oppression, famine, floods, locusts, and warfare. Sudan is among the poorest countries in the world and its citizens the least literate. Civil war has raged in Sudan nearly continuously since independence from Britain in 1956. The religious war between the Islamic fundamentalists in the north, and the diverse African ethnic groups, many of whom are Christian, in the south, has devastated the country and its people.

The Islamic government in the north has a long history of persecution of the Sudanese citizenry, especially southerners and Christians. Using famine as a weapon of war, military leaders in the capital of Khartoum have repeatedly withheld internationally donated food and relief supplies in the regions of the south already devastated by drought and fighting. In 1988 alone, more than 250 000 Sudanese died of starvation. By 1989, inflation had risen by 80%, and the debt to $13 billion, and yet there was no plan by the government to rebuild the country. The corruption of the country's leaders prevented aid from such organizations as the United Nations, United States Agency for International Development and numerous non-governmental organizations (NGOs) reaching rebel-held areas. The cities swelled with refugees fleeing the devastated countryside, and millions of Sudanese fled to the neighboring countries of Ethiopia, Uganda, Kenya, and Egypt. In 1993, it was estimated that 4 750 000 Sudanese found refuge in other countries, excluding the greater than 1 300 000 who died in the flight. From these camps, nearly

Refugee and Immigrant Health: A Handbook for Health Professionals, Charles Kemp and Lance A. Rasbridge. Published by Cambridge University Press. © C. Kemp and L. A. Rasbridge 2004.

20 000 refugees from Sudan have been accepted for resettlement in the United States (Central Intelligence Agency, 2003; Immigration and Refugee Services of America (IRSA), 2002; Johnstone & Mandryk, 2001).

History of immigration

There are several different subpopulations of refugees from Sudan. The largest number in the USA are refugees from the south of Sudan, composed of various minority ethnic groups fleeing religious and political persecution, warfare, and starvation. Additionally, there are political dissenters from the north who escaped from the oppressive Muslim fundamentalist regime in Khartoum. Many of these fled to neighboring countries, especially Ethiopia, to escape forced conscription, or in fewer cases, religious persecution, in particular against Baha'is. The United Nation's High Commissioner for Refugees (UNHCR) assisted these refugees in Ethiopia (IRSA, 2002).

Refugees from the south of Sudan come from the three different geographical regions: the Bahr-el Ghazal, the Upper Nile, and Equatoria, the latter containing Juba, the capital of the south. There is tremendous cultural diversity, not only between the Sunni Moslem north and the animist (traditional) and Christian south, but also within the southern region itself. Tribal affinity among the "Nilotic" groups (a reference to the thin physique and common ancestral language of those groups living along the Nile) is the norm, with infrequent intermarriage. Many ethnic languages are not mutually intelligible, although English, and to a lesser extent, Arabic, are the most widespread languages.

There are at least ten different ethnic groups from the south that are represented as resettled refugees in the USA. The largest in number are the Nuer. Formerly a pastoralist group, the Nuer have witnessed great destruction and strife as they are located most closely to the Arab-occupied areas along the Upper Nile. The Nuer live over a wide area and are divided into about ten subgroups or clans. There are several dialects of the Nuer language, and many speak Arabic as well. Three other ethnic groups of lesser number also came from the Upper Nile region and are resettled in the USA: the Anuak, Bor, and the Shilluk.

Next to the Nuer, the second largest Sudanese population in the USA are the Dinka, who represent the majority group in southern Sudan. They originated primarily from the Bahr-el Ghazal region of Southwestern Sudan, where they were pastoralists and agriculturalists. They speak Dinka, and secondarily Arabic and English. Like the Nuer, there is much diversity within the Dinka, with at least two dozen recognized subgroups, as well as great contrast between the missionized and pagan groups. Some other groups coming from this region include the Balanda and the Ndogo.

Finally, there are Sudanese refugees who originally lived in the Equatoria region in southernmost Sudan: the Azande, the Moru, and the Madi. All three groups were primarily agriculturalists, and are now predominantly Christian.

In 1991, a special group of about 3000 young men known as the "Lost Boys" of Dinka and other ethnicities were resettled *en masse* in the United States (Church World Service, 2003). These refugees fled Sudan over a decade previously to escape forced conscription, and after a perilous journey through several countries, had been living in the Kakuma refugee camp in Kenya.

Culture and social relations

In terms of social etiquette, there are some generalized distinctions between the Islamic north and the African south. For example, for Muslims, when greeting, men shake hands with men, but it is not culturally appropriate for men to shake hands with women, except within the family. Respect should always be afforded to the man as the household head, but typically mothers will be more knowledgeable about children's health and can be addressed directly, especially with southern families, where the rules of interaction are less rigid. Separation of the sexes is common to the Muslim north, and even homes are divided into male and female areas.

Muslim women from northern Sudan may be quite reluctant to be examined by a male physician, although most southern Sudanese women will view this as a medical necessity. In general, great diplomacy must be used in exchanges on gynecological matters. Sudanese women will frequently use euphemisms when referring to genitalia, or when English is poor, to avoid the topic completely.

Especially among the southern groups, relative age is of great importance in interpersonal relationships, determining not only the terms of address but also the manner of acting with others. For example, men of the same "age set" will call each other "brother" and will act informally with one another. Alternatively, someone older than you is afforded utmost respect, and is referred to as "uncle" or "aunty," or even "father" or "mother" if related by blood.

Marriage is typified as a sort of contract between the families involved, with the final approval left to the girl's side. Especially in the south, the groom's family is required to pay a dowry to the bride's family, usually in the form of heads of cattle, to compensate them for the lost labor of their daughter. The exchange in the north is usually more in the form of money. While in the north there is preferential marriage to cousins and other relatives, in the south marriages are exogamous, meaning that the union can only be between peoples of different clans or villages, formalizing political alliances within the tribe as well. The wife does not take the husband's name. There are strict formalities regarding the interaction between the man and his in-laws. The newlyweds initially reside with the wife's family, until after the first child is born and weaned, at which time they move to the husband's village. Great emphasis is placed on the woman's ability to bear and raise children, hence birth control is typically antithetical to this cultural value. Divorce is possible but discouraged because of the exchange of property involved. Widowed women become the responsibility of the deceased's younger brother. Polygamy is practiced and is a sign of wealth and prestige in the north, but is uncommon in southern Sudan.

Communications

As mentioned, Sudan is quite diverse linguistically, especially in the southern regions, where each tribe has its own language and sometimes several dialects. However, rudimentary Arabic language is spoken by almost all Sudanese, as it is the common language of commerce and discourse between tribes. In southern Sudan, English is only spoken by the educated minority. English was the official language until independence in 1956, when it was replaced by Arabic by the Khartoum government.

Literacy is very low, especially since schooling has been disrupted by chronic warfare and strife. Dinka and Nuer are written languages, "romanized" by missionaries in this century, but can only be read by those with some schooling. Literacy in Arabic is less than the tribal languages, and English lower still. Hence, except with the educated, it is not beneficial to use written health or other materials.

Religion

About 70% of the population of Sudan are Sunni Muslims, the vast majority in the north. About one-quarter of the peoples practice only "indigenous beliefs," and the remainder are Christian, both groups being found mainly in the south (Gray-Fisher 1994). While the Christians are a small but rapidly growing minority (in the south, Christians have increased from 5% in 1960 to as much as 70% in 2000), they tend to be the most educated. This Christian community is disproportionately represented in the resettled population, as their claims to asylum were the most well founded. They tend to be rather fervent in their Christian beliefs here (Gray-Fisher 1994; Johnstone & Mandryk, 2001).

There is widespread belief in Sudanese culture, especially among southerners, in the spiritual realm and its manifestations on health and illness, although the beliefs vary greatly from one tribe to the next. The Nuer, for example, believe in a pantheon of Gods and spirits, both supernatural beings and spirits of animals, especially birds.

During periods of epidemics or even individual health crises, oracles are sought out to identify the offended spirits and determine the proper recourse. Frequently an offering is presented or an animal is sacrificed in order to appease or drive away the evil spirit. A typical Dinka ceremony involves a spiritual elder praying over and then sacrificing a special white chicken in the presence of the afflicted. There is also a widespread belief in the concept of the "evil eye," where a malevolent person possessing supernatural powers can cast a spell on someone just by gazing upon them.

These spiritual beliefs and practices are observed mostly by non-Christians in the south and are sometimes sources of contention with the Christian community. In most cases, other available medical resources are resorted to when spiritual healing does not bring about the desired outcome.

Health beliefs and practices

There are multiple herbal and "traditional" remedies used by Sudanese (although lack of availability limits their use here in the USA) (Rasbridge, 2000). For example, a widely used cure for migraine headaches is a certain chalky compound (clay, mixed with certain leaves and water) that is rubbed over the head. To relieve the symptoms of malaria, there is a certain root chewed like a stick. One common form is called *visi ri*, a bitter shrub that bends its shoot to follow the sun. I have heard the testimonial of a highly educated southern Sudanese who swears this cure is more effective than chloroquine and other Western drugs.

There are also certain leaves that are boiled and consumed to relieve malarial sweats, and the same mixture is used to treat stomach disorders. For wounds, there are special leaves found in the bush which are tied over the wound like a plaster. These leaves may sometimes be burned and the ashes spread over the wound site. Parasitism is very common amongst Sudanese, especially tapeworms, amoebas, bilharzia (schistosoma), and roundworm (ascaris). To cure infection from ascaris, leaves and roots are boiled to produce a bitter liquid, which when swallowed expels the worms. Thread worm infection, under the skin, is treated by slowly rolling the emerging worm on a stick until the whole worm comes out.

All these curative measures are particularly relied upon where there is no access to clinics. Most of these cures are not commonly used by resettled refugees, as they are not readily available in the West, nor are the specialists who are sometimes required to make them.

Resettled Sudanese in the West experience numerous difficulties in accessing medical care, although to different degrees depending on background factors like educational level and prior exposure to biomedical care in Sudan. Language and cultural obstacles are obvious barriers, but also factors like name and birth date discrepancies, and the general lack of previous medical documentation, greatly confound the encounter. Most Sudanese have not had well care or medical check-ups in Sudan and therefore present with medical conditions of which they were previously unaware. Common undiagnosed cases include diabetes, hypertension, food allergies, severe cases of depression, vision and hearing loss, and parasitism. Also, dental problems are significant, especially as food habits change here. Several tribes, such as the Dinka perform various types of dental extractions or teeth filing as male puberty rites, and it is not uncommon for southern Sudanese men in the West to seek cosmetic dental care in order "not to look different."

Sudanese routinely share over-the-counter medications or borrow prescription medicines from others for cases of similar symptomatology. This is a result of coping with chronic shortages of medicines and severely limited care facilities in Sudan, and it circumscribes expensive medical costs in the USA. Similarly, Sudanese also tend to discontinue Western medicines as soon as symptoms resolve rather than completing the full course of treatment. Education on self-treatment and the importance of completed therapy is imperative for this population.

Pregnancy and childbirth

(The following information pertains mostly to the southern Sudanese, and in some cases is specific to Nuer culture. References to northern Sudanese culture are noted.) During pregnancy, women frequently eat a special kind of clay, which is rather salty. When chewed, this type of clay is believed to increase the appetite and decrease the nausea associated with pregnancy. There are not really any specific food restrictions during pregnancy which are not otherwise observed, such as a universal taboo against eating snake.

Most deliveries are in the home, attended by village midwives. First-born boys are afforded special attention, and are usually raised in the maternal family's village. Virtually all children breastfeed for about 2 years. Soft porridge made from sorghum and soups of boiled meat are believed to stimulate breast milk production. At delivery, a cow or goat is frequently slaughtered to ensure enough meat for the postpartum period. Weaning typically occurs when the child is walking, or is otherwise ready as judged by the parents.

Apart from cow's milk, a soft porridge made from fermented sorghum, mixed with a sour fruit, is commonly used as a weaning food (as well as a food for the infirm or elderly). In the general diet, sorghum is the most common starch, prepared in many different ways. Vegetables and greens, both wild and cultivated, make up a large proportion of the traditional diet, with meats including beef, goat, sheep, freshwater fish, and chicken (although chickens are generally more valued for egg production).

The system of naming children is rather complex. In some groups the child is named after the male lines, but traced either through the mother's or father's ancestry. A similar system gives the child the last name of the paternal grandfather's first name, the middle name being the father's first name, and the first or given name selected by the father. Christian children often have Biblical names and Sudanese names, used interchangeably. First names, when used, are commonly preceded by a title, like "Mr."

Birth dates are also quite confusing, as most southerners do not follow the Georgian calendar and at best know only the year and season of birth, and few tribal groups kept official records. In many cases, birth certificates have been lost or destroyed. In resettlement, commonly, a default date of January 1 is selected (Power & Shandy, 1998). As age is a critical criterion for resettled refugees in receiving benefits and enrolment in school, incorrect birthdates can be a significant barrier for Sudanese refugees (Gray-Fisher, 1994). Moreover, ambiguity in birthdates for children can confound immunization schedules and growth assessment for healthcare providers.

Childrearing is traditionally the responsibility of all the women in the village; while the father takes considerable pleasure in his children, discipline is the responsibility of the mother. In southern Sudan, while childhood is characteristically carefree, puberty as seen as the passage into adulthood and its responsibilities and is a marked occasion for both sexes. For girls, passage from childhood to adulthood is marked by the first menstruation, at which time the mother prepares her for her soon-to-be role as mother and home-manager. At this time, some tribes, especially Dinka, receive body decoration on the torso, done by cutting (scarification) or tattoos with henna.

For males, there is a complicated set of rituals through which an entire village age-set progresses, culminating in ritualized cutting of lines or striations across the forehead, especially among Dinka and Nuer. There is also a common traditional practice of teeth-pulling among the Dinka. Other groups have other types of rituals, often involving cutting marks. Circumcision is common among some groups, especially in the Equatorial region, but typically for hygenic rather than for religious or cultural reasons. However, there is much variation even within groups.

In northern Sudan, circumcision for males occurs shortly after birth in accordance with Islamic tradition. Female genital cutting (FGC) is practiced (89% females overall, with most (82%) having Type III done), sometimes under crude conditions, ostensibly to keep the girls chaste (Toubia, 1999). Type III (infibulation) consists of the removal of the clitoris, the adjacent labia (majora and minora), followed by the pulling of the scraped sides of the vulva across the vagina. The sides are then secured with thorns or sewn with catgut or thread. A small opening to allow passage of urine and menstrual fluid is left. An infibulated woman must be cut open to allow for intercourse on her wedding night, and the opening may then be closed again afterwards to secure fidelity to her husband. Less severe forms of FGC are also practiced in northern Sudan (Toubia, 1999).

End of life

For Muslim Sudanese from the north, issues surrounding dying and death closely approximate the customs and beliefs of other Muslims like Somalis or Iraqis (Kemp & Rasbridge, 2001; Sheikh, 1998). Burial takes place as soon as possible. The body is taken to the mosque to be ritually cleaned and blessed by an Imam. The body is then carried to the previously prepared grave in a funeral procession. Mourning lasts between 3 and 7 days. Widows wear black clothes indefinitely, but may remarry.

For the southern Sudanese, as mentioned, there is strong belief in the spirits of past ancestors and that spirits in general can be the cause of illness and misfortune. Death is seen as the will of a spirit or God and is surrounded by the supernatural. Accordingly, there are important rituals observed by the various southern Sudanese groups during end-of-life events.

At death, the family, relatives, and other villagers, especially elders, gather around the body, usually in groups separated by sex. It is considered inappropriate for children to view the corpse. All southern Sudanese bury the deceased rather than cremate. Traditionally, the corpse is washed by the family and wrapped in a mat of woven grass or a cow skin and buried. There are no cemeteries *per se* but rather portions of family land that are set aside as sacred. The grave is sometimes marked with a certain plant.

The family mourns in isolation in the family home for about 40 days. This period would be typically followed by a ceremony where elders sacrifice a sheep in order to "cleanse" the mourning spirits that have befallen the family. From time to time, especially in periods of strife or hardship, elders perform a ceremony of animal sacrifice around a family "totem" or wooden statue that symbolizes the spirits of the deceased. However, these types of practices decrease in southern Sudan in the face of increasing Christian conversion.

When a wife dies, the husband is free to remarry, typically after a year or so. In the case of a deceased husband, the widow still remains part of the husband's family and may even be taken as a wife by the deceased's brother. Children born of such a union will be named for the deceased husband. For property inheritance, there is rarely a legal will, but transmission of property is usually discussed by the family before the death of the elder. Otherwise, the elder son or less frequently the elder daughter makes the decisions about inheritance.

In the USA, southern Sudanese are confronted with a myriad of new cultural traditions and options in the care and treatment of the infirm. If children still believe strongly in traditions, they should care for the elderly in the home. However, there would probably not be strong objections to nursing home placement in this culture if it were necessitated because of full-time jobs, etc. Similarly, there is unlikely to be strong opposition to withdrawal of life support, as there is general deference to and respect of the opinion of the Western physician. However, there may be overriding influence by the individual family and the community of elders in general. There is not any dominant cultural proscription against informing a patient of a terminal illness, although the family elder should certainly be approached first. As one Dinka man told us, "Dinka are brave people, we are prepared to die from sickness and war."

Health problems and screening

The healthy life expectancy or HALE in Sudan is 45.5 years (decreased from 2000–2001) and the full life expectancy is 56 years (Population Reference Bureau, 2002; World Health Organization (WHO), 2002a). Infectious diseases are the leading documented causes of death and disability in Sudan. Health risks for new Sudanese immigrants or refugees (Hawn & Jung, 2003; Kemp, 2002; WHO, 2002a) include:

- amebiasis
- anthrax
- boutonneuse fever (African tick fever)
- chikungunya
- cholera
- dracunculiasis (Guinea worm disease)
- echinococcosis (hydatid disease)
- filariasis – Bancroftian filariasis and Malayan filariasis, loiasis or loa loa (usually found in tropical Africa, but potential exists), onchocerciasis (usually found in tropical Africa, but potential exists)
- hemorrhagic fevers (HFs): Lassa HF, Marburg and Ebola HFs, Crimean–Congo HF, Chikungunya fever, dengue fever and dengue HF, and Rift Valley fever
- hookworm
- leishmaniasis
- leprosy
- malaria (including multi-drug resistant)
- malnutrition
- measles
- plague
- relapsing fevers (tick-borne)

- sexually transmitted infections, including HIV/AIDS, cervical cancer, chancroid, chlamydia, gonorrhea, granuloma inguinale, lymphogranuloma venereum, syphilis
- sickle cell disease or sickle cell hemoglobinopathies
- strongylodiasis
- trachoma
- trematodes (liver-dwelling: clonorchiasis and opisthorchiasis; blood-dwelling: schistosomiasis or bilharzias; intestine-dwelling; and lung-dwelling)
- tuberculosis (including multi-drug resistant)
- typhoid and paratyphoid fever (sometimes termed enteric fever)
- typhus
- yaws (frambesia)
- post-traumatic Stress Disorder

Acknowledgements

Mayen Ater, Professor Nyamlell Wakoson and Hamid Abdalla.

REFERENCES

Central Intelligence Agency (2003). *World Factbook* (revised 2003). Retrieved March 22, 2003 from www.cia.gov/cia/publications/factbook.

Church World Service (2003). *The Lost Boys of Sudan.* Accessed online www.churchworldservice.org.

Gray-Fisher, D. M. (1994). *The Land of the Black* (Infogram on the Democratic Republic of the Sudan). Iowa Department of Human Services, Bureau of Refugee Services.

Immigration and Refugee Services of America (2002). *Refugee Reports, 23.* Retrieved April 2, 2003 from www.refugees.org.

Johnstone, P. & Mandryk, J. (2001). *Operation World: 21st Century Edition.* Waynesboro, GA: Paternoster USA.

Kemp, C. (2002). *Infectious Diseases of Refugees and Immigrants.* Retrieved May 4, 2003 from www.baylor.edu/~Charles_Kemp/Infectious_Diseases.htm.

Kemp, C. and Rasbridge, L. A. (2001). Culture and the end of life: East African cultures, Part II, Sudan. *Journal of Hospice and Palliative Nursing,* **34,** 100–12.

Population Reference Bureau (2002). *2002 World Population Data Sheet.* Retrieved May 12, 2003 from http://www.prb.org/pdf/WorldPopulationDS02_Eng.pdf.

Power, D. V. & Shandy, D. J. (1998). Sudanese refugees in a Minnesota family practice clinic. *Family Medicine,* **30,** 185–9.

Rasbridge, L. A. (2000). *Sudanese Refugees.* Retrieved April 4, 2001 from www.baylor.edu/~Charles_Kemp/refugee_health.htm.

Sheikh, A. (1998). Death and dying – a Muslim perspective. *Journal of the Royal Society of Medicine*, **9**, 138–40.

Toubia, N. (1999). *Caring for Women with Circumcision*. New York: Rainbo Publications. Also available on-line at www.rainbo.org.

World Health Organization (2002). *World Health Report*. Retrieved June 5, 2003 from http://www.who.int/whr/2002/en/.

36

Thailand

Nitaya Thammasithiboon and Charles Kemp

Introduction

Thailand is in mainland Southeast Asia and is bordered on the north by Burma and Laos, on the east by Laos and Cambodia, on the west by Burma, and in the south by the Gulf of Thailand (East), Andaman Sea (West), and a short border with Malaysia. Thailand includes a tropical, monsoonal central and southern area, a drier plateau area (Khorat) to the east, tropical mountains in the north and west, and a hot and humid southern peninsula. Of the 62.6 million people living in Thailand, 75% are Thai, 14% Chinese, and 11% other. About 10% of the total population of Thailand lives in the Bangkok (capital) metropolitan area (Central Intelligence Agency (CIA), 2003; National Statistical Office Thailand, 2000; Population Reference Bureau (PRB), 2002).

Thailand (literally, free land) has been a unified kingdom since the 14th century. Known as Siam until 1939, Thailand is the only Southeast Asian country never colonized by a European country. The Thai government has been a constitutional monarchy since 1932, with the king having enormous popularity and wielding great personal influence, while the military holds much of the power.

History of immigration

During the 1960s and 1970s many Thai immigrants came as students to the United States and other Western countries. A large American military presence in Thailand during the Vietnam War also played a role in increasing immigration to the West. There have been no refugees from Thailand, though many Cambodian, Lao, and Burmese refugees have passed through Thailand.

Refugee and Immigrant Health: A Handbook for Health Professionals, Charles Kemp and Lance A. Rasbridge. Published by Cambridge University Press. © C. Kemp and L. A. Rasbridge 2004.

Culture and social relations

Thai culture is concretely family and religion oriented. When possible, the extended family lives together in a compound or adjoining properties. Within the family, respect for elders is a strong positive value, with grandparents revered and looked to for guidance in traditions and customs. Respect for elders (*kreng chai*) extends beyond the family to elders in general, and especially to teachers and monks.

Outwardly, men hold the power in the family and are expected to be the bread-winners. Men also have far more sexual freedom than do women; purchasing sex is common among Thai men. Men may also have more than one wife. Women, on the other hand, hold strong behind-the-scenes power and hold the deeds to much of the property in Thailand. Despite increasing numbers of Thai women working outside the home (especially among overseas immigrants), traditional gender roles remain largely unchanged. Even employed women are expected to keep house, cook, and otherwise maintain traditional roles along with newer roles (Roselieb & Wilde, 2003).

In Thai tradition, sons are cherished, as they are the ones to stay in the household and support the family. Daughters, on the other hand, will eventually leave the household to be with their husband, and therefore may not be equally valued in the family.

"Saving face" (*ku na*) or maintaining personal dignity and integrity is important in all relationships. To criticize or treat another with disrespect results in both parties losing face; for the person on the receiving end, the loss is greater. To lose face in front of others creates immense distress for Thai people. Thai culture also puts great value on equanimity (*chai yen*). The expression of strong feelings – especially negative – is a cause for loss of face. It is not relevant whether one is right or wrong, but that the feelings are openly expressed. The famous Thai expression, *mai pen rai* (it doesn't matter or never mind) is a means of dealing constructively with interpersonal stress or conflict – or simply with the difficulties inherent in life.

Communications

The Thai language – at least to the Western ear – is usually extraordinarily soft and musical. Communications usually are characterized by pleasant and solicitous formality and an acute sense of social status. Communications tend to be indirect and smiling is highly valued under most circumstances.

The traditional greeting is called *wai*, and is done by placing one's hands together as if in prayer. The person of lower social status holds her or his hands higher and the person of higher social status holds her or his hands lower. A person of lower social status may also bow as she or he *wai*s. A person of higher social status does not necessarily *wai* in response to a person of lower status, and a monk never responds with a *wai*. Younger people and those of lower status always greet first.

As noted earlier, communication of strong feelings is in poor taste. This includes hearty laughter, loud talk, back-slapping, and especially expression of negative feelings. Staring into another's eyes is also rude, and touching another adult's shoulders and especially head is unpardonably rude. Pointing, showing the bottom of one's foot, or calling with upraised finger is insulting to Thai people. Bringing attention to oneself is in very poor taste among Thai people.

Religion

Religion permeates Thai culture, with Buddhism the religion of 95% of Thai people, followed by Islam (3.8%), and Christianity (0.5%) (Central Intelligence Agency, CIA, 2002). Images of the Buddha and other religious figures are found on every Thai street and in almost every home. Virtually all Thai Buddhists follow Theravada Buddhism, the "lesser vehicle." In the villages, much of the education is through temples. Throughout Thailand and among Thai people worldwide, monks play essential roles in decision-making and other aspects of daily life (Buddha Dharma Education Association 1992–2003).

Many Thais also concurrently practice animism or spiritism in which supernatural forces are perceived as causing suffering and problems of life; as well as a means of alleviating suffering and trouble. Evidence of the pervasiveness of these practices is seen in the presence of spirit houses (*san phra phum*) at most homes and businesses. These spirit houses range from a simple and small (0.25 meter square) house on top of a 4–5 foot pole to an elaborate edifice three or more meters square. The houses may be decorated with figures of people, furniture, elephants, and the like, and daily offerings of incense, flowers, and candles are made at the house.

Another aspect of Thai spirituality is the incorporation of (Hindu) Brahmanism in Buddhism. Representations of Hindu gods (e.g. Brahma, Vishnu, Rama, and Indra) are found inside and outside many Buddhist temples and in homes and at businesses. One of the best known of these is the statue of Lord Brahma at the Erawan Hotel, where there is a never-ending stream of worshippers at the shrine.

It is of little use to try to understand who believes what (or more accurately, how much of what) among Thais with respect to Buddhism, spiritism, and Brahmanism. Beliefs are intertwined with one another, often unspoken, not always perceived, and subject to change with circumstances. Suffice it to say that syncretism is operational; for many Thais, the rejection of other religions as practiced by Christians and Muslims is strange indeed.

Health beliefs and practices

Traditional Thai beliefs about health and illness are based on the idea that spiritual and physical harmony should exist within the self and between the self and nature or the outside world. When there is harmony, an optimal state of health occurs and when there is disharmony, illness or poor health results. Traditionally and in keeping with Buddhist philosophy, Thais see no separation between self and nature.

The use of amulets and other magico-religious objects is common among Thais. Specific monks or temples (*wats*) are thought to possess and be able to transmit healing and other powers through ritual, amulets, and other means. Overseas, Thai who are ill or distressed may return to Thailand to consult such a monk or obtain an especially powerful amulet. Buddha images (sometimes enclosed in clear plastic) are worn on a chain around the neck by many Thai people. White thread tied them around the wrist is also common – especially among travelers.

Traditional healers and herbalists practice in rural Thailand and among the poor in cities. At the same time, Thailand has a sophisticated medical system and modern biomedical care is available for those able to afford it. The many government-operated clinics and hospitals are not sufficient to meet health needs of the populace (Roselieb & Wilde, 2003).

Health and related issues of interest to healthcare providers in the West include the following (Phaosavasdi *et al.*, 2001; Roselieb & Wilde, 2003):

- The head is the most sacred part of the body and being touched on the head is distressing to Thai people. Before touching a patient's head, one should explain the reason and then limit the examination to what is necessary.
- When bathing and drying off, Thai people do not use the same towel for the whole body. The correct way is to use one for the upper part (the head) and another for the lower parts.
- Preserving modesty is very important during an interview or physical examination, especially for Thai females.
- Among the more elderly Thais living outside of their culture, it is important for the healthcare provider to understand that eye contact is avoided out of respect and not meant to be impolite or evasive.
- Doctors and nurses are highly respected – especially by older people – and may both be referred to as *Khun Mo*.
- Even in healthcare situations, many Thais will not say outright what is wrong or bothering them, hence, it is important to ask specific questions. Complaining of health problems may be seen by some as bringing attention to themselves, hence is avoided.

- The reluctance to complain (and probably other factors) results in some patients delaying treatment well past when other people would likely seek treatment.

Traditional healthcare/treatments or indigenous practices are, in many cases, adapted from traditional Chinese medicine (TCM). The degree to which TCM is integrated into Thai health beliefs is shown in the very common practice of Thai pharmacies having a Western biomedical side of the store and a TCM side. Many books have been written on these types of herbal medicines and therefore only a brief summary of the more common uses will be explained.

- *Yaa klaang baan* (a root and stem of bawraphet, a type of wood climber) is used for fever reduction.
- *Raak chaa phluu* (Piper root) is used for stomach ailments.
- *Yaa hawn* (fragrant or aroma medicine such as Monkey Holding a Peach) is used as a balm for muscle pain or headaches.
- *Mara* (bitter melon) is used for myalgia and general fatigue.
- Opium is used for analgesia.
- Ginkgo biloba is used for cardiac and pulmonary problems.

Culture-bound syndromes found among the Thai (American Psychiatric Association, APA, 2000; Jilek & Jilek-Aall, 1985) include the following.

- *Rook-joo* is the Thai term for *Koro*, the intense anxiety that the genitals (or in females, vulva and nipples) will retract into the body and cause death.
- *Baah-ji* is the Thai term for what is more commonly known as *latah*, a hypersensitivity to intense fright or anxiety characterized by echolalia, echopraxia, command obedience, and dissociative or trance-like behavior.

Pregnancy and childbirth

Traditionally, there are food and behavior changes involved in pregnancy, including avoidance of spicy or oily foods. In Thailand, in rural areas, birth is assisted by a midwife or female relative. In the cities, most births occur in hospitals. Among overseas Thai, prenatal care is valued and sought early in the pregnancy.

Thai women tend to be stoic during birth, yet readily accept analgesia if certain that no harm will come to the baby. Postpartum, neither the mother nor the baby should be exposed to cold or wind, e.g., as would happen if the hair were shampooed. Mother and baby are kept warm, and in the case of the mother, the custom of "lying by fire" is used to maintain warmth. "Cold" foods, exercise, and emotional turmoil are avoided and sexual abstinence is common. With a clear preference for "human milk" over "animal milk," breastfeeding is the norm in Thailand and overseas. As is true in much of the world, Thai babies sleep with the parents until another child is born or the child is deemed to be old enough to sleep alone (Kaewsarn *et al.*, 2003; Rice & Naksook, 1998).

End of life

Devout Thai Buddhists approach death and suffering with equanimity. The family (if available) is likely to be deeply involved in the process; if there is no family available, a Thai patient living in the West is likely to return to Thailand for the end of life. Maintaining awareness during the process of dying is very important, hence analgesia may be refused in favor of a clear sensorium. The home is the preferred place of death, but since Thai patients are not always informed by the family of their prognosis, the patient may sometimes prefer the hospital in hope of a cure.

After death, the body is kept at home for at least a day – preferably longer for ceremonies and attendance by family and friends. Ceremonies are conducted by monks in the home immediately following death and at the temple for specified periods after death. Cremation is the means of disposing of the body and except for Chinese from Thailand, burial is not acceptable (Roselieb & Wilde, 2003).

Health problems and screening

The healthy life expectancy or HALE in Thailand is 46.4 years and the full life expectancy is 56 years (Population Reference Bureau, 2002; World Health Organization (WHO), 2002). Infectious diseases are the leading causes of death and disability in Thailand. Thailand is one of 22 countries worldwide with a "high burden" of tuberculosis (WHO, 2003). Note, however, that there is an enormous disparity in health status between educated or wealthy Thai who are likely to emigrate as opposed to poor people who are less likely to go overseas. Health risks for new Thai immigrants (CIA, 2003; Hawn & Jung, 2003; Kemp, 2002; WHO, 2002) include:

- amebiasis
- angiostrongyliasis
- anthrax
- capillariasis
- chikungunya
- cholera
- cryptococcosis
- cryptosporidiosis
- cysticercosis (tapeworm)
- dengue fever
- encephalitis (Japanese)
- filariasis (Bancroftian filariasis and Malayan filariasis)
- gnathostomiasis

- helminthiasis (ascariasis, echinococcosis/hydatid disease, schistosomiasis)
- hepatitis B (14% carriage rate)
- hookworm
- lactose intolerance
- leishmaniasis
- leprosy
- leptospirosis
- malaria, including multi-drug resistant (MDR) from *Plasmodium falciparum* resistant parasites and especially from malaria re-infection.
- melioidosis
- mycetoma
- sexually transmitted infections, including HIV/AIDS (1.8%–2.15% positivity rate among adults), chancroid, chlamydia, gonorrhea, granuloma inguinale, lymphogranuloma venereum, syphilis
- strongylodiasis
- thalassemias
- trematodes (liver-dwelling: clonorchiasis and opisthorchiasis; blood-dwelling: schistosomiasis or bilharzias; intestine-dwelling; and lung-dwelling: paragonimiasis)
- tropical sprue
- tuberculosis (including multi-drug resistant)
- typhus
- yaws (frambesia)

REFERENCES

American Psychiatric Association (APA) (2000). *Diagnostic and Statistical Manual of Mental Disorders*, 4th edn, text revision. Washington, DC: author.

Central Intelligence Agency (CIA). (2003). *World Factbook*. Author. Retrieved July 3, 2003 from http://www.cia.gov/cia/publications/factbook/geos/ni.html.

Hawn, T. R. & Jung, E. C. (2003). Health screening in immigrants, refugees, and internationally adopted orphans. In *The Travel and Tropical Medicine Manual*, 3rd edn., ed. E. C. Jong and R. McMullen, pp. 255–65. Philadelphia, PA: W. B. Saunders.

Jilek, W. G. & Jilek-Aall, L. (1985). The metamorphosis of 'culture-bound' syndromes, *Social Science and Medicine*, **21**, 205–10.

Kaewsarn, P., Moyle, W., & Creedy, D. (2003). Traditional postpartum practices among Thai women. *Journal of Advanced Nursing*, **41**, 358–66.

Kemp, C. (2002). *Infectious Diseases*. Retrieved April 12, 2003 from http://www3.baylor.edu/~Charles_Kemp/Infectious_Disease.htm.

National Statistical Office Thailand (2000). *Population and Housing Census 2000*. Retrieved July 4, 2003 from http://www.nso.go.th/pop2000/prelim_e.htm.

Phaosavasdi, S., Taneepanichskul S., Tannirandorn, Y., Hongladarom, S., & Wilde, H. (2001). New World and transcultural impact on Thai medical practices and professional behavior. *Journal of the Medical Association of Thailand*, **84**, 1650–2.

Population Reference Bureau (2002). *2002 World Population Data Sheet.* Retrieved May 12, 2003 from http://www.prb.org/pdf/WorldPopulationDS02_Eng.pdf.

Rice, P. L. & Naksook, C. (1998). Child rearing and cultural beliefs and practices amongst Thai mothers in Victoria, Australia: Implications for the sudden infant death syndrome. *Journal of Paediatrics and Child Health*, **34**, 320–4.

World Health Organization (2002). *World Health Report.* Retrieved June 5, 2003 from http://www.who.int/whr/2002/en/.

    (2003). *Global TB Control Report 2003.* Retrieved June 1, 2003 from http://www.who.int/gtb/publications/globrep/index.html.

37

Vietnam

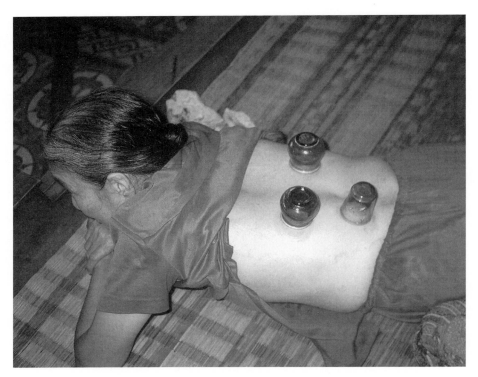

Traditional healing technique (cupping or *giac*) common among Vietnamese (this patient), Laotians, Cambodians, and other Asians. (Photograph by courtesy of Lance A. Rasbridge.)

Refugee and Immigrant Health: A Handbook for Health Professionals, Charles Kemp and Lance A. Rasbridge. Published by Cambridge University Press. © C. Kemp and L. A. Rasbridge 2004.

Introduction

Vietnam is in Southeast Asia and is bordered on the north by China, on the west by Laos and Cambodia, to the east by the Gulf of Tonkin and to the south by the South China Sea. The country ranges from tropical to monsoonal and from mountainous (most of the land) to marsh and flatlands. Almost 90% of the people are ethnic Vietnamese, followed by Thai-Dai (4.8%), Mon-Khmer (4.1%), Hmong/Mein (1.6%), and ethnic Chinese (1.6%) (Johnstone & Mandryk, 2001).

The recent history of Vietnam is well known. Along with Cambodia and Laos, Vietnam was a French colony (French Indochina) until the French defeat at Dien Bien Phu in 1954. The country was then partitioned into communist North Vietnam and noncommunist South Vietnam. The first large wave of Vietnamese refugees was composed of Catholics and others fleeing the north to the south in 1954. Almost immediately, North Vietnam began a political and guerilla war campaign to unite the country. The USA became gradually involved in the early 1960s, with US involvement peaking in the late 1960s and ending in 1973. What is referred to in Vietnam as "the American War" ended with the fall of Saigon in 1975. An immediate outflow of refugees ensued.

History of immigration

Since the fall of Vietnam in 1975, approximately 1.6 million Vietnamese have resettled in other countries and 250 000 died at sea trying to leave (Radio Australia, n.d.). Despite appearances to outsiders, the Vietnamese population as a whole is heterogeneous in many respects. This heterogeneity is represented largely by the refugee "wave" in which the individual or family arrived in the West.

- The first group of refugees to come to the West in 1975 were educated and urban professionals (and their families) who were airlifted directly from Saigon, most to the United States. This group has for the most part gone on to resume their professional lives in the USA, Australia, and France.
- The second wave of Vietnamese refugees, arriving from the late 1970s through the mid-1980s, included a much higher proportion of merchants, farmers and other rural Vietnamese who escaped Communist Vietnam in small boats. These "boat people" suffered extreme hardship and loss through the refugee process, often remaining in harsh refugee camps for years.
- The third wave, continuing to arrive to the present, come to the West under more "orderly" programs, typically on the basis of their statuses as political prisoners in Vietnam, offspring of Vietnamese women and American fathers, or through family reunification with previously resettled family members. The first of these two categories (prisoners and "Amerasians") suffered great hardship and discrimination in Vietnam.

And finally, there are Vietnamese born in the West and growing up in diverse environments ranging from inner-city gang territory to upper-class neighborhoods and first tier universities.

Culture and social relations

Vietnam has been strongly influenced by China for over 1000 years, and among the most important cultural patterns emerging from this influence are (a) a strongly held respect for learning and the learned and (b) familism, the valuing of family welfare over individual or community welfare, with deep respect paid to ancestors, elders, and the family unit. Extended families are common, but nuclear families are increasing as acculturation continues. In some cases, families have found a middle ground between extended and nuclear families, with younger generations supporting and remaining deeply invested in older generations, yet maintaining separate (but often nearby) residences.

Decision-making in health and other matters is usually the responsibility of the oldest male. However, an older woman may wield even more influence within the family. In more traditional families, the welfare of the family is clearly the overriding concern in all decisions. In younger, nuclear families, individualism is more highly valued. In nearly all cases, the oldest male has the greatest involvement in interacting with persons and institutions outside the family (Galanti, 2000). Conflict within the family is avoided – as is conflict with others.

Communications

Vietnamese language is a tonal language similar to those of China, but the written script has been romanized. French was spoken by older, highly educated, urban Vietnamese and of course, those Vietnamese now living in France. Names are formally written and frequently spoken by family name, middle name, and then given name. Touching members of the same sex, including men holding hands, is perfectly acceptable, but public affection or even touching between the sexes is discouraged. Shaking hands between men is common. Traditionally, the head is considered the "house of the soul" and should not be touched, although this custom is waived in the course of a medical examination. Alternatively, the sole of the foot is considered profane and would never be directed at another individual. Direct eye contact or physical positioning of elevation over one's superior is considered forward and impolite by some traditional Vietnamese.

Religion

In pre-war Vietnam, about 10% of the population was Catholic. This percentage is probably slightly higher among refugees in the USA, as Catholics are singled out for persecution by the communist regime. However, the vast majority of Vietnamese follow Buddhist precepts, particularly as influenced by Confucianism. Buddhism on the whole is best understood not as a religion in the Western sense but more a religious philosophy; it impacts profoundly on all aspects of Vietnamese life, including healthcare beliefs and practices.

Buddhism teaches that life is a cycle of suffering and rebirth; if one lives life in adherence to the Buddhist path, one can expect less suffering in future existences. Buddhism stresses disconnection to the present, especially materialism and self-aggrandizement. Suffering, however, is inevitable and pain and illness are sometimes endured and health-seeking remedies delayed because of this belief. Similarly, preventive health care has little meaning in this philosophy. See Chapter 5 for a discussion of Buddhism.

Also, as is common to Confucianism, Vietnamese Buddhists profess profound respect for elders and those in authority. This means that more traditional Vietnamese in the West will rarely be confrontational with others. In disagreement, a "face-saving" measure of avoidance or superficial acceptance is preferred to questioning or defiance, especially of those in positions of superiority, such as doctors and teachers.

Healthcare beliefs and practices

Illness is frequently understood in three different, although overlapping, models. The first, the least common, is what could be considered supernatural or spiritual, in which illness can be brought on by a curse or sorcery, or nonobservance of a religious ethic. Traditional medical practitioners are common in Vietnamese culture, both in the West and in Vietnam. Some are specialists in the more magico-religious realm, and these may be called upon to exorcise a bad spirit, for example, via chanting, a magical potion, or consultation from and recitation of ancient Western texts.

The use of amulets and other forms of spiritual protection are also commonly employed by Vietnamese. For example, babies and children commonly wear *bua*, an amulet of cloth blessed by a monk or containing a Buddhist verse worn on a string around the wrist or neck. For spiritual illness of a more Buddhist etiology, religious practices may be intensified, such as the burning of incense at the home altar to appease the ancestors, or a Buddhist monk may be consulted for prayer.

The second major concept in understanding illness is a widespread belief that the universe is composed of opposing elements held in balance; consequently, health is a state of balance between these forces, known as *Am* and *Duong* in Vietnamese, based on the more familiar concepts of *yin* and *yang* in China. Specific to health, these forces are frequently translated as "hot" and "cold," although it is important to understand that these concepts are not necessarily referring to temperature. Illness results when there is an imbalance of these "vital" forces. The imbalance can be a result of physiological state, such as pregnancy or fatigue, or it can be brought on by extrinsic factors like diet or over-exposure to "wind," one of the body forces or "humors." Balance can be restored by a number of means, including diet changes to compensate for the excess of "hot" or "cold," western medicines and injections, and traditional medicines, herbs and medical practices. These practices and medications include the following.

- Coining (*cao gio* or "catch the wind"). A coin dipped in mentholated oil is vigorously rubbed across the skin in a prescribed manner, causing a mild dermabrasion. This practice is believed to release the excess force "wind" from the body and hence restore balance.
- Cupping (*giac*). A series of small, heated glasses are placed on the skin, forming a suction that leaves a red circular mark, drawing out the bad force.
- Pinching (*bat gio*). Similar to coining and cupping, the contusion caused by pinching the skin allows the force to leave the body. The temporary marks produced by *bat gio* should not be confused with abuse or injury.
- Steaming (*xong*). A mixture of medicinal herbs is boiled, the steam is inhaled, and the body bathed.
- Balm. Various medicated oils or balms, like Tiger balm or Monkey Holding a Peach, are rubbed over the skin.
- Acupuncture. Specialized practitioners insert thin steel needles into specific locations known as vital-energy points. Each of these points has specific therapeutic effects on the corresponding organs.
- Acupressure or massage. Fingers are pressed at the same points as with acupuncture, and together with massage, stimulate these points to maximize their therapeutic effects.
- Herbs. Various medicinal herbs are boiled in water in specific proportions or mixed with "wine" and consumed, for example, in the postpartum, to restore balance.
- Patent medicines. These powdered medicines come packaged usually from Thailand or China and are mixed or boiled with water and taken for prescribed ailments.
- Minor bloodletting (*Le*). The forehead (between the brows) is pricked using a small, sharp object, such as a safety pin, and one or more drops of blood are squeezed out for the purpose of letting out "bad blood."

The third concept of illness among Vietnamese includes "Western" concepts of disease causation, like the germ theory. There is widespread understanding, for example, that disease can come from contaminants in the environment, even if concepts of microbiology or virology are not fully grasped. Concomitantly, through decades of French occupation and then the American influence, even the most rural Vietnamese has come to know the life-saving power of antibiotics.

When Vietnamese enter a Western healthcare setting, they do so frequently with the goal to relieve symptoms. In general, the Vietnamese patient expects a medicine to cure the illness immediately. When a medication is not prescribed initially, the patient is likely to seek care elsewhere. In addition to the myriad of traditional healers and other traditional medicines and practices available to resettled Vietnamese, Western pharmaceuticals, especially vitamins and even antibiotics, are obtainable, either through specialized "injectionists," or from relatives in other countries where some of these medicines are available without prescriptions.

Vietnamese frequently discontinue medicines after their symptoms disappear; similarly, if symptoms are not present, then illness is not thought to be present. Long-term medications like anti-hypertensives, and treatments that cause distress, like chemotherapy, must be prescribed with culturally sensitive education. It is quite common for Vietnamese patients to amass large quantities of half-used prescription drugs, some of which are shared with friends and may also make their way back to Vietnam.

Western medicines, especially oral medications, are held in general to be "hot" medicines, in their effect on the balance of the body. When oral medications are prescribed for a condition such as skin lesions, which is understood traditionally as a hot illness with the excess force erupting through the skin, a compliance issue may result. Similarly, Vietnamese commonly believe that Western pharmaceuticals are developed for Americans and Europeans, and hence dosages are too strong for more slightly built Vietnamese, resulting in self-adjustment of dosages. Patient and family education, then, is a high priority.

As mentioned above, Vietnamese hold great respect for those with education, especially physicians. The doctor is considered the expert on health; therefore, the expectation is that diagnosis and treatment should happen at the first visit, with little examination or personally invasive laboratory or other diagnostic tests. In fact, a doctor who probes a great deal into symptoms may be held incompetent by some traditional Vietnamese for not being able to diagnose readily. Similarly, extensive discussion and explanation with the patient and/or family may be viewed with some degree of perplexity. In a traditional Vietnamese doctor–patient relationship, there is little sharing of information or explanation of illness or treatment.

Commonly, laboratory procedures involving the drawing of blood are feared and even resisted by Vietnamese, who believe the blood loss will make them sicker and that the body cannot replace what was lost. Surgery is particularly feared for this reason. Overall, as health is believed to be a function of balance, surgery would be considered an option only of last resort, as the removal of an organ would irreparably alter the internal balance.

Food also affects balance and health, with some foods being *am* or "hot" and others *duong* or "cold" – though neither designation necessarily refers to the temperature or degree of spiciness. In illness the most commonly taken food is rice soup. Examples of *am* foods are green beans, leafy vegetables, bananas, cantaloupes, papaya, and tofu. *Duong* foods include bean sprouts, pepper, onions, ginger, garlic, high protein food, mango, watermelon, logan, and pineapple.

It is common for Vietnamese to view health and illness from a variety of different perspectives, sometimes simultaneously. In other words, it is not uncommon for a sick person to interpret their illness as an interaction of spiritual factors, internal balance inequities, and even an infective process. Accordingly, Vietnamese will combine diagnostic and treatment elements from all three models in order to get the maximum health benefits.

Vietnamese traditionally do not have a concept of mental illness as discrete from somatic illness, and hence are reluctant to utilize Western-based psychological and psychiatric services. Instead, most mental health issues such as depression or anxiety fall into this spiritual health realm and are treated accordingly. Similarly, physical expression of spiritually based illnesses (somatization) is common, and treatments overlap with the realms of health understanding.

Pregnancy and childbirth

The humoral system of balance discussed above is perhaps most apparent in the beliefs and practices surrounding pregnancy and parturition among Vietnamese women. Intrinsically, pregnancy is regarded as a humorally "hot" period, primarily because of fetal development, weight gain, and the cessation of menses. Certain foods considered *am* or "hot" are proscribed during this period, lest the equilibrium be thrown so unbalanced as to cause miscarriage. In fact, traditional abortifacients are believed to work precisely in this manner, and there are several herbal medicines for this purpose available in the West. Prenatal medical care is certainly not the norm in rural Vietnam, but is common among Vietnamese in the West. Some traditional beliefs concerning pregnancy are still widespread, such as the prohibition against heavy lifting, raising the hands over the head, or sexual relations late in pregnancy, all of which are believed to harm the fetus (D'Avanzo, 1992).

According to traditional Chinese medical principles, women are *yin* in nature, with more of the cold principle and thus are more susceptible to illnesses that result from an excess of cold – particularly at childbirth (Pillsbury, 1978). Immediate warming of the body after delivery is thought to be paramount to stave off long-term deleterious consequences of this susceptibility, ranging from wrinkled skin to arthritis to death. In the traditional context, a recently delivered woman reclined on a bamboo-slatted bed over a bucket of hot coals. While this practice is not performed in the West, other practices, such as steam baths, dietary consumption of "hot" foods, and in particular, the consumption of humorally "hot" medicines such as herb-wine tonic, are common. There are also sexual and work taboos in the postpartum, for at least 1 month but sometimes longer.

The more traditional mothers are opposed to any form of cutting, such as episiotomies, circumcision, or even cesarean section, as the spirit of the body could escape at these points (D'Avanzo, 1992). More universally, Vietnamese tend to be very superstitious around the postnatal period, fearing, for example that praising a newborn or even speaking her or his given name may attract malevolent spirits.

At birth a child is said to be 1 year old. Breastfeeding was the norm, for 2 years or more, in Vietnam, but less time in the West. Childrearing is rather permissive for the first few years of life and is often the responsibility of a slightly older sibling (Geissler, 1998).

End of life

As with other patients and families, a terminal illness in a Vietnamese family often brings old personal or family issues into sharp and immediate focus (Dinh *et al.*, 2000). Language difficulties and constraints on communicating about personal issues outside the family may result in great difficulty in establishing a therapeutic relationship. On the other hand, reminiscing about the war years, or perhaps even more therapeutic, about the time before the war destroyed Vietnam, may be easier with hospice or palliative care staff than with family – who may have tired of old stories. In most cases, family, especially women, will be very involved in care.

The involvement of clergy is different in Buddhist (and often, Vietnamese Catholic) tradition than in Western religions. It is unusual for Buddhist monks to visit a home before a person dies. A person's life in the present is a sum of her or his life in the past, hence there is little to accomplish with a home visit by clergy – no soul to save, so to speak. Nevertheless, religious practice and ritual in the home (and hospital, which should be encouraged by staff) is an integral part of daily life in many families, and thus of great importance to a person who is dying.

Discussing a terminal prognosis with the patient is usually resisted by the family. Common reasons given include "bad luck," i.e., talking about it might make it happen and talking about dying will cause the patient to lose hope. This creates conflict between fundamental Western ethical concepts of patient autonomy (especially informed consent), veracity, and fidelity on the one hand, and deeply held cultural values on the other.

Pain and other symptoms and suffering are often endured with greater equanimity among Vietnamese and other Buddhists than others. There are no proscriptions among Vietnamese against any treatment, including, in most cases, double effect treatment (that which life may be shortened in the effort to control symptoms). Euthanasia is not acceptable. Organ transplant and autopsy are not prohibited in

Buddhism. Removal of life support is usually accepted, when careful explanation and gentle recommendations are given.

Aftercare practices are not dissimilar to Western practices. The family often wishes to stay with the body for some period of time. If death occurs at home and a ceremony is held at home, the body is washed and kept for a day or more.

Contrary to popular concepts of Vietnamese and other Asians as inscrutable or less demonstrative, the expression of grief is often open and strong, including crying and wailing. White is the color of mourning. Burial is preferred, but cremation is also practiced, and in some cases, the ashes are sent back to Vietnam for interment near other deceased family.

Health problems and screening

Significant numbers of Vietnamese have extensive experience with war and war-related trauma. Many men, and not a few women, have been exposed to extreme violence and other trauma and are thus at high risk for post-traumatic stress disorder (PTSD) and depression (Kemp & Rasbridge, 2000; Silove *et al.*, 1997). All Vietnamese over age 25 experienced the loss of country and, to a large extent, loss of culture, and thus may experience chronic sorrow. Over time, Vietnamese are at risk for more chronic problems like hypertension, heart disease, cancer and diabetes.

The healthy life expectancy or HALE in Vietnam is 58.6 years and the full life expectancy is 68 years (Population Reference Bureau, 2002; World Health Organization (WHO), 2002). Infectious diseases are the leading causes of death and disability in Vietnam. Vietnam is one of 22 countries worldwide with a "high burden" of tuberculosis (WHO, 2003). Health risks for new Vietnamese immigrants (Hawn & Jung, 2003; Kemp, 2002; WHO, 2002) include:

- amebiasis
- angiostrongyliasis
- anthrax
- capillariasis
- chikungunya
- cholera
- cryptococcosis
- cryptosporidiosis
- cysticercosis (tapeworm)
- dengue fever
- encephalitis (Japanese)
- filariasis: Bancroftian filariasis and Malayan filariasis
- gnathostomiasis
- helminthiasis (ascariasis, echinococcosis/hydatid disease, schistosomiasis)

- hepatitis B (14% carriage rate)
- hookworm
- leishmaniasis
- leprosy
- leptospirosis
- malaria, including multidrug resistant (MDR) from *Plasmodium falciparum* resistant parasites and especially from malaria re-infection
- melioidosis
- mycetoma
- sexually transmitted infections, including HIV/AIDS, chancroid, chlamydia, gonorrhea, granuloma inguinale, lymphogranuloma venereum, syphilis
- strongylodiasis
- thalassemias
- trematodes (liver-dwelling: clonorchiasis and opisthorchiasis; blood-dwelling: schistosomiasis or bilharzias; intestine-dwelling; and lung-dwelling: paragonimiasis)
- tropical sprue
- tuberculosis (including multi-drug resistant)
- typhus
- yaws (frambesia)
- post-traumatic stress disorder
- chronic non-infectious diseases

REFERENCES

D'Avanzo, C. E. (1992). Bridging the cultural gap with Southeast Asians. *Maternal Child Nursing*, **17**, 204–8.

Dinh, A, Kemp, C. & Rasbridge, L. (2000). Culture and the end of life: introduction (to a series) and Vietnamese health beliefs and practices related to the end of life. *Journal of Hospice and Palliative Nursing*, **2**, 109–17.

Galanti, G. A. (2000). Vietnamese family relationships. *Western Journal of Medicine*, **172**, 415–16.

Geissler, E. M. (1998). *Cultural Assessment*, 2nd edn. Mosby: St. Louis.

Hawn, T. R. & Jung, E. C. (2003). Health screening in immigrants, refugees, and internationally adopted orphans. In *The Travel and Tropical Medicine Manual*, 3rd edn., ed E. C. Jong and R. McMullen, pp. 255–65. Philadelphia, PA: W. B. Saunders.

(2000). *Refugee Health – Immigrant Health*. Retrieved August 18, 2000 from http://www.baylor.edu/~Charles_Kemp/refugee_health.htm.

Kemp, C. E. (2002). *Infectious Diseases*. Retrieved April 12, 2003 from http://www3.baylor.edu/~Charles_Kemp/Infectious_Disease.htm.

Pillsbury, B. (1978). "Doing the month": Confinement and convalescence of Chinese women after childbirth. *Social Science and Medicine*, **12**, 11–22.

Population Reference Bureau. (2002). *2002 World Population Data Sheet.* Retrieved May 12, 2003 from http://www.prb.org/pdf/WorldPopulationDS02_Eng.pdf.

Radio Australia (n.d.). *Unfinished Journeys: Vietnam.* Retrieved August 10, 2003 from http://www.goasiapacific.com/specials/journeys/numbers_vietnam.htm.

Silove, D., Sinnerbrink, I. Field, A., Manicavasagar, V., & Steel, Z. (1997). Anxiety, depression, and PTSD in asylum-seekers: associations with pre-migration trauma and post-migration stressors. *British Journal of Psychiatry*, **170**, 351–7.

World Health Organization (2002). *World Health Report.* Retrieved June 5, 2003 from http://www.who.int/whr/2002/en/.

(2003). *Global TB Control Report 2003.* Retrieved June 1, 2003 from http://www.who.int/gtb/publications/globrep/index.html.

Part III

Appendices

Appendix A
Relief organizations and sources of information

These are listed together because many serve several purposes. See chapter references for sources of information on specific populations and issues.

American Friends Service Committee
Relief, social action
1501 Cherry St.
Philadelphia, PA 19102
www.afsc.org

American Jewish Joint Distribution Committee
Relief, social action
711 Third Ave. 10th Floor
New York, NY 10017
www.jdc.org

American Refugee Committee
Relief, social action, information
430 Oak Grove St.
Suite 204
Minneapolis, MN 55403
http://www.archq.org/

Baptist World Alliance
Relief, religious
405 North Washington St.
Falls Church, VA 22046
http://www.bwanet.org/

CARE
Relief
10–13 Rushworth St.
London SE1 0RB
United Kingdom
http://www.careinternational.org/

Catholic Relief Services
Relief, social action, religious
209 West Fayette St.
Baltimore, MD 21201-3443
www.catholicrelief.org

Centers for Disease Control and Prevention
Information, public health
1600 Clifton Rd.
Atlanta, GA 30333
http://www.cdc.gov/

Central Intelligence Agency
Information, more
World Factbook
http://www.cia.gov/cia/publications/factbook/index.html

Church World Service
Relief, social action, religious-based
28606 Phillips St.
PO Box 968
Elkhart, IN 46515
www.churchworldservice.org

CountryWatch.com
Information only
Two Riverway, Suite 1770
Houston, TX 77056
http://www.countrywatch.com/

Cross-Cultural Health Care Program
Information only
270 So. Hanford St., Suite 100

Seattle, WA 98134
http://www.xculture.org/index.cfm

Cultural Diversity
Information only
http://www.health.qld.gov.au/hssb/cultdiv/cultdiv/home.htm

Cultural Survival
Information only
215 Prospect St.
Cambridge, MA 02139
http://www.cs.org/

Cultural Profiles Project
Information only
Online only
http://cwr.utoronto.ca/cultural/

Ethnomed
Information only
Online only
http://ethnomed.org/ethnomed/index.html

Global Health Council
Professional organization
http://www.globalhealth.org/

Human Rights Watch
Information, advocacy
350 Fifth Ave., 34th Floor
New York, NY 10118-3299
http://www.hrw.org/

InterAction
Advocacy, information, clearinghouse (employment)
1717 Massachusetts Ave., NW, Suite 701
Washington, DC 20036
http://www.interaction.org/

International Career Employment Center
Expensive and extensive newsletter, but worth it for serious job-seekers
http://www.internationaljobs.org/

International Committee of the Red Cross
Relief
19 avenue de la Paix
CH 1202 Geneva
http://www.icrc.org/

International Rescue Committee
Relief and resettlement
122 East 42nd St.
New York, NY 10168
http://www.theirc.org/

American Jewish Joint Distribution Committee
Relief
PO Box 372
847-A Second Ave.
New York, NY 10017
http://www.jdc.org/

Médécins Sans Frontières
(Doctors Without Borders)
Relief
124–132 Clerkenwell Rd.
London EC1R 5DJ
United Kingdom
www.uk.msf.org

Mercy Corps International
Relief
3015 SW First
Portland, OR 97201
www.mercycorps.org

Oxfam Great Britain
Relief, social action
274 Banbury Rd.

Oxford OX2 7DZ
United Kingdom
http://www.oxfam.org.uk/

Oxfam America
Relief, social action
26 West St.
Boston MA 02111
www.oxfamamerica.org

Pan American Health Organization
Information, projects, public health
http://www.paho.org/

Peace Corps
Public health, social action
The Paul D. Coverdell Peace Corps Headquarters
1111 20th St. NW
Washington, DC 20526
www.peacecorps.gov

Physicians for Human Rights
Advocacy
http://www.phrusa.org/

Population Reference Bureau
Information only
1875 Connecticut Ave., NW
Suite 520
Washington, DC 20009-5728
http://www.prb.org/

Refugee Health – Immigrant Health
Information only
http://www.baylor.edu/~Charles_Kemp/refugee_health.htm

Relief Web
Information only
http://www.reliefweb.int

Save the Children
Relief, social action
54 Wilton Rd
Westport, CT 06880
www.savethechildren.org

World Concern
Relief, social action
19303 Fremont Ave. N.
Seattle, WA 98133
www.worldconcern.org

World Relief
Relief, religious
7 East Baltimore St.
Baltimore MD 21202
www.worldrelief.org

World Vision
Relief, religious
PO Box 9716
Federal Way, WA 98063-9716
www.worldvision.org

United Nations Children's Fund (UNICEF)
Relief, social action, information
http://www.unicef.org/

United Nations High Commissioner for Refugees
Relief, social action, information
Case Postale 2500
CH-1211 Genève 2 Dépôt
Suisse
http://www.unhcr.org/

US Committee for Refugees
Relief, social action, advocacy, information
1717 Massachusetts Ave. NW
Suite 200
Washington, DC 20036
http://www.refugees.org/

World Health Organization
Public/international health, information
Avenue Appia 20
1211 Geneva 27
Switzerland
http://www.who.int/

Appendix B
Universal Declaration of Human Rights

Adopted and proclaimed by General Assembly resolution 217 A (III) of 10 December 1948

Preamble

Whereas recognition of the inherent dignity and of the equal and inalienable rights of all members of the human family is the foundation of freedom, justice and peace in the world,

Whereas disregard and contempt for human rights have resulted in barbarous acts which have outraged the conscience of mankind, and the advent of a world in which human beings shall enjoy freedom of speech and belief and freedom from fear and want has been proclaimed as the highest aspiration of the common people,

Whereas it is essential, if man is not to be compelled to have recourse, as a last resort, to rebellion against tyranny and oppression, that human rights should be protected by the rule of law,

Whereas it is essential to promote the development of friendly relations between nations,

Whereas the peoples of the United Nations have in the Charter reaffirmed their faith in fundamental human rights, in the dignity and worth of the human person and in the equal rights of men and women and have determined to promote social progress and better standards of life in larger freedom,

Whereas Member States have pledged themselves to achieve, in co-operation with the United Nations, the promotion of universal respect for and observance of human rights and fundamental freedoms,

Whereas a common understanding of these rights and freedoms is of the greatest importance for the full realization of this pledge, **Now, Therefore THE GENERAL ASSEMBLY proclaims THIS UNIVERSAL DECLARATION OF HUMAN RIGHTS** as a common standard of achievement for all peoples and all nations, to the end that every individual and every organ of society, keeping this Declaration constantly in mind, shall strive by teaching and education to promote respect for these rights and freedoms and by progressive measures, national and international, to secure their universal and effective recognition and observance, both among the peoples of Member States themselves and among the peoples of territories under their jurisdiction.

Article 1

All human beings are born free and equal in dignity and rights. They are endowed with reason and conscience and should act towards one another in a spirit of brotherhood.

Article 2

Everyone is entitled to all the rights and freedoms set forth in this Declaration, without distinction of any kind, such as race, colour, sex, language, religion, political or other opinion, national or social origin, property, birth or other status. Furthermore, no distinction shall be made on the basis of the political, jurisdictional or international status of the country or territory to which a person belongs, whether it be independent, trust, non-self-governing or under any other limitation of sovereignty.

Article 3

Everyone has the right to life, liberty and security of person.

Article 4

No one shall be held in slavery or servitude; slavery and the slave trade shall be prohibited in all their forms.

Article 5

No one shall be subjected to torture or to cruel, inhuman or degrading treatment or punishment.

Article 6

Everyone has the right to recognition everywhere as a person before the law.

Article 7

All are equal before the law and are entitled without any discrimination to equal protection of the law. All are entitled to equal protection against any discrimination in violation of this Declaration and against any incitement to such discrimination.

Article 8

Everyone has the right to an effective remedy by the competent national tribunals for acts violating the fundamental rights granted him by the constitution or by law.

Article 9

No one shall be subjected to arbitrary arrest, detention or exile.

Article 10

Everyone is entitled in full equality to a fair and public hearing by an independent and impartial tribunal, in the determination of his rights and obligations and of any criminal charge against him.

Article 11

(1) Everyone charged with a penal offence has the right to be presumed innocent until proved guilty according to law in a public trial at which he has had all the guarantees necessary for his defense.

(2) No one shall be held guilty of any penal offence on account of any act or omission which did not constitute a penal offence, under national or international law, at the time when it was committed. Nor shall a heavier penalty be imposed than the one that was applicable at the time the penal offence was committed.

Article 12

No one shall be subjected to arbitrary interference with his privacy, family, home or correspondence, nor to attacks upon his honour and reputation. Everyone has the right to the protection of the law against such interference or attacks.

Article 13

(1) Everyone has the right to freedom of movement and residence within the borders of each state.

(2) Everyone has the right to leave any country, including his own, and to return to his country.

Article 14

(1) Everyone has the right to seek and to enjoy in other countries asylum from persecution.

(2) This right may not be invoked in the case of prosecutions genuinely arising from non-political crimes or from acts contrary to the purposes and principles of the United Nations.

Article 15

(1) Everyone has the right to a nationality.

(2) No one shall be arbitrarily deprived of his nationality nor denied the right to change his nationality.

Article 16

(1) Men and women of full age, without any limitation due to race, nationality or religion, have the right to marry and to found a family. They are entitled to equal rights as to marriage, during marriage and at its dissolution.

(2) Marriage shall be entered into only with the free and full consent of the intending spouses.

(3) The family is the natural and fundamental group unit of society and is entitled to protection by society and the State.

Article 17

(1) Everyone has the right to own property alone as well as in association with others.

(2) No one shall be arbitrarily deprived of his property.

Article 18

Everyone has the right to freedom of thought, conscience and religion; this right includes freedom to change his religion or belief, and freedom, either alone or in community with others and in public or private, to manifest his religion or belief in teaching, practice, worship and observance.

Article 19

Everyone has the right to freedom of opinion and expression; this right includes freedom to hold opinions without interference and to seek, receive and impart information and ideas through any media and regardless of frontiers.

Article 20

(1) Everyone has the right to freedom of peaceful assembly and association.

(2) No one may be compelled to belong to an association.

Article 21

(1) Everyone has the right to take part in the government of his country, directly or through freely chosen representatives.

(2) Everyone has the right of equal access to public service in his country.

(3) The will of the people shall be the basis of the authority of government; this will shall be expressed in periodic and genuine elections which shall be by universal

and equal suffrage and shall be held by secret vote or by equivalent free voting procedures.

Article 22

Everyone, as a member of society, has the right to social security and is entitled to realization, through national effort and international co-operation and in accordance with the organization and resources of each State, of the economic, social and cultural rights indispensable for his dignity and the free development of his personality.

Article 23

(1) Everyone has the right to work, to free choice of employment, to just and favourable conditions of work and to protection against unemployment.
(2) Everyone, without any discrimination, has the right to equal pay for equal work.
(3) Everyone who works has the right to just and favourable remuneration ensuring for himself and his family an existence worthy of human dignity, and supplemented, if necessary, by other means of social protection.
(4) Everyone has the right to form and to join trade unions for the protection of his interests.

Article 24

Everyone has the right to rest and leisure, including reasonable limitation of working hours and periodic holidays with pay.

Article 25

(1) Everyone has the right to a standard of living adequate for the health and well-being of himself and of his family, including food, clothing, housing and medical care and necessary social services, and the right to security in the event of unemployment, sickness, disability, widowhood, old age or other lack of livelihood in circumstances beyond his control.
(2) Motherhood and childhood are entitled to special care and assistance. All children, whether born in or out of wedlock, shall enjoy the same social protection.

Article 26

(1) Everyone has the right to education. Education shall be free, at least in the elementary and fundamental stages. Elementary education shall be compulsory. Technical and professional education shall be made generally available and higher education shall be equally accessible to all on the basis of merit.
(2) Education shall be directed to the full development of the human personality and to the strengthening of respect for human rights and fundamental freedoms.

It shall promote understanding, tolerance and friendship among all nations, racial or religious groups, and shall further the activities of the United Nations for the maintenance of peace.

(3) Parents have a prior right to choose the kind of education that shall be given to their children.

Article 27

(1) Everyone has the right freely to participate in the cultural life of the community, to enjoy the arts and to share in scientific advancement and its benefits.

(2) Everyone has the right to the protection of the moral and material interests resulting from any scientific, literary or artistic production of which he is the author.

Article 28

Everyone is entitled to a social and international order in which the rights and freedoms set forth in this Declaration can be fully realized.

Article 29

(1) Everyone has duties to the community in which alone the free and full development of his personality is possible.

(2) In the exercise of his rights and freedoms, everyone shall be subject only to such limitations as are determined by law solely for the purpose of securing due recognition and respect for the rights and freedoms of others and of meeting the just requirements of morality, public order and the general welfare in a democratic society.

(3) These rights and freedoms may in no case be exercised contrary to the purposes and principles of the United Nations.

Article 30

Nothing in this Declaration may be interpreted as implying for any State, group or person any right to engage in any activity or to perform any act aimed at the destruction of any of the rights and freedoms set forth herein.

Index